Pediatric Dermatology

Editor

KARA N. SHAH

PEDIATRIC CLINICS
OF NORTH AMERICA

www.pediatric.theclinics.com

Consulting Editor
BONITA F. STANTON

April 2014 • Volume 61 • Number 2

ELSEVIER

1600 John F. Kennedy Boulevard ● Suite 1800 ● Philadelphia, Pennsylvania, 19103-2899

http://www.theclinics.com

THE PEDIATRIC CLINICS OF NORTH AMERICA Volume 61, Number 2
April 2014 ISSN 0031-3955, ISBN-13: 978-0-323-29480-5

Editor: Kerry Holland
Developmental Editor: Casey Jackson

The Pediatric Clinics of North America (ISSN 0031-3955) is published bimonthly by Elsevier Inc., 360 Park Avenue South, New York, NY 10010-1710. Months of issue are February, April, June, August, October, and December. Periodicals postage paid at New York, NY and additional mailing offices. Subscription prices are $200.00 per year (US individuals), $493.00 per year (US institutions), $270.00 per year (Canadian individuals), $657.00 per year (Canadian institutions), $325.00 per year (international individuals), $657.00 per year (international institutions), $100.00 per year (US students and residents), and $165.00 per year (international and Canadian residents and students). To receive students/resident rare, orders must be accompanied by name of affiliated institution, date of term, and the signature of program/residency coordinator on institution letterhead. Orders will be billed at individual rate until proof of status is received. Foreign air speed delivery is included in all *Clinics* subscription prices. All prices are subject to change without notice. **POSTMASTER:** Send address changes to *The Pediatric Clinics of North America*, Elsevier Health Sciences Division, Subscription Customer Service, 3251 Riverport Lane, Maryland Heights, MO 63043. **Customer Service: 1-800-654-2452 (US and Canada). From outside of the US and Canada: 1-314-447-8871. Fax: 1-314-447-8029. For print support, E-mail: JournalsCustomerService-usa@elsevier.com. For online support, E-mail: JournalsOnlineSupport-usa@elsevier.com.**

Reprints. For copies of 100 or more, of articles in this publication, please contact the Commercial Reprints Department, Elsevier Inc., 360 Park Avenue South, New York, NY 10010-1710. Tel.: 212-633-3874; Fax: 212-633-3820; E-mail: reprints@elsevier.com.

The Pediatric Clinics of North America is also published in Spanish by McGraw-Hill Inter-americana Editores S.A., Mexico City, Mexico; in Portuguese by Riechmann and Affonso Editores, Rua Comandante Coelho 1085, CEP 21250, Rio de Janeiro, Brazil; and in Greek by Althayia SA, Athens, Greece.

The Pediatric Clinics of North America is covered in *MEDLINE/PubMed (Index Medicus), Excerpta Medica, Current Contents, Current Contents/Clinical Medicine, Science Citation Index, ASCA, ISI/BIOMED,* and *BIOSIS.*

Printed in the United States of America.

PROGRAM OBJECTIVE
The goal of the *Pediatric Clinics of North America* is to keep practicing physicians and residents up to date with current clinical practice in pediatrics by providing timely articles reviewing the state-of-the-art in patient care.

TARGET AUDIENCE
All practicing pediatricians, physicians and healthcare professionals who provide patient care to pediatric patients.

LEARNING OBJECTIVES
Upon completion of this activity, participants will be able to:
1. Review pediatric vitiligo.
2. Discuss the diagnosis and management of diaper dermatitis.
3. Recognize cutaneous bacterial infections due to staphylococcus aureus and streptococcus pyogenes in infants and children.

ACCREDITATION
The Elsevier Office of Continuing Medical Education (EOCME) is accredited by the Accreditation Council for Continuing Medical Education (ACCME) to provide continuing medical education for physicians.

The EOCME designates this enduring material for a maximum of 15 *AMA PRA Category 1 Credit*(s)™. Physicians should claim only the credit commensurate with the extent of their participation in the activity.

All other health care professionals requesting continuing education credit for this enduring material will be issued a certificate of participation.

DISCLOSURE OF CONFLICTS OF INTEREST
The EOCME assesses conflict of interest with its instructors, faculty, planners, and other individuals who are in a position to control the content of CME activities. All relevant conflicts of interest that are identified are thoroughly vetted by EOCME for fair balance, scientific objectivity, and patient care recommendations. EOCME is committed to providing its learners with CME activities that promote improvements or quality in healthcare and not a specific proprietary business or a commercial interest.

The planning committee, staff, authors and editors listed below have identified no financial relationships or relationships to products or devices they or their spouse/life partner have with commercial interest related to the content of this CME activity:
Leslie Castelo-Soccio, MD, PhD; Derek H. Chu, MD; Jeffrey S. Gerber, MD, PhD; Danielle Hawkins, MD; Elena B. Hawryluk, MD, PhD; A. Hernandez-Martin, MD; Kerry Holland; Brynne Hunter; Indu Kumari; Beatriz Larru, MD, PhD; Sandy Lavery; Ronald M. Laxer, MDCM; Jill McNair; Marilyn G. Liang, MD; Lucero Noguera-Morel, MD; Lindsay Parnell; Elena Pope, MD; Kara N. Shah, MD, PhD; Aimee C. Smidt, MD; Bonita F. Stanton, MD; Tracy Ting, MD, MS; Megha Tollefson, MD; Antonio Torrelo, MD; Sierra Wolter, MD, FAAD.

The planning committee, staff, authors and editors listed below have identified financial relationships or relationships to products or devices they or their spouse/life partner have with commercial interest related to the content of this CME activity:
Harper N. Price, MD, FAAD, FAAP is on speakers bureau for Galderma S.A; is consultant/advisor for Anacor Pharmaceuticals Inc.
Katherine B. Püttgen, MD is a consultant/advisor for Laboratoires Pierre Fabre.
Adam I. Rubin, MD is a textbook author for Atlas and Synopsis of Lever's Histopathology of the Skin 3rd ed; and has an employment affiliation with the University of Pennsylvania.
Helen Shin, MD is a consultant/advisor for Onset Dermatologics.
Nanette B. Silverberg, MD has a research grant from AstellasPharma, Inc.

UNAPPROVED/OFF-LABEL USE DISCLOSURE
The EOCME requires CME faculty to disclose to the participants:
1. When products or procedures being discussed are off-label, unlabelled, experimental, and/or investigational (not US Food and Drug Administration (FDA) approved); and
2. Any limitations on the information presented, such as data that are preliminary or that represent ongoing research, interim analyses, and/or unsupported opinions. Faculty may discuss information about pharmaceutical agents that is outside of FDA-approved labelling. This information is intended solely for CME and is not intended to promote off-label use of these medications. If you have any questions, contact the medical affairs department of the manufacturer for the most recent prescribing information.

TO ENROLL

To enroll in the *Pediatric Clinics of North America* Continuing Medical Education program, call customer service at 1-800-654-2452 or sign up online at http://www.theclinics.com/home/cme. The CME program is available to subscribers for an additional annual fee of USD 290.

METHOD OF PARTICIPATION

In order to claim credit, participants must complete the following:

1. Complete enrolment as indicated above.
2. Read the activity.
3. Complete the CME Test and Evaluation. Participants must achieve a score of 70% on the test. All CME Tests and Evaluations must be completed online.

CME INQUIRIES/SPECIAL NEEDS

For all CME inquiries or special needs, please contact elsevierCME@elsevier.com.

Contributors

CONSULTING EDITOR

BONITA F. STANTON, MD
Vice Dean for Research and Professor of Pediatrics, School of Medicine, Wayne State University, Detroit, Michigan

EDITOR

KARA N. SHAH, MD, PhD
Medical Director, Division of Pediatric Dermatology, Cincinnati Children's Hospital; Associate Professor, Pediatrics and Dermatology, University of Cincinnati College of Medicine, Cincinnati, Ohio

AUTHORS

LESLIE CASTELO-SOCCIO, MD, PhD
Assistant Professor, Section of Dermatology, Department of Pediatrics, The Children's Hospital of Philadelphia, Philadelphia, Pennsylvania

DEREK H. CHU, MD
Resident, Department of Dermatology, Hospital of the University of Pennsylvania, Philadelphia, Pennsylvania

JEFFREY S. GERBER, MD, PhD
Division of Infectious Diseases, The Children's Hospital of Philadelphia, Perelman School of Medicine, University of Pennsylvania; Center for Pediatric Clinical Effectiveness, The Children's Hospital of Philadelphia, Philadelphia, Pennsylvania

DANIELLE M. HAWKINS, MD
Department of Dermatology, University of New Mexico, Albuquerque, New Mexico

ELENA B. HAWRYLUK, MD, PhD
Clinical Fellow, Harvard Medical School; Dermatology Program, Boston Children's Hospital, Boston, Massachusetts

ÁNGELA HERNÁNDEZ-MARTÍN, PhD
Department of Dermatology, University Hospital of the Infant Jesus, Madrid, Spain

BEATRIZ LARRU, MD, PhD
Division of Infectious Diseases, The Children's Hospital of Philadelphia, Perelman School of Medicine, University of Pennsylvania, Philadelphia, Pennsylvania

RONALD M. LAXER, MDCM
Staff Rheumatologist and Professor, Departments of Paediatrics and Medicine, The Hospital for Sick Children, University of Toronto, Toronto, Ontario, Canada

MARILYN G. LIANG, MD
Assistant Professor, Harvard Medical School; Dermatology Program, Boston Children's Hospital, Boston, Massachusetts

LUCERO NOGUERA-MOREL, MD
Department of Dermatology, University Hospital of the Infant Jesus, Madrid, Spain

ELENA POPE, MD, MSc
Head, Section of Dermatology and Associate Professor, Department of Paediatrics, The Hospital for Sick Children, University of Toronto, Toronto, Ontario, Canada

HARPER N. PRICE, MD, FAAD, FAAP
Fellowship Director and Chief of Division, Department of Dermatology, Phoenix Children's Hospital, Phoenix, Arizona

KATHERINE B. PÜTTGEN, MD
Interim Director, Division of Pediatric Dermatology, Assistant Professor, Departments of Dermatology and Pediatrics, Johns Hopkins University School of Medicine, Baltimore, Maryland

ADAM I. RUBIN, MD
Assistant Professor of Dermatology, Pediatrics, and Pathology and Laboratory Medicine, Hospital of the University of Pennsylvania, The Children's Hospital of Philadelphia, Perelman School of Medicine at the University of Pennsylvania, Philadelphia, Pennsylvania

HELEN T. SHIN, MD
Chief, Pediatric Dermatology, The Joseph M. Sanzari Children's Hospital, Hackensack University Medical Center, Hackensack, New Jersey; Assistant Clinical Professor, Departments of Dermatology and Pediatrics, New York University School of Medicine, New York, New York.

NANETTE B. SILVERBERG, MD
Department of Dermatology, St. Luke's-Roosevelt Hospital Center, Icahn School of Medicine at Mount Sinai; Clinical Professor of Dermatology, Columbia University College of Physicians and Surgeons, New York, New York

AIMEE C. SMIDT, MD
Departments of Dermatology and Pediatrics, University of New Mexico, Albuquerque, New Mexico

TRACY V. TING, MD, MS
Assistant Professor, Division of Pediatric Rheumatology, Cincinnati Children's Hospital Medical Center, Cincinnati, Ohio

MEGHA M. TOLLEFSON, MD
Assistant Professor, Departments of Dermatology and Pediatrics, Mayo Clinic, Rochester, Minnesota

ANTONIO TORRELO, MD, PhD
Department of Dermatology, University Hospital of the Infant Jesus, Madrid, Spain

SIERRA WOLTER, MD, FAAD
Department of Dermatology, Phoenix Children's Hospital, Phoenix, Arizona

Contents

 Video of Pruritus in atopic dermatitis accompanies this article

Atopic dermatitis (AD) is a common chronic inflammatory skin condition characterized by intense pruritus and a waxing and waning course. AD often presents in infancy and childhood and can persist throughout adulthood. The exact cause of AD is unknown, but it likely reflects an interplay between genetic and environmental factors. AD affects up to 20% of children in the United States, and prevalence may be increasing. Treatment can be effective in alleviating symptoms but serves only to manage the disease, not cure it. Appropriate therapy can also prevent significant complications, such as infection, sleep disturbance, behavioral problems, and growth impairment.

Psoriasis is increasing in both children and adults. The association of comorbidities, specifically obesity and other components of the metabolic syndrome, are also increasing. The precise cause is unknown but genetic and complex immunologic factors play a role in the development of the disease and its comorbidities. There are multiple clinical variants, and the severity of the disease can range from mild localized lesions in most patients to severe generalized involvement in some. Most patients with mild to moderate disease can be controlled with topical treatments.

Although pediatric melanoma is a rare disease, diagnosis and management of pigmented lesions in the pediatric population, particularly dysplastic nevi and Spitz nevi, can be challenging. In this article, we provide an overview of pigmented lesions in children, including melanoma and management of melanoma risk factors and melanocytic nevi in the pediatric population. Congenital melanocytic nevi, Spitz nevi, dysplastic and acquired nevi, and changes over time are reviewed. We discuss considerations for excision and management of pigmented lesions in children.

This article presents an overview of diaper dermatitis for the pediatric community. The pathogenesis, differential diagnosis, and management of this common condition in infancy are reviewed. This information will assist in making the appropriate diagnosis and managing this irritant contact dermatitis of the diaper area. With conservative management, most cases of irritant diaper dermatitis are self-limited. When the condition persists, one must consider other diagnoses.

Propranolol has replaced corticosteroids as preferred first-line therapy for the management of infantile hemangiomas (IH). The topical β-blocker timolol is now an alternative to oral propranolol and watchful waiting for smaller IH. Research in the last decade has provided evidence-based data about natural history, epidemiology, and syndromes associated with IH. The most pressing issue for the clinician treating children with IH is to understand current data to develop an individualized risk stratification for each patient and determine the likelihood of complications and need for treatment. This article emphasizes the nuances of complicated clinical presentations and current treatment recommendations.

Cutaneous adverse drug reactions (ADRs) constitute a major pediatric health problem frequently encountered in clinical practice, and represents a diagnostic challenge. Children are more susceptible than adults to errors in drug dosage because of their smaller body size; moreover, ADRs can mimic other skin diseases of children, especially viral exanthems. Most ADRs with cutaneous involvement are mild and resolve on withdrawal of the causative drug. The most common forms of cutaneous ADRs, maculopapular exanthems and urticarial reactions, have excellent outcomes. Less frequent but more severe reactions may incur a risk of mortality.

Alopecia in childhood is a source of high concern, frustration, and anxiety. Delineating types of alopecia and those that are chronic or potentially related to underlying medical problems is important. There are 5 common types of hair loss in children: alopecia related to tinea capitis, alopecia areata spectrum/autoimmune alopecia, traction alopecia, telogen effluvium, and trichotillomania/trichotillosis. Hair-cycle anomalies including loose anagen syndrome can lead to sparse-appearing hair. Rarer reasons for alopecia in children include pressure-induced alopecia, alopecia related to nutritional deficiency or toxic ingestion, and androgenetic alopecia. Congenital lesions should be considered for areas of localized alopecia occurring at birth.

PEDIATRIC CLINICS OF NORTH AMERICA

NOW AVAILABLE FOR YOUR iPhone and iPad

Foreword

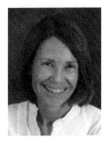

Bonita F. Stanton, MD
Consulting Editor

What pediatrician would not thrill at the opportunity to have a six-month mini-residency in pediatric dermatology! Dr Shah and the cast of outstanding dermatologists who have compiled these 13 superb articles are not quite offering us that—but something pretty close.

This issue is a beautifully written compendium of state-of-the-art descriptions of some of the most common and/or most important (and at times vexing) dermatologic disorders presenting to pediatricians. I know that this issue will be in my clinical office and I suspect that over time the pages will become quite well-worn in each of your copies. Updates on very common but nonetheless very important topics (such as sunburns, diaper dermatitis, nail disorders, atopic dermatitis, and cutaneous fungal and bacterial infections) will be helpful on a daily basis. Less common but certainly presenting in every pediatric practice are children with morphea and lichen sclerosus et atrophicus, cutaneous vasculitis, infantile hemangiomas, psoriasis, and pediatric vitiligo. The volume is very informative, clearly written, and complete with superb illustrations.

So maybe some year you will be able to do that six-month mini-residency, but in the meantime, you will be well-versed in state-of-the-art practice regarding pediatric dermatologic disorders.

Bonita F. Stanton, MD
School of Medicine
Wayne State University
1261 Scott Hall
540 East Canfield, Suite 1261
Detroit, MI 48201, USA

E-mail address:
bstanton@med.wayne.edu

Pediatr Clin N Am 61 (2014) xiii
http://dx.doi.org/10.1016/j.pcl.2014.01.001
0031-3955/14/$ – see front matter © 2014 Published by Elsevier Inc.

Preface

Pediatric Dermatology for the Primary Care Provider

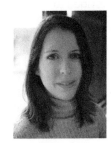

Kara N. Shah, MD, PhD
Editor

It is my great pleasure to highlight selected topics in Pediatric Dermatology in this issue of *Pediatric Clinics of North America*. Dermatologic concerns, including rashes, birthmarks, and skin infections, are very common in children and adolescents and are a frequent reason for ambulatory visits to pediatric primary care providers. In addition, referrals to Dermatology are one of the most common subspecialty referrals made by pediatric primary care providers and were the third most common subspecialty referral, behind Ophthalmology and Orthopedics, in a review of referral practices from a large network of private pediatric practices affiliated with the Children's Hospital of Boston.[1]

In the United States, access to pediatric dermatologists and general dermatologists with interest and expertise in pediatric dermatology is limited. In a recent survey conducted in collaboration with the AAP Committee on Pediatric Workforce, 81.6% of primary care pediatricians reported a lack of access to pediatric dermatologists, ranking behind only subspecialty care access to child/adolescent psychiatrists and developmental-behavioral pediatricians.[2]

Specific barriers to subspecialty care include long wait times for subspecialty appointments and significant distance from subspecialty care. However, a recent review of data from the National Ambulatory Medical Care Survey for the years 2002 to 2006 revealed that a significant proportion of care provided to children and adolescents by subspecialists, including dermatologists, was for routine follow-up or preventative care for common conditions, suggesting that at least a proportion of this care could be provided by the primary care provider.[3]

Although there are multiple factors contributing to the large demand for pediatric dermatology subspecialty care, one of these factors is the paucity of pediatric dermatology education provided during pediatric residency training, in particular, to pediatric residents intending to practice primary care. Unfortunately, despite the fact that dermatologic issues are common in pediatric practice, there are no ACGME

Pediatr Clin N Am 61 (2014) xv–xvi
http://dx.doi.org/10.1016/j.pcl.2014.01.002
0031-3955/14/$ – see front matter © 2014 Elsevier Inc. All rights reserved.

requirements for education in pediatric dermatology during pediatrics residency training and limited or no access to teaching faculty in pediatric dermatology in many residency programs, and therefore, most pediatrics residents receive little or no formal training in pediatric dermatology.

Educational opportunities for pediatric residents and primary care providers that contribute to increased competence in pediatric dermatology are an important component of improving the quality and efficiency of dermatologic care provided to children and adolescents. The 13 articles that comprise this issue have been selected to capture a significant proportion of the most common skin diseases that are seen in children and adolescents. They are intended to provide practical information on diagnosis and initial management that can be performed by the primary care provider and to provide a framework for allowing for more active involvement by the primary care provider with regards to ongoing management of these conditions. From atopic dermatitis to vitiligo, the pediatric primary care provider is guaranteed to see these conditions in their practice. Of note, pediatric acne, despite being a very common skin disease in children and adolescents, was not included due to the recently published guidelines entitled, "Evidence-based Recommendations for the Diagnosis and Treatment of Pediatric Acne," which are an excellent resource for the pediatric primary care provider.[4]

Pediatric dermatology is a diverse and exciting field. Although given the breadth and depth of skin disease seen in children and adolescents it can be somewhat intimidating, a working knowledge of the more common skin conditions is well within the scope of care that can be provided by the primary care provider, thus ensuring that all children and adolescents receive appropriate initial evaluation and management of these disorders.

Kara N. Shah, MD, PhD
Director, Division of Pediatric Dermatology
Cincinnati Children's Hospital
3333 Burnet Avenue
MLC 3004
Cincinnati, OH 45229, USA

Pediatrics and Dermatology
University of Cincinnati College of Medicine
Cincinnati, OH 45229, USA

E-mail address:
Kara.Shah@cchmc.org

REFERENCES

1. Vernacchio L, Muto JM, Young G, et al. Ambulatory subspecialty visits in a large pediatric primary care network. Health Serv Res 2012;47(4):1755–69.
2. Pletcher BA, Rimsza ME, Cull WL, et al. Primary care pediatricians' satisfaction with subspecialty care, perceived supply, and barriers to care. J Pediatr 2010; 156(6):1011–5, 1015.e1.
3. Valderas JM, Starfield B, Forrest CB, et al. Routine care provided by specialists to children and adolescents in the United States (2002-2006). BMC Health Serv Res 2009;9:221.
4. Eichenfield LF, Krakowski AC, Piggott C, et al. Evidence-based recommendations for the diagnosis and treatment of pediatric acne. Pediatrics 2013;131(Suppl 3): S163–86.

Atopic Dermatitis

Sierra Wolter, MD, Harper N. Price, MD*

KEYWORDS

- Atopic dermatitis • Eczema • Pruritus • Diagnosis • Complications
- Management recommendations

KEY POINTS

- Atopic dermatitis (AD) is a chronic inflammatory skin condition characterized by intense pruritus.
- Patients with AD require periodic physician assessment of disease state, comorbidities, and complications.
- Treatment of AD requires a multimodal approach using intensive patient education, anti-inflammatories, antibacterial intervention, and psychological support.

 Video of Pruritus in atopic dermatitis accompanies this article at http://www.pediatric.theclinics.com/

OVERVIEW

Atopic dermatitis (AD) is a common chronic inflammatory skin condition characterized by intense pruritus and a waxing and waning course. This condition most often presents in infancy and childhood and can persist, in one form or another, throughout adulthood. The exact cause of AD is unknown, but it likely reflects an interplay between genetic and environmental factors. AD affects up to 20% of children in the United States, and the prevalence may be increasing.[1] Treatment can be very effective in alleviating symptoms but serves only to manage the disease, not cure it. Appropriate therapy can also prevent significant complications, such as infection, sleep disturbance, behavioral problems, and growth impairment.

EPIDEMIOLOGY

Population studies have demonstrated an increasing prevalence of AD throughout the world. In the United States, it affects approximately 10% to 20% of children younger than 18 years, and these numbers are rising. Affected children are more likely to be black, urban, and living in homes with higher education levels.[1] As a chronic disease,

Department of Dermatology, Phoenix Children's Hospital, 1919 East Thomas Road, Phoenix, AZ 85006, USA
* Corresponding author.
E-mail address: hprice@phoenixchildrens.com

Pediatr Clin N Am 61 (2014) 241–260
http://dx.doi.org/10.1016/j.pcl.2013.11.002
0031-3955/14/$ – see front matter © 2014 Elsevier Inc. All rights reserved.

AD has a significant impact on health care resource utilization, similar to asthma or diabetes. There were an estimated 7.4 million outpatient physician visits for AD during the 7-year-period between 1997 and 2004, amounting to an estimated health care cost of US $364 million to $3.8 billion annually.[2,3]

PATHOPHYSIOLOGY

The exact cause of AD is unknown. However, it is generally agreed that AD results from a combination of genetic and environmental factors. Twin studies support a high rate of concordance; identical twins have a 7-fold increased risk for AD, and fraternal twins have a 3-fold increased risk.[4]

Healthy skin acts as a barrier to both outside influences and transepidermal water loss. Current theory holds that a genetically compromised barrier allows for penetration of environmental factors (irritants, allergens, and bacteria) with resultant immune dysregulation. A mutation in the filaggrin gene, responsible for an important component of the barrier, can be found in up to 10% of people of European ancestry.[5] Filaggrin is an epidermal protein that acts as waterproof "mortar" between keratinocytes in the outermost layer of the skin. Mutations in this protein cause ichthyosis vulgaris and are positively associated with more severe or persistent AD.[6]

Other prevalent theories of pathogenesis in AD focus on immune dysfunction. One observation in support of the role of immune dysfunction is that many primary immunodeficiency syndromes are characterized by early onset of diffuse eczematous eruptions and are caused by genetic mutations resulting in disruption of various immune functions, such as hyper-immunoglobulin E (IgE) syndrome, severe combined immunodeficiency, Wiskott-Aldrich syndrome, and Omenn syndrome. In the 1980s, a popular theory, termed the "hygiene hypothesis," emerged in an attempt to explain the fact that atopy tends to affect individuals from developed nations and those in a higher socioeconomic status.[7] This hypothesis asserts that the lack of childhood exposure to infectious agents results in an immune response favoring atopy, whereas early exposure to infectious agents triggers a T helper 1 (T_H1) response, thus diverting the immune system away from a T helper 2 (T_H2) "atopic" response. There is somewhat conflicting data in support of this hypothesis, and in truth, the interplay between T_H1 and T_H2 is likely more complex than previously thought.[8,9] More rigorous studies into causation are needed.

PREVENTION AND PROGNOSIS

Many studies have investigated primary prevention strategies and their effect on AD. These studies have examined the effect of early exposure to environmental and dietary factors such peanuts, eggs, soy, and animal dander or early supplementation of probiotics, breast milk, and vitamin D as related to development of AD.[10,11] There is currently no convincing evidence that any of these strategies are helpful.

The natural history of AD is variable. Based on population studies, a significant proportion of affected children "outgrow" the disease, as only 1% to 3% of adults are affected.[12] Patients with the most severe disease are more likely to have persistent disease.[13]

PRESENTATION
History

Pruritus, or itch, is defined as an unpleasant sensation that provokes the desire to scratch. A history of pruritus is required to establish the diagnosis of AD. Young infants, who are not yet capable of coordinating scratching behavior, will exhibit fussiness and poor sleep associated with excessive movement or squirming. Older infants and children will scratch and rub at their skin, often incessantly and particularly at night (Video 1).

Most patients manifest symptoms in the first year of life, with the remainder usually presenting before the age of 10 years.[14] Parental or sibling history of atopy supports the diagnosis of AD and is a strong risk factor for the development of the disease.[15]

Physical Examination

In infants, involvement of the face, neck, and extensor extremities (elbows, knees) is characteristic. Infantile eczema on the cheeks can appear more acute with a pseudo-vesicular or "weepy" appearance (**Fig. 1**). This condition is often misdiagnosed as impetigo. Persistent, bright red plaques may develop on the cheeks and chin at the time of teething and introduction of solid food, likely related to chronic irritation from saliva and foods. Infants may also have a more diffuse variant, but often with characteristic sparing of the diaper area. Scalp dermatitis is common and linear excoriations are common at this site, even with minimal skin involvement.

With increasing age, children tend to develop the classic flexural patches and plaques on the antecubital and popliteal fossae (**Fig. 2**). Hand and foot plantar dermatitis is also quite common (**Fig. 3**). In more severe cases, thickened plaques are seen on the dorsal hands, feet, and knees, often with a lichenified or leathery appearance, with prominent skin lines (**Figs. 4–6**) Children with darker skin typically have perifollicular hyperpigmented or hypopigmented rough 1- to 2-mm papules that can coalesce into broad, near-diffuse plaques, most prominent on the extensor surfaces (**Fig. 7**). This can give the skin a "pebbled" or spotty appearance (**Fig. 8**). This variant is often termed papular eczema. The nummular variant can be seen on the extremities as coin-shaped crusted or exudative plaques.

The surrounding skin is often dry and flaky, and there may be platelike ichthyosis of the distal extremities, especially in older children. Postinflammatory hyperpigmentation or hypopigmentation representing prior areas of disease activity is common and more obvious in darker-skinned individuals or those with tanned skin. Excoriations and erosions are nearly universal and are often the result of scratching or an indication of bacterial colonization (**Fig. 9**).

Superinfection is common, especially in children with more severe skin disease. Periauricular erosions and fissures overlying eczematous plaques provide a clue to staphylococcal colonization or infection. Isolated or adjacent pustules can be seen. Thick purulent crust, periocular involvement, or punched out ulcerations are often

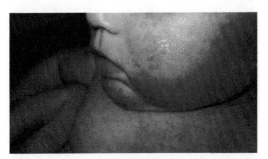

Fig. 1. Infantile atopic dermatitis with facial involvement. (*Courtesy of* Ronald Hansen, MD, Phoenix, AZ.)

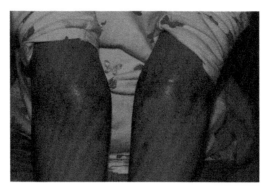

Fig. 2. Childhood atopic dermatitis with classical involvement of antecubital fossae.

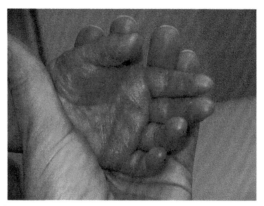

Fig. 3. Palmar involvement in atopic dermatitis.

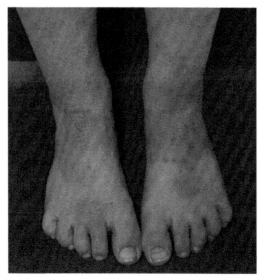

Fig. 4. Dorsal foot involvement in atopic dermatitis.

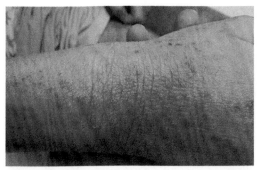

Fig. 5. Lichenification in severe atopic dermatitis.

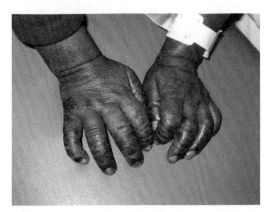

Fig. 6. Severe atopic dermatitis of the dorsal hands.

Fig. 7. Papular atopic dermatitis.

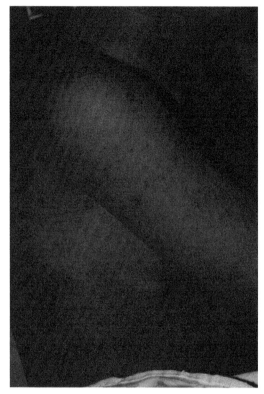

Fig. 8. Diffuse perifollicular atopic dermatitis.

seen in streptococcal infections.[16] Monomorphic punched out ulcers or vesicopustules within eczematous plaques, with or without fever, can indicate a superimposed herpes simplex viral (HSV) infection, more commonly known as eczema herpeticum (**Fig. 10**).

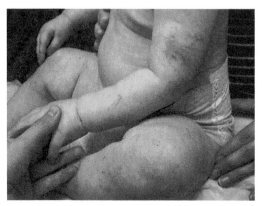

Fig. 9. Excoriations.

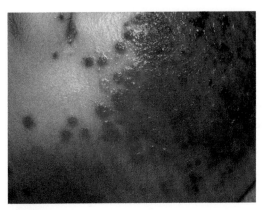

Fig. 10. Eczema herpeticum.

Supporting Features

Other physical examination findings can support the diagnosis of AD. These findings are not specific to AD and can be seen with other atopic disorders or in isolation. One of the most common coexistent conditions is keratosis pilaris, which is common on the upper outer arms and cheeks but can be seen diffusely over the extremities, shoulders, and back (**Fig. 11**). Ichthyosis vulgaris, often in association with hyperlinear palms, is present in approximately 25% of patients.[17] Many other skin and eye findings are more commonly seen in patients with AD (**Box 1**).

Comorbidities

AD is part of the atopic diathesis accompanied by asthma and seasonal allergies. AD generally precedes the development of asthma and allergic rhinitis and is thought to be the first step of the "atopic march." Children with eczema have a 2- to 3-fold increased risk of developing asthma and allergic rhinitis later in life.[18,19]

DIFFERENTIAL DIAGNOSIS

AD is the most common chronic skin condition seen in children. The distribution and appearance are the most distinguishing features. A family or personal history of atopy supports the diagnosis. There are several clues that should alert the clinician to an alternate diagnosis or a complicating feature of preexisting AD (**Table 1**).

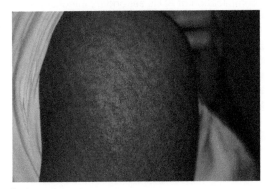

Fig. 11. Keratosis pilaris.

Box 1
Diagnosis of atopic dermatitis in children

Major Features
Pruritus
Typical age-specific distribution and morphology
Chronic or relapsing dermatitis
Personal or family history of atopy

Minor or Associated Features

Xerosis (dry skin)	Elevated IgE levels
Keratosis pilaris	Cheilitis
Pityriasis alba	Eye findings (conjunctivitis, keratoconus, anterior
Periauricular fissures	subcapsular cataracts)
Ichthyosis and palmar hyperlinearity	Periorbital darkening
Susceptibility to cutaneous infections	Dennie-Morgan lines (infraorbital fold)
Perifollicular accentuation (dark-skinned patients)	
Hand and foot dermatitis	
Scalp dermatitis	

Data from Hanifin JM, Rajka G. Diagnostic features of atopic eczema. Acta Dermatol Venereol Suppl 1980;92:44–7; and Hanifin JM. Atopic dermatitis in infants and children. Pediatr Dermatol 1991;38(4):763–89.

WORKUP/DIAGNOSIS

AD is a clinical diagnosis, based on physical findings and supportive history (see **Box 1**).

Histology

Histology of AD is not specific to this condition and resembles most other eczematous eruptions. Therefore, biopsy is not indicated unless other causes remain on the differential diagnosis (eg, psoriasis, pityriasis rubra pilaris, and mycosis fungoides).

Laboratory Studies

There are no specific laboratory studies needed to establish the diagnosis of AD, but certain tests can be helpful in identifying complications and comorbid conditions.

COMPLICATIONS
Infection

The most common complication of AD is secondary infection, occurring as a result of a disrupted epidermal barrier and altered immune response. Children with AD are more frequently colonized with *Staphylococcus aureus* than their healthy counterparts. The rates of colonization vary among studies and regions and range between 40% and 93% of patients with AD, as compared to 24% to 30% of healthy children.[20–25] Even in the absence of overt superinfection, *Staphylococcus* is thought to serve as a *superantigen*, acting as a significant driver of disease, and thus may be correlated with more severe skin disease.[26] True soft tissue infections also occur, affecting 40% to 60% of all patients with AD during their lifetime.[23,27,28] At least a portion of these infections are caused by drug-resistant organisms, such as methicillin-resistant *Staphylococcus aureus*, although regional variability exists.[21] Streptococcal superinfection is an emerging problem in AD. This problem is often underrecognized but is associated with higher rates of invasive infection, bacteremia, and need for hospitalization than staphylococcal infections.[16] Eczema herpeticum is a feared complication, and in one

Table 1
Differential diagnosis of atopic dermatitis

Disease	Patient	Physical Examination	Key Features	Diagnosis	Other
Seborrheic dermatitis	Newborns (under 2 mo of age) and teens	Symmetric, *well-demarcated*, flexural bright red plaques with *greasy scale* (unlike the dry scale of AD)	Unlike AD, it is usually *asymptomatic* and can involve the *diaper area*	Clinical	May overlap with infantile psoriasis, which initially affects the diaper area
Tinea (capitis, faciei, corporis)	Any age	Well-demarcated scaly plaques; may be annular with more scale at the periphery	Usually *asymptomatic or* mildly pruritic	Fungal scrapings and culture	Can become more widespread with topical steroid use
Allergic contact dermatitis	Any age (although usually school age or older)	Unusually distributed eczematous papules or plaques, usually occurring at sites of exposure	May produce an "id" reaction" characterized by widespread pruritic papules far from the site of initial exposure	Clinical, may be confirmed by patch testing	Nickel dermatitis is characterized by periumbilical or periauricular involvement
Scabies	Any age	Polymorphic (papules, vesicles, pustules, nodules); often on intertriginous sites (finger and foot webs, groin)	Spares the face	Clinical. Scabies preparation from linear burrows can confirm presence of the mite	Counsel families that pruritus and eczematous eruption commonly persist for months after successful treatment
Immune deficiencies	Infants and toddlers	Early, severe, and widespread eczematous eruption	Also with growth impairment, frequent skin and systemic infections; may have dysmorphic features	Genetic testing; some role for serologic testing (complete blood cell count and immunoglobulin levels); referral to appropriate specialists	Includes Wiskott-Aldrich syndrome, Omenn syndrome, hyper-IgE syndrome, SCID
Deficiencies (zinc, biotin, essential fatty acids, kwashiorkor)	Premature infants; patients on restrictive diets, TPN, or with malabsorption	Periorificial, acral and perianal scaling, erosions, and desquamation	Associated irritability, alopecia, diarrhea, and infections (especially *Candida* infections)	Serum zinc, essential fatty acid, and biotin levels; alkaline phosphatase and albumin; genetic testing	Genetic or the result of dietary deficiency; if dietary, must screen for concurrent deficiencies

Abbreviations: IgE, immunoglobulin E; SCID, severe combined immunodeficiency; TPN, total parenteral nutrition.

retrospective study, 57% of affected patients required hospitalization and intravenous antiviral therapy.[29] A significant portion of these patients will develop repeat infections. Herpetic keratitis can also occur and cause permanent ocular scarring.

If there is a suspicion for superinfection, skin swabs should be performed to confirm the presence of infection and to direct antimicrobial therapy. For bacterial infection, cultures can be obtained by firmly rubbing the swab tip on moist or eroded areas of the skin. To increase culture yield with dry or crusted areas, the tip can be moistened with culture media or plain water before application. Adherent crusts can be gently dislodged to swab the underlying skin surface. Studies to confirm herpes infection depend on local laboratory availability and include Tzanck smear, HSV polymerase chain reaction, viral culture, and HSV DFA (direct fluorescent antibody). As time is of the essence in eczema herpeticum, often the best test is that which can give a result most quickly. The test is performed by rupturing an intact vesicle or pustule and then scraping the roof *and* the base vigorously. Serologic studies (HSV immunoglobulin G and immunoglobulin M) may be of value in rare cases and are generally not recommended to establish a diagnosis. Periocular involvement should prompt a full evaluation by an ophthalmologist.

Psychosocial Impact

Itch is the most important and debilitating symptom in AD. Consequently, it can have the largest impact on the lives of those with AD. Although itch occurs at all hours of the day, it is often worst at night. Scratching behavior increases as well, and sleep suffers as a result. Studies that have used a combination of polysomnography, parent and patient surveys, actigraphy (measurement of movement), and video monitoring of patients with AD during sleep have repeatedly shown decreased sleep efficiency and total sleep time with increased nighttime awakenings.[30,31] Patients with AD spend an average of 11 to 84 minutes a night scratching.[32] Increased severity of skin disease correlates to increased sleep disruption.

Parental surveys have demonstrated that nearly 60% of children with AD have impairment of their ability to perform daytime activities, particularly in school performance.[33] Neurocognitive testing of children with AD demonstrated deficits in verbal comprehension, perceptual reasoning, and working memory when compared with controls.[34] Several recent meta-analyses have established a positive association between AD and attention-deficit/hyperactivity disorder (ADHD) symptoms. Pooled data from several studies suggest a 43% increased risk for a child with AD to display clinical ADHD symptoms when compared with a child without AD.[35,36] There is some evidence that children with AD *and* sleep disturbance have the highest risk of developing ADHD.[37]

Caring for a child with AD is more financially and emotionally stressful than caring for a child with insulin-dependent diabetes.[38] Parents of children with AD spend an average of 2 to 3 hours per day administering treatment at home and lose an average of 1 to 2 hours of sleep per night. The disease also places considerable financial burdens on families because of prescription medication costs, medical visits, and time off work to care for the child's disease.

THERAPEUTIC RECOMMENDATIONS

A successful treatment plan revolves around parent and patient education about the disease, basic skin care, and methods to reduce the frequency and severity of disease flares. Certain elements of the care plan can be standardized to all patients, whereas other elements should be individualized to account for the patient's severity and extent of disease. It is also important to incorporate patient preference, lifestyle constraints, and specific expectations and phobias into the plan so that these issues can

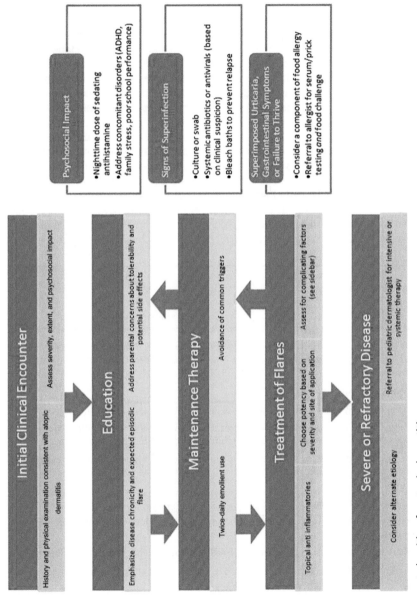

Fig. 12. Treatment algorithm for atopic dermatitis.

be addressed early, thereby increasing patient compliance and adherence to treatment (**Fig. 12**).

Parent and Patient Counseling

Parent and patient education is essential to the management of AD (**Box 2**). First and foremost, the physician must prepare the parent for the chronicity of the disease. Families should understand that therapy is directed at controlling, not curing, the disease. The physician must also explain that the disease is characterized by periods of remission and flares and treatment regimens must be adjusted to the stage of the disease. A care plan can be divided into maintenance and flare management strategies, which allows the parent to interpret the stage of the disease and to manage flares at home. This approach has the advantage of limiting the child's overall exposure to topical corticosteroids (CSs) and helps to overcome parental fears about potential side effects.

Good Skin Care

Daily bathing is important for removing bacteria, gentle exfoliation, and improving hydration of the skin. Parents should be instructed to apply an ointment-based, dye-free, fragrance-free emollient over the child's entire body immediately after the bath to reduce transepidermal water loss. Parent and patient preference in products should be solicited and reevaluated at each visit. Older children may avoid certain products because they are too greasy, whereas younger children may complain of a stinging or burning sensation with alcohol-containing products, such as diluted lotions. Alternate

---

Box 2
Patient and parent education

Good Daily Skin Care

- Bath or shower daily in warm (not hot) water for 10 to 15 minutes maximum. Use minimal soap.
- Apply a thick, nonfragranced moisturizer all over twice daily. This can be applied right after the bath after gently patting the skin dry. The best moisturizers come in tubs and are thick and greasy.

Avoidance of Triggers

- Eczema is usually worsened by cold and dry weather, harsh detergents, and fragrances.
- Avoid products that have added fragrances or additives (this includes lotions, detergents, fabric softeners, perfumes) and look for products that are labeled fragrance free.
- It can be very difficult to pinpoint specific environmental triggers (eg, dust, pet dander, pollen, food) in most patients with eczema. Try to avoid those that seem to clearly cause flares of skin disease.

Treatment of Eczema Flares

- Treat the red, itchy, and rough areas with the topical medicines until they are smooth and itch free.
- Always apply medicines to the areas that need them before applying a moisturizer all over.
- Prescription topical medications are tailored to match the severity of the eczema and the part of the body they are used on, so use as prescribed.

When to Call the Doctor

- Call the doctor if there are areas of crusting, scabbing, or oozing or sores that do not heal. The presence of such areas can be a sign of infection.
- If using the topical medications as prescribed and the eczema has not improved.

products should be suggested to improve patient compliance. It should be stressed that moisturizers only work in preventing severity of flares when they are applied regularly.

Avoidance of Triggers

Harsh detergents, dry weather, and fragrances are known to exacerbate disease in most patients with AD and should be avoided. Aeroallergens, such as animal dander, pollens, and dust mites, may worsen AD in a subset of patients, particularly those with asthma or rhinitis. It is difficult for most patients to completely avoid environmental triggers, and doing so may not resolve or improve the underlying disease.[39]

Specific foods may act as triggers for a limited number of patients with AD. The most common skin manifestations of food allergy are IgE mediated and include acute urticaria and angioedema. Mixed IgE- and cell-mediated food allergies may play a role in some patients with AD, manifesting as what is commonly known as *late eczematous reactions* or worsening of existing eczema.[40] One study by Breuer and colleagues[41] found that although 45% of patients with AD developed late eczematous reactions with food challenge, only 12% of these positive reactions were seen in isolation. Most of these late eczematous reactions were accompanied by an immediate-type reaction, such as urticaria. In this study, food-specific IgE levels had only a 64% positive predictive value of clinically observed food reaction.

Many patients with AD have elevated baseline IgE levels, and nearly 80% will have positive food-specific IgE titers.[42] The clinical relevance of a positive test result must be explored before dietary restrictions are recommended. Confirming the presence and clinical impact of food allergens is difficult, but should include a good patient history (including relevant food exposures), specific allergen testing of implicated foods, *and* confirmatory food challenge testing. An estimated 35% to 40% of patients with AD will have a relevant food allergy with food challenge, most commonly to egg, milk, and/or peanut.[43] A 2008 Cochrane review[44] showed no benefit of typical elimination diets, however, in *unselected* participants with AD. Therefore, a switch to elemental formulas or avoidance of eggs or milk is not recommended unless confirmatory testing is performed. Clinicians and parents should be cautioned against extreme elimination diets because these have resulted in severe malnutrition in several patients with AD, most notably in infants.[45,46]

Topical CSs

Emollients and trigger avoidance alone are rarely sufficient in controlling flares of AD. Topical CSs have been the mainstay in treatment of AD since they were first synthesized in 1951. CSs have been proven to be effective in decreasing inflammation and thereby reducing the severity and duration of flares, reducing bacterial colonization, and improving sleep.

The choice of topical CS depends on several factors, including age of the patient, site of application, and distribution and severity of the disease. Topical CSs are divided into 7 classes based on their vasoconstrictive properties. Class I CSs represent the strongest potency; class 7, the lowest potency. The difference in potency between classes is dramatic and not linear (**Box 3**). For example, clobetasol propionate, a class 1 CS, is 1800 times more potent than hydrocortisone, a class 7 CS.[47] A common misperception among patients is that the percentage on the CS label following the drug name corresponds to the strength or potency of the medication. To increase patient understanding, it may be helpful for the physician to visually list prescribed medications on a ladder of potency, so that families understand, for example, that triamcinolone acetonide 0.1% is much stronger than hydrocortisone 1%. This may also help to explain why certain CSs are used on certain parts of the body and avoided on other sites.

Box 3
Topical corticosteroid potency classes[a]

Class 1: Superpotent
- Clobetasol ointment 0.05%
- Halobetasol propionate 0.05%

Class 2: Potent
- Fluocinonide 0.05%
- Desoximetasone 0.25%

Class 3: Upper Midstrength
- Fluticasone propionate 0.005%
- Mometasone furoate 0.1%

Class 4: Midstrength
- Fluocinolone acetonide 0.025%
- Triamcinolone acetonide 0.1%

Class 5: Lower Midstrength
- Desonide 0.05%
- Triamcinolone acetonide 0.025%

Class 6: Low Potency
- Alclometasone dipropionate 0.05%

Class 7: Least Potent
- Hydrocortisone 2.5%
- Hydrocortisone 1%

[a] Ointment formulation.

Physicians should be comfortable with the use of at least one CS in the major potency classes (mild, moderate, moderate-high, and high potency) for prescribing. As a general rule, the clinician should choose the least potent CS that is effective at quickly decreasing the severity of disease flare. Potency should be tailored to site of application and severity of disease (**Table 2**). General guidelines for patients and families should include the following: (1) medications should be applied twice daily to the red, rough, and itchy areas of the skin; (2) topical medications should be applied before application of a bland emollient; and (3) treatment with topical medications should continue until the affected skin is smooth, no longer red, and itch free.

Various strategies exist to control disease flares (designated as disease maintenance).[48] Some advocate more prolonged use of lower potency preparations, with occasional medication "holidays." Others recommend intermittent or rotational strategies, such as twice-weekly application of low- to medium-potency preparations to disease-prone areas. Others prescribe a "topical steroid burst" for severe flares, with the use of a higher-potency medication for a few days followed by a medium-potency steroid for a week followed by a lower-potency medication, as needed only for maintenance. With any prescribed strategy, parent education about goals of therapy is tantamount to success, and follow-up is needed to monitor response and potential side effects of therapy.

Table 2
Pharmacologic treatment of atopic dermatitis

	Examples	Suggested Use	Key Points
Antiinflammatories			
Topical corticosteroids	Low potency (hydrocortisone 2.5%)	Face and folds (groin, axillae)	Ointment formulation preferred
	Midpotency (triamcinolone 0.1%)	Body involvement	Instruct patient to use medication on rough, raised, itchy areas until smooth and itch free
	Potent (fluocinonide) Superpotent (clobetasol)	Lichenified and thickened areas on hands and feet	Typically do *not* need to set time limits for duration of use, unless using a "topical steroid burst" therapy model
Topical calcineurin inhibitors	Pimecrolimus and tacrolimus	Practical for maintenance therapy or mild flares on the face and folds, to minimize risk of steroid atrophy	
Oral Corticosteroids	Rarely necessary and known to cause rebound symptoms after cessation		
Adjunctive Therapies			
Oral Antihistamines	Hydroxyzine, diphenhydramine, doxepin	Sedating antihistamines are given at bedtime to promote good sleep	
Oral Antibiotics	Cephalexin, clindamycin, doxycycline	For active infection or with severe flares of AD and signs of significant colonization	Always perform culture of site to direct therapy
Topical Antibacterials	Mupirocin	Rarely effective as monotherapy (because of widespread colonization) but may be used intranasally in conjunction with bleach baths for MRSA eradication	
Bleach Baths	Dilute sodium hypochlorite (regular bleach) 0.005%	One-eighth to one-fourth cup in a half tub of water (half cup in full tub), soak neck down for 10–15 min, repeat 2–3 times weekly	Chlorhexidine wash is an alternative for children or teens who prefer showering

Abbreviation: MRSA, methicillin-resistant Streptococcus aureus.

There are few long-term, well-designed studies that examine the true incidence of side effects with topical CS use. When used appropriately, the risk of local and systemic effects of topical CS is thought to be quite low. Risk of skin atrophy (characterized by striae, telangiectasia, and epidermal thinning) increases with excessive use. Excessive use is characterized by prolonged duration of therapy, high-potency preparations, and use on thin-skinned areas (face or intertriginous sites) or under occlusion. Excessive use of topical CS periocularly is thought to cause glaucoma and cataracts. Risk of systemic side effects, namely, adrenal suppression, is quite low but increases in younger children and infants.[49] For this reason, the use of class 1 corticosteroids is typically avoided in very young children.[50]

It is important to address parental concerns about the potential risks of topical CS use and place the true risk of adverse reactions into perspective. CS phobia can lead to poor patient compliance and lack of response to treatment. A recent multicenter survey of patients with AD and parents of children with AD revealed that more than 80% of responders expressed fears about using topical CSs and 36% of responders admitted to nonadherence to treatment.[51]

Even in the absence of CS phobia, adherence to topical regimens in AD is low. One small study of 26 children with AD used electronic stealth monitoring of medication use and found an overall adherence rate of only 32% to recommended topical therapy. Better adherence was associated with a greater decrease in disease severity. Adherence rates doubled around the time of office visits, but decreased rapidly thereafter.[52]

It is therefore important to address parental and patient (when age-appropriate) concerns about side effects at each visit, establish close follow-up appointments to increase compliance and adherence to therapy, and continue to explore and address reasons for treatment failure.

Topical Calcineurin Inhibitors

Topical calcineurin inhibitors (TCIs) have been used to treat AD for over a decade, and have been studied extensively in children. TCIs, which include tacrolimus (Protopic©) and pimecrolimus (Elidel©), function via local inhibition of immune cells at the site of application. TCIs have been proved to be effective in multiple randomized controlled trials in the treatment of AD in children and are approved for use as second-line therapy for intermittent use in children older than 2 years.[53] One advantage of TCIs over topical CSs is that they do not cause atrophy or ocular complications, making them particularly useful for chronic or recurrent facial or intertriginous AD involvement.[50] The most commonly observed side effect is a localized burning sensation, which usually resolves with continued use.[48] In 2006, the US Food and Drug Administration placed a black box warning on the label based on a theoretical risk of increased skin malignancy and lymphoma. Although long-term studies are lacking, there is currently no data in support of this theory.[50,53,54] The role of TCIs in the management of AD is still evolving.

Adjuvant Therapy

Many patients may benefit from treatment of bacterial colonization.[50] "Bleach baths" have recently become the standard of care for managing recurrent infections in many dermatology practices (see **Table 2**). Huang and colleagues[55] studied a series of 31 patients with moderate to severe AD and signs of bacterial infection. All patients were treated with a course of cephalexin and then randomized to receive bleach baths with intranasal mupirocin or placebo, and eczema severity scores were assessed for 3 months. Although posttreatment *Staphylococcus* cultures gave positive results for all patients, patients in the treatment arm demonstrated improvement of their eczema in areas of the body that were submerged.

Wet wraps are a form of adjuvant therapy that have been in use for many decades and tend to be particularly helpful for children with moderate to severe AD experiencing a severe or diffuse flare.[56] This treatment can be performed in several ways but typically involves stepwise wetting of the skin, application of a topical CS (often triamcinolone acetonide 0.1% ointment or cream), and application of a "wet" layer (eg, tight-fitting damp pajamas) followed by a "dry" layer (eg, loose pajamas). Ideally the wet layer is rewetted every 2 to 3 hours, or the process is repeated twice a day.

These treatments can be administered in the hospital, or at home, and can be continued safely for up to a week or two at a time. A retrospective study from Mayo clinic demonstrated an improvement in all 218 hospitalized children receiving wet wrap treatment at their institution.[57]

Although helpful for comorbidities, such as allergic rhinoconjunctivitis, there is little role for oral antihistamine therapy in AD. Daily nonsedating antihistamines do not reduce pruritus or disease flares in children with AD. Longer-acting, sedating oral antihistamines given before bedtime are helpful to promote sleep and thus prevent the nighttime scratch-wake cycle.[50] Topical antihistamines should be avoided because these can cause allergic or irritant contact dermatitis.

Referral to Specialists

The first step in managing patients with recalcitrant disease is to rule out other causes, such as immunodeficiency, and to assess for complicating factors, such as allergic contact dermatitis. Patients with true persistent chronic disease, severe flares, or other complicating factors (eg, frequent superinfection or significant psychosocial distress) may benefit from suppressive immunotherapy. Therapies used in these cases include phototherapy, cyclosporine, azathioprine, mycophenolate mofetil, and methotrexate. Referral to a specialist with experience with systemic treatments for pediatric patients with AD should ensue so that these options can be discussed with the family, because these therapies are not without risks and require safety monitoring and follow-up visits. Professional psychological evaluation with subsequent support and treatment may be necessary for some children or families. Referral to internet resources such as www.nationaleczema.org may be helpful for some older children and families.

SUMMARY

AD is a chronic inflammatory skin condition characterized by pruritus and a waxing and waning course. It is common in childhood, but can persist into adulthood. Treatment can be very effective at alleviating symptoms and is essential in preventing complications, including infection, sleep disturbance, behavioral complications, and psychosocial stress. Topical treatment is the mainstay of therapy, with systemic therapy often reserved for severe cases. Parent and patient education is essential in managing this chronic disease.

SUPPLEMENTARY DATA

Supplementary data related to this article can be found online at http://dx.doi.org/10.1016/j.pcl.2013.11.002.

REFERENCES

1. Shaw TE, Currie GP, Koudelka CW, et al. Eczema prevalence in the United States: data from the 2003 National Survey of Children's Health. J Invest Dermatol 2011; 131(1):67–73.
2. Horii KA, Simon SD, Liu DY, et al. Atopic dermatitis in children in the United States, 1997-2004: visit trends, patient and provider characteristics, and prescribing patterns. Pediatrics 2007;120(3):e527–34.
3. Mancini AJ, Kaulback K, Chamlin SL. The socioeconomic impact of atopic dermatitis in the United States: a systematic review. Pediatr Dermatol 2008; 25(1):1–6.

4. Thomsen SF, Ulrik CS, Kyvik KO, et al. Importance of genetic factors in the etiology of atopic dermatitis: a twin study. Allergy Asthma Proc 2007;28(5): 535–9.

5. Sandilands A, Terron-Kwiatkowski A, Hull PR, et al. Comprehensive analysis of the gene encoding filaggrin uncovers prevalent and rare mutations in ichthyosis vulgaris and atopic eczema. Nat Genet 2007;39:650–4.

6. Henderson J, Northstone K, Lee SP, et al. The burden of disease associated with filaggrin mutations: a population-based, longitudinal birth cohort study. J Allergy Clin Immunol 2008;121(4):872–7.e9.

7. Strachan DP. Hay fever, hygiene, and household size. BMJ 1989;299(6710): 1259–60.

8. Elston DM. The hygiene hypothesis and atopy: bring back the parasites? J Am Acad Dermatol 2006;54(1):172–9.

9. Flohr C, Yeo L. Atopic dermatitis and the hygiene hypothesis revisited. Curr Probl Dermatol 2011;41:1–34.

10. Batchelor JM, Grindlay DJ, Williams HC. What's new in atopic eczema? An analysis of systematic reviews published in 2008 and 2009. Clin Exp Dermatol 2010; 35(8):823–7 [quiz: 827–8].

11. Kramer MS, Kakuma R. Maternal dietary antigen avoidance during pregnancy or lactation, or both, for preventing or treating atopic disease in the child. Cochrane Database Syst Rev 2012;(9):CD000133.

12. Schultz Larsen F, Hanifin J. Epidemiology of atopic dermatitis. Immunol Allergy Clin North Am 2002;22(1):1–24.

13. Hanifin JM. Atopic dermatitis in infants and children. Pediatr Clin North Am 1991;38(4):763–89.

14. Kristal L, Klein PA. Atopic dermatitis in infants and children. An update. Pediatr Clin North Am 2000;47(4):877–95.

15. Fergusson DM, Horwood LJ, Shannon FT. Parental asthma, parental eczema and asthma and eczema in early childhood. J Chronic Dis 1983;36(7):517–24.

16. Sugarman JL, Hersh AL, Okamura T, et al. A retrospective review of streptococcal infections in pediatric atopic dermatitis. Pediatr Dermatol 2011;28(3): 230–4.

17. Uehara M, Hayashi S. Hyperlinear palms: association with ichthyosis and atopic dermatitis. Arch Dermatol 1981;117(8):490–1.

18. von Kobyletzki LB, Bornehag CG, Hasselgren M, et al. Eczema in early childhood is strongly associated with the development of asthma and rhinitis in a prospective cohort. BMC Dermatol 2012;12:11. http://dx.doi.org/10.1186/1471-5945-12-11.

19. van der Hulst AE, Klip H, Brand PL. Risk of developing asthma in young children with atopic eczema: a systematic review. J Allergy Clin Immunol 2007;120(3): 565–9.

20. Suh L, Coffin S, Leckerman KH, et al. Methicillin-resistant *Staphylococcus aureus* colonization in children with atopic dermatitis. Pediatr Dermatol 2008; 25(5):528–34.

21. Tang CS, Wang CC, Huang CF, et al. Antimicrobial susceptibility of *Staphylococcus aureus* in children with atopic dermatitis. Pediatr Int 2011;53(3):363–7.

22. Balma-Mena A, Lara-Corrales I, Zeller J, et al. Colonization with community-acquired methicillin-resistant *Staphylococcus aureus* in children with atopic dermatitis: a cross-sectional study. Int J Dermatol 2011;50(6):682–8.

23. Hoeger PH, Ganschow R, Finger G. Staphylococcal septicemia in children with atopic dermatitis. Pediatr Dermatol 2000;17(2):111–4.

24. Nakamura MM, Rohling KL, Shashaty M, et al. Prevalence of methicillin-resistant *Staphylococcus aureus* nasal carriage in the community pediatric population. Pediatr Infect Dis J 2002;21(10):917–22.
25. Hussain FM, Boyle-Vavra S, Daum RS. Community-acquired methicillin-resistant *Staphylococcus aureus* colonization in healthy children attending an outpatient pediatric clinic. Pediatr Infect Dis J 2001;20(8):763–7.
26. Breuer K, Kapp A, Werfel T. Bacterial infections and atopic dermatitis. Allergy 2001;56(11):1034–41.
27. David TJ, Cambridge GC. Bacterial infection and atopic eczema. Arch Dis Child 1986;61(1):20–3.
28. White MI, Noble WC. Consequences of colonization and infection by *Staphylococcus aureus* in atopic dermatitis. Clin Exp Dermatol 1986;11(1):34–40.
29. Luca NJ, Lara-Corrales I, Pope E. Eczema herpeticum in children: clinical features and factors predictive of hospitalization. J Pediatr 2012;161(4):671–5.
30. Wahlgren CF. Itch and atopic dermatitis: an overview. J Dermatol 1999;26(11): 770–9.
31. Camfferman D, Kennedy JD, Gold M, et al. Eczema and sleep and its relationship to daytime functioning in children. Sleep Med Rev 2010;14(6):359–69.
32. Monti JM, Vignale R, Monti D. Sleep and nighttime pruritus in children with atopic dermatitis. Sleep 1989;12(4):309–14.
33. Paller AS, McAlister RO, Doyle JJ, et al. Perceptions of physicians and pediatric patients about atopic dermatitis, its impact, and its treatment. Clin Pediatr (Phila) 2002;41(5):323–32.
34. Camfferman D, Kennedy JD, Gold M, et al. Sleep and neurocognitive functioning in children with eczema. Int J Psychophysiol 2013;89(2):265–72.
35. Schmitt J, Apfelbacher C, Heinrich J, et al. Association of atopic eczema and attention-deficit/hyperactivity disorder - meta-analysis of epidemiologic studies. Z Kinder Jugendpsychiatr Psychother 2013;41(1):35–42 [quiz: 42–4].
36. Gee SN, Bigby M. Atopic dermatitis and attention-deficit/hyperactivity disorder: is there an association? Arch Dermatol 2011;147(8):967–70.
37. Romanos M, Gerlach M, Warnke A, et al. Association of attention-deficit/hyperactivity disorder and atopic eczema modified by sleep disturbance in a large population-based sample. J Epidemiol Community Health 2010;64(3):269–73.
38. Su JC, Kemp AS, Varigos GA, et al. Atopic eczema: its impact on the family and financial cost. Arch Dis Child 1997;76(2):159–62.
39. Krakowski AC, Eichenfield LF, Dohil MA. Management of atopic dermatitis in the pediatric population. Pediatrics 2008;122(4):812–24.
40. Mansoor DK, Sharma HP. Clinical presentations of food allergy. Pediatr Clin North Am 2011;58(2):315–26, ix.
41. Breuer K, Heratizadeh A, Wulf A, et al. Late eczematous reactions to food in children with atopic dermatitis. Clin Exp Allergy 2004;34(5):817–24.
42. Hill DJ, Heine RG, Hosking CS, et al. IgE food sensitization in infants with eczema attending a dermatology department. J Pediatr 2007;151(4):359–63.
43. Greenhawt M. The role of food allergy in atopic dermatitis. Allergy Asthma Proc 2010;31(5):392–7.
44. Bath-Hextall F, Delamere FM, Williams HC. Dietary exclusions for established atopic eczema. Cochrane Database Syst Rev 2008;(1):CD005203. http://dx.doi.org/10.1002/14651858.CD005203.pub2.
45. Katoh N, Hosoi H, Sugimoto T, et al. Features and prognoses of infantile patients with atopic dermatitis hospitalized for severe complications. J Dermatol 2006; 33(12):827–32.

46. Keller MD, Shuker M, Heimall J, et al. Severe malnutrition resulting from use of rice milk in food elimination diets for atopic dermatitis. Isr Med Assoc J 2012; 14(1):40–2.

47. Olsen EA, Cornell RC. Topical clobetasol-17-propionate: review of its clinical efficacy and safety. J Am Acad Dermatol 1986;15(2 Pt 1):246–55.

48. Dohil MA, Eichenfield LF. A treatment approach for atopic dermatitis. Pediatr Ann 2005;34(3):201–10.

49. Charman C, Williams H. The use of corticosteroids and corticosteroid phobia in atopic dermatitis. Clin Dermatol 2003;21(3):193–200.

50. Paller AS, Simpson EL, Eichenfield LF, et al. Treatment strategies for atopic dermatitis: optimizing the available therapeutic options. Semin Cutan Med Surg 2012;31(Suppl 3):S10–7.

51. Aubert-Wastiaux H, Moret L, Le Rhun A, et al. Topical corticosteroid phobia in atopic dermatitis: a study of its nature, origins and frequency. Br J Dermatol 2011;165(4):808–14.

52. Krejci-Manwaring J, Tusa MG, Carroll C, et al. Stealth monitoring of adherence to topical medication: adherence is very poor in children with atopic dermatitis. J Am Acad Dermatol 2007;56(2):211–6.

53. Kalavala M, Dohil MA. Calcineurin inhibitors in pediatric atopic dermatitis: a review of current evidence. Am J Clin Dermatol 2011;12(1):15–24.

54. Callen J, Chamlin S, Eichenfield LF, et al. A systematic review of the safety of topical therapies for atopic dermatitis. Br J Dermatol 2007;156(2):203–21.

55. Huang JT, Abrams M, Tlougan B, et al. Treatment of *Staphylococcus aureus* colonization in atopic dermatitis decreases disease severity. Pediatrics 2009; 123(5):e808–14.

56. Devillers AC, Oranje AP. Wet-wrap treatment in children with atopic dermatitis: a practical guideline. Pediatr Dermatol 2012;29(1):24–7.

57. Dabade TS, Davis DM, Wetter DA, et al. Wet dressing therapy in conjunction with topical corticosteroids is effective for rapid control of severe pediatric atopic dermatitis: experience with 218 patients over 30 years at mayo clinic. J Am Acad Dermatol 2012;67(1):100–6.

Diagnosis and Management of Psoriasis in Children

Megha M. Tollefson, MD

KEYWORDS

- Psoriasis • Pediatric • Obesity • Metabolic syndrome • Topical steroids
- Quality of life

KEY POINTS

- The incidence and prevalence of psoriasis is increasing in the pediatric population.
- There is increasing evidence that childhood psoriasis is associated with the metabolic syndrome.
- Variants of psoriasis in childhood include chronic plaque type, scalp, guttate, inverse, diaper, and nail.
- Topical medications should be used to treat most cases of mild to moderate disease.

INTRODUCTION

Overview

Psoriasis is a common chronic scaly inflammatory condition that primarily affects the skin. In this article, what is known about the pathophysiology of the disease, its epidemiology, and overall prognosis are reviewed. The different presentations that can be seen in children as well as clues to clinical diagnosis are discussed. Although thought to primarily be a skin disorder, recent research has linked psoriasis to several comorbidities that are presented below. Finally, skin-directed therapies, which should be helpful in most patients with mild to moderate psoriasis, are discussed.

Pathophysiology

The pathophysiology behind psoriasis is not completely understood. It is thought to be an immune-mediated inflammatory disease of the skin that has a genetic predisposition. Activation of several T cells, Th-1, Th-17, and Th-22, resulting in production of specific cytokines, such as interferon-γ, tumor necrosis factor, IL-17, IL-22, and IL-23, has recently been discovered to play an important role in the development of the disease.[1,2] These cytokines then activate keratinocytes, leading to increased

Departments of Dermatology and Pediatrics, Mayo Clinic, 200 First Street South West, Rochester, MN 55905, USA
E-mail address: Tollefson.Megha@mayo.edu

Pediatr Clin N Am 61 (2014) 261–277
http://dx.doi.org/10.1016/j.pcl.2013.11.003
0031-3955/14/$ – see front matter © 2014 Elsevier Inc. All rights reserved.

inflammatory cells and products at the skin site.[3] Epidermal hyperplasia and proliferation of keratinocytes are also a hallmark of psoriasis, which may be due to induction by activated T lymphocytes via inflammatory cytokine response and to an increase in cell cycle turnover.[4]

There is also a known genetic component to psoriasis; those with a first-degree relative with psoriasis have an approximately 5-fold increased risk of developing the disease as compared with the general population,[5] and many children with psoriasis have a first-degree relative with the disease.[6,7] Furthermore, monozygotic twins have a higher concordance rate than dizygotic twins of developing psoriasis.[8] Several candidate chromosomal regions, termed PSORS1 to PSORS10, have been linked to a risk of developing psoriasis.[9] There is a strong association of the HLA-Cw6 allele with early-onset disease. Several other gene regions, including those encoding some of the implicated interleukins, have also been identified in some affected populations.[3] Although attempts to identify precise etiologic factors continue, it has become apparent that development of the disease results from a complex interplay of both genetic and environmental factors.

Epidemiology

Psoriasis is one of the most common inflammatory skin conditions affecting both children and adults. The worldwide prevalence of psoriasis is estimated at approximately 4%, with ranges from 0% to 8.5% depending on the population studied.[10] In children prevalence is estimated to be as high as 0.71%, with increasing prevalence as age increases to a high of 1.2% at age 18.[11] Incidence of the disease is steadily increasing with a 2-fold increase in both children and adults since 1970.[12] Approximately one-third of patients develop the disease in childhood, with a median age of 10.6 years at first diagnosis. Although psoriasis can develop at any age, cases of congenital psoriasis are extremely rare[13] but up to 27% of children may develop it before age 2.[7] There does not seem to be a gender bias in childhood; when all subtypes of psoriasis are considered, boys and girls develop the disease at equal rates.[7,12]

Prognosis

Psoriasis is a life-long condition that tends to have a chronic relapsing course. Fortunately, most affected children will have mild disease. Often, mild disease is well-controlled with topical medications requiring intermittent treatment. Some patients with psoriasis are able to achieve complete remission that may last several years. Children are more likely than adults to have the guttate form of psoriasis (described below); those with guttate psoriasis may clear their skin completely without recurrence, develop disease again with streptococcal infection, or go on to develop chronic plaque-type psoriasis. A minority of children with psoriasis unfortunately may worsen with age and may have more severe and widespread involvement, requiring more aggressive treatment.

CLINICAL FEATURES
History

The history and presenting symptoms may differ depending on the age of the child and type of psoriasis. Infants with psoriasis most commonly present with a persistent diaper rash that has been refractory to multiple treatments. Older children may present with an asymptomatic scaly rash and/or with refractory or severe dandruff or "cradle cap."[7] Many children with psoriasis are asymptomatic but many may also present with pruritus and decreased sleep as a result; this is particularly true with psoriasis of the scalp. Patients that present with guttate psoriasis may have had a preceding strepto-coccal infection of the throat or perianal area.[14]

There are several possible triggers and exacerbating factors of psoriasis in children and include trauma or irritation of the skin, known as the Koebner phenomenon,[15] infection, most commonly streptococcal infection resulting in guttate psoriasis,[14,16] emotional stress,[17] and medications (**Box 1**).[18] Although lithium and β-blocker medi-cations are known to trigger psoriasis in adults, these medications are less relevant in childhood psoriasis.[19]

It has recently been discovered that overweight and obesity are a strong risk factor for the development of childhood in psoriasis.[20] As overweight and obesity are quickly increasing in the pediatric population, this may in part explain the increasing incidence and prevalence of childhood psoriasis.

Physical Examination

The classic psoriatic lesion is a well-demarcated pink-red plaque with overlying silvery-white scale. Removal of this scale by mechanical factors often results in pinpoint bleeding, known as the Auspitz sign.[21] When compared with adults with pso-riasis, children tend to have more facial and flexural (especially diaper) involvement and have smaller, thinner plaques, which may lead to some diagnostic confusion.[7,22] Clinical morphology and symptoms may vary according to the subtype and location on the body of the disease as discussed below and in **Table 1**.

- The most common type of psoriasis in both adults and older children is chronic plaque psoriasis (**Fig. 1**); up to 75% of children with psoriasis have the plaque variant.[7,12] In this variant of psoriasis, typical well-defined psoriatic lesions are most commonly found on the extensor extremities, but may also be seen on the scalp, trunk, flexures, and face (**Fig. 2**). Less commonly, plaque psoriasis can have a follicular or annular morphology.[22]
- Scalp psoriasis may be seen in isolation or in association with chronic plaque dis-ease. The scalp is often the first site of involvement in children.[23] Scalp lesions are well-defined and scaly and can have varying amounts of underlying erythema (**Fig. 3**). The occipital scalp and the hairline are common areas of scalp involve-ment. Scalp scale may be quite thick, also called tinea amiantacea (**Fig. 4**), and can have associated matting down of the hair, scale surrounding the hair shaft, and resulting nonscarring alopecia. In cases with alopecia, the hair usually re-turns when disease control is achieved. Scalp psoriasis may be particularly pruritic.

Box 1
Triggers and exacerbating factors of pediatric psoriasis

Trauma or local skin irritation (Koebner phenomenon)

Infection

   Streptococcal pharyngitis

   Perianal streptococcus

Emotional stress

Medications

   Antimalarials

   Rebound effect after systemic steroids

Table 1
Psoriasis variants, associated clinical findings, and differential diagnosis

Type	Age Group	Clinical Findings	Differential Diagnosis
Chronic plaque	Any age	Well-defined erythematous plaques, silvery white scale Auspitz sign Extensor surfaces, trunk, periumbilical May be follicular or annular	Nummular eczema Atopic dermatitis Tinea corporis Pityriasis rubra pilaris
Scalp	Any age	Well-defined erythematous scaly plaques Tinea amiantacea Often extends onto forehead	Seborrheic dermatitis Tinea capitis Atopic dermatitis
Guttate	Children, adolescents, young adults	Small, "drop-like" <1 cm erythematous scaly papules Trunk, extremities, face, scalp	Pityriasis rosea Tinea corporis Pityriasis rubra pilaris Nummular eczema
Inverse	Younger children	Erythematous plaques with little scale, possible maceration Flexural areas and face	Intertrigo Seborrheic dermatitis Erythrasma Contact dermatitis
Diaper/napkin	Ages 0–2	Well-defined bright red plaques in diaper area Little scale, may be macerated Involves inguinal folds	Irritant contact dermatitis Allergic contact dermatitis Intertrigo Candidal diaper dermatitis Acrodermatitis enteropathica
Nail	Any age, more common in older children and adults	Pitting, onycholysis, oil spots, subungual hyperkeratosis, trachyonychia May or may not have skin signs of psoriasis	Onychomycosis Pityriasis rubra pilaris Lichen planus
Pustular	Older children and adults	Superficial sterile pustules on erythematous skin May have annular configuration May be localized to palmoplantar areas	Candida infection Dyshidrotic eczema Staphylococcal scalded skin syndrome Blistering dactylitis Tinea infection
Erythrodermic	Any age	Generalized erythema Minimal scale Very rare	Staphylococcal scalded skin syndrome Pityriasis rubra pilaris Cutaneous T-cell lymphoma Atopic dermatitis

- Guttate psoriasis is the second-most common type of psoriasis seen in children, with a frequency rate of 15% to 30% of all children with psoriasis.[6,12,24] This type of psoriasis is characterized by abrupt onset of "droplike" papular lesions of up to 1 cm in size that are symmetrically distributed over the trunk, limbs, and face (**Fig. 5**). It may be preceded by throat or perianal streptococcal infection.[14] Guttate psoriasis may resolve spontaneously within 3 to 4 weeks, although many patients may go on to develop chronic plaque psoriasis.[6,24]

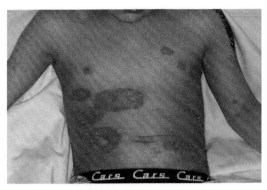

Fig. 1. Chronic plaque psoriasis on the trunk.

- Involvement with psoriasis primarily in the flexural areas and on the face is called inverse psoriasis. This type of psoriasis is more common in children than adults. The morphology of the lesions, particularly in the flexural locations, is often distinct from chronic plaque psoriasis as there can be maceration of the plaques and very little overlying scale due to moisture.
- Diaper or napkin psoriasis is another common variant of psoriasis almost exclusively seen in infancy. Well-defined brightly erythematous plaques that may be macerated are usually seen (**Fig. 6**). The inguinal folds are usually involved (unlike in irritant contact dermatitis), and erythematous scaly psoriatic lesions may be seen in other locations of the body (**Fig. 7**).[7] Diaper psoriasis can be particularly difficult to treat and commonly resolves with toilet-training.
- Nail psoriasis is less common in children than in adults but can be seen in up to 40% of children with psoriasis.[24] Nail changes that may be seen are pitting, overall roughness (trachyonychia), onycholysis (distal separation of the nail plate from the nail bed), oil spots, and subungual hyperkeratosis (**Fig. 8**). These changes can be seen in isolation, can precede, coincide with, or come after the onset of skin psoriasis. Nail involvement of psoriasis is very difficult to treat.
- Pustular psoriasis is a rare variant whereby sterile superficial pustules are seen in localized or generalized fashion (**Fig. 9**). Those with generalized pustular psoriasis may be systemically ill with fever and malaise. Although pustular psoriasis is more common in adults,[12] an annular configuration of pustules is seen more commonly in children than adults.[25] The pustular variant of psoriasis is often mistaken for infection.

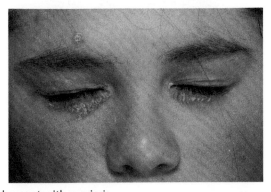

Fig. 2. Facial involvement with psoriasis.

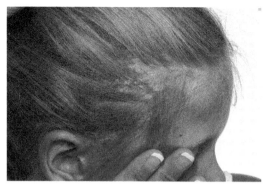

Fig. 3. Scalp psoriasis.

- Erythrodermic psoriasis is another rare variant characterized by greater than 90% body surface area involvement with erythema. Scaling may be minimal. This type of psoriasis is extremely rare.

Several clinical tools can be used to calculate the severity of skin disease. The Psoriasis Area and Severity Index and Physician Global Assessment are the most commonly used tools in clinical trials. Severity is also often based on body surface area, the presence of comorbidities, and the impact on quality of life (QOL).

Co-morbidities

Although psoriasis is primarily a disorder of the skin, there is increasing evidence that the disease has multiple comorbidities, even in children (**Box 2**). Because it is an

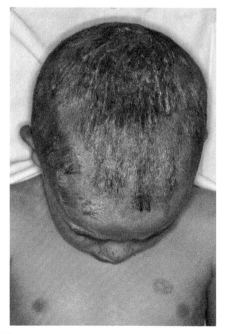

Fig. 4. Tinea amiantacea.

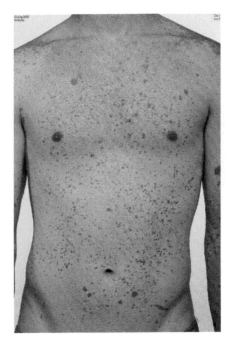

Fig. 5. Guttate psoriasis.

immune-mediated inflammatory disease, one theory is that chronic low-level inflammation also leads to the multiple nonskin comorbidities.[26]

The most widely recognized comorbidity is that of psoriatic arthritis. Estimates of the prevalence of psoriatic arthritis in all patients with psoriasis have ranged from 5% to 40%.[27] Prevalence rates in children are unknown. It is thought that the onset of skin disease precedes the onset of joint disease by an average of 10 years, but in approximately 15% of patients the joint disease precedes the skin disease.[28] The peak of onset of psoriatic arthritis in childhood is between ages 9 and 12,[29] and up to 20% of arthritis in childhood is psoriatic arthritis.[30] Patients with psoriatic arthritis most commonly present with oligoarthritis involving small joints such as the joints of the hands and feet. Involvement of the digits may characteristically present with

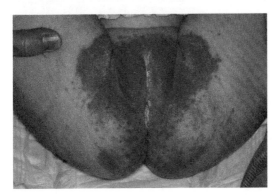

Fig. 6. Diaper psoriasis.

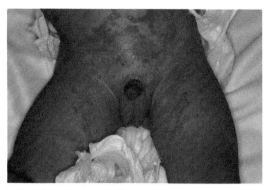

Fig. 7. Diaper psoriasis with typical psoriatic papules and plaques elsewhere.

sausagelike swelling. The presence of psoriatic arthritis may be an indication for aggressive treatment, but the overall prognosis for children who develop psoriatic arthritis is generally good.

It has recently been discovered that pediatric patients with psoriasis are twice as likely to have comorbidities as those that do not have psoriasis. Increased rates of hyperlipidemia (2-fold), obesity (2-fold), hypertension (2-fold), diabetes mellitus (2-fold), rheumatoid arthritis, and Crohn disease (3- to 4-fold) have been seen in

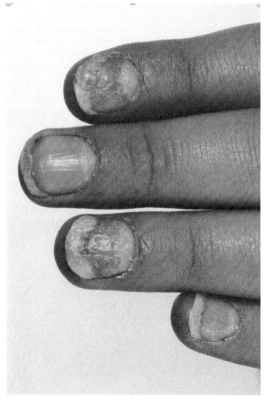

Fig. 8. Nail psoriasis with pitting, oil spots, and onycholysis.

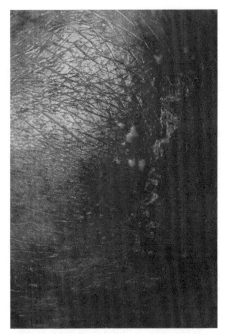

Fig. 9. Pustules with underlying erythema in pustular psoriasis.

children with psoriasis.[11,31,32] Alarmingly, even when controlling for weight and body mass index, children with psoriasis have higher blood lipids and increased frequency of the metabolic syndrome than those that do not have psoriasis.[20,33]

Psoriasis has been established as a risk factor for the development of cardiovascular disease in adulthood. A study done in women demonstrated it to be an independent predictor for nonfatal cardiovascular disease among women, and that those who were diagnosed with psoriasis at a younger age or who had a longer duration of disease had a particularly high risk.[34] This finding is pertinent to children because it indicates that pediatric patients with psoriasis may be at increased risk of cardiovascular disease in adulthood, possibly because of increased rate of the metabolic syndrome.

DIFFERENTIAL DIAGNOSIS

The differential diagnosis of psoriasis can be quite varied depending on the types and locations of the disease (see **Table 1**). It can be mistaken for other inflammatory

| **Box 2** |
| **Comorbidities of pediatric psoriasis** |
| Psoriatic arthritis |
| Overweight and obesity |
| Hyperlipidemia |
| Diabetes mellitus |
| Rheumatoid arthritis |
| Crohn disease |

conditions such as contact dermatitis (irritant or allergic), nummular eczema, atopic dermatitis (some patients may have both atopic dermatitis and psoriasis), dyshidrotic eczema, lichen planus, seborrheic dermatitis, pityriasis rosea, and pityriasis rubra pilaris. Infectious conditions may also mimic psoriasis including tinea infections, blistering dactylitis, intertrigo, candida infection, onychomycosis, and erythrasma. Other entities on the differential diagnosis include acrodermatitis enteropathica, staphylococcal scalded skin syndrome, and cutaneous T-cell lymphoma.

DIAGNOSTIC RECOMMENDATIONS

The diagnosis is usually made clinically, although specific investigations may be helpful with atypical presentations, when the diagnosis is unclear, to evaluate for identifiable triggers, and in the evaluation for comorbidities (**Table 2**).

Laboratory Studies

There are no specific laboratory investigations that are found in patients with most forms of psoriasis. In children who are suspected to have streptococcal infection, particularly those with guttate psoriasis, the appropriate site (throat, perianal) should be cultured for the presence of group A β-hemolytic streptococcus. In patients with severe generalized pustular psoriasis, a complete blood count and chemistries should be considered because they may have a leukocytosis with neutrophilia on complete blood count, abnormal electrolyte values, and impaired renal or hepatic function. Patients suspected to have psoriatic arthritis may have an elevated erythrocyte sedimentation rate, C-reactive protein, and a negative rheumatoid factor. Weight, height, and body mass index should be recorded and charted on all children with psoriasis. In those at risk for the metabolic syndrome, appropriate components should be evaluated with fasting lipid profile, blood pressure measurement, and fasting blood sugar.

Radiology

Imaging is not necessary and not helpful in most patients with psoriasis. The exception is in suspected psoriatic arthritis. Patients suspected to have psoriatic arthritis should have radiographs of involved joints. Positive findings may include bone demineralization, joint space narrowing, articular erosions, and soft tissue swelling around the joints.[35,36]

Histology

Chronic and established lesions of psoriasis may show several histologic features compatible with the disease. The usual histologic features are parakeratosis of the

Table 2
Diagnostic tests to consider in pediatric psoriasis

Laboratory	Height, weight, body mass index, blood pressure in all patients Guttate—culture swab from appropriate location for group A streptococcus Pustular, generalized—consider CBC, chemistries, Cr, LFTs Psoriatic arthritis—ESR, CRP, RF Concern for metabolic syndrome—fasting blood glucose and lipid profile, blood pressure measurement
Radiology	Radiographs of affected joints in those suspected to have psoriatic arthritis
Histology	Consider skin biopsy in cases of uncertain diagnosis or atypical presentation

Abbreviations: CBC, complete blood count; Cr, creatinine; CRP, C-reactive protein; ESR, erythrocyte sedimentation rate; LFTs, liver function tests; RF, rheumatoid factor.

stratum corneum with intracorneal neutrophilic collections (Munro microabscesses), acanthosis or thickening of the epidermal layer of skin, thickening of the suprapapillary epidermis, and absence of the granular layer. In some variants such as diaper or guttate psoriasis, or in early lesions, all of the typical findings may not be seen.

THERAPEUTIC RECOMMENDATIONS

Psoriasis is a chronic condition without a cure. For that reason it can be extremely frustrating to treat and requires diligent compliance to a treatment regimen. Anticipatory guidance and education of the patient and family is an important component in addition to the prescribed treatment regimen. Although complete clearance of the disease for a period of time is possible, that is not always necessary, as having a few asymptomatic lesions may be acceptable.

Pharmacologic Treatment

In most children, particularly those with mild to moderate disease, topical skin-directed treatment is sufficient (**Tables 3** and **4**). Below, the most commonly used topical medications in children with psoriasis, most of which are used off-label, are reviewed.[37,38] Often, combinations of treatments are used to treat psoriasis so that efficacy can be increased while limiting toxicity. The vehicle of the treatment is also an important consideration. Occlusive ointments are often more effective that creams or lotions but may be less esthetically pleasing particularly in the adolescent population. Solutions, oils, and foams are best for hair-bearing sites such as the scalp. Most topical medications should be applied twice daily to affected areas.

- Topical steroids are the most commonly prescribed medication and are generally first-line for the treatment of active areas of childhood psoriasis.[37,39] Topical steroids are anti-inflammatory and antiproliferative and reduce itching, scaling, and erythema; benefit from their use in psoriasis has been demonstrated in several clinical trials.[40,41] They are available in a wide variety of strengths, with multiple different products for every class of strength and are available in every vehicle. In general, low potency medications are used in the flexures and in areas with thin skin. High-potency medications are usually used in areas of thick skin, such as the palms and soles. When used appropriately, they are extremely safe, but potential side effects include local telangiectasias, atrophy, and striae of the skin, and if extensively applied, suppression of the adrenal axis. Intermittent or rotational use can limit potential side effects of long-term use. Oral steroids should not be used in the treatment of psoriasis, not only because of risk of significant adverse effects from the medication, but also because there is a significant risk of rebound psoriasis, including pustular and erythrodermic forms with accompanying systemic and life-threatening symptoms.
- Vitamin D analogues, calcipotriene and calcitriol, are safe and effective in the topical treatment of psoriasis and act by inhibiting the proliferation of keratinocytes.[42] They are available in cream, ointment, and solution forms. In practice, they may be used as monotherapy but are usually used in conjunction with topical steroids for synergistic and steroid-sparing effects.[43] Although no formal guidelines exist, use of up to 45 g/wk/m^2 does not seem to affect serum calcium levels.[42] Localized irritation of the skin is the most common side effect.[44]
- Tars are one of the oldest treatment modalities for psoriasis. The most frequently used forms are crude coal tar and a more esthetically pleasing modified preparation called liquor carbonis detergens.[45] Although the mechanism of action has not been precisely delineated, tars have an antipruritic and antiproliferative effect

Table 3
Topical treatments for childhood psoriasis

Medication	Mechanism of Action	Available Vehicle(s)	Adverse Effects	Other Considerations
Topical steroids	Anti-inflammatory, antiproliferative	Lotion, cream, ointment, gel, solution, oil, foam	Skin atrophy, striae, acneiform eruption, telangiectasias, adrenal axis suppression	Mild potency for face, flexures, groin Moderate potency for trunk, extremities High potency for palms, soles, scalp
Vitamin D analogues: calcipotriene, calcitriol	Inhibition of keratinocyte proliferation	Cream, ointment, solution	Local skin irritation, if excessive doses hypercalcemia	Often used in conjunction with topical steroids for synergistic effect
Tars: crude coal tar, LCD	Antiproliferative Antipruritic	Cream, lotion	Irritation, folliculitis, photosensitivity	Best for areas of thick plaque, often adjunctive
Anthralin (dithranol)	Anti-inflammatory Antiproliferative	Cream, lotion	Irritation, staining of skin and clothing	Best for areas of thick skin or thick plaque, can use in short contact, often adjunctive
Topical calcineurin inhibitors: tacrolimus, pimecrolimus	Inhibition of T-cell activation and proliferation, immunomodulatory	Ointment, cream	Stinging, burning, pruritus	Most useful in treatment of face, flexures, groin
Tazarotene	Reduces inflammation, restores normal epidermal proliferation	Cream, gel	Irritation	Best as adjunctive treatment of thick plaques not in sensitive areas, useful for nail psoriasis Category X

Abbreviation: LCD, liquor carbonis detergens.

Table 4
Treatment recommendations by psoriasis type and site

Type/Site	First-Line	Second-Line
Chronic plaque	Topical steroids	
Face, flexures, groin	Low potency (hydrocortisone 1, 2.5%, desonide 0.05%)	Topical calcineurin inhibitors (tacrolimus, pimecrolimus)
Trunk, extremities	Moderate potency (triamcinolone 0.1%, mometasone 0.1 cream)	Vitamin D analogues (calcipotriene, calcitriol) Anthralin Tar Tazarotene
Scalp	Moderate- to high-potency topical steroids	Vitamin D analogues Tar
Guttate	Antistreptococcal antibiotics if active infection Topical steroids	Vitamin D analogues
Diaper	Low potency topical steroids	Topical calcineurin inhibitors Vitamin D analogues (use with caution)
Nail	Moderate- to high-potency topical steroids	Tazarotene

on psoriasis.[46] These medications are often compounded into a variety of vehicles. They may be used as monotherapy but are most often used in conjunction with topical steroids, keratolytics, and phototherapy, with use primarily reserved for areas of thick plaque. Odor and staining of skin and clothing can be limitations to the use of tar. Potential side effects are folliculitis, irritant dermatitis, and photosensitivity. Although concern has been raised for the theoretical increased risk of cancer in patients treated with tar, this has not found to be true in dermatology patients.[47,48]

- Anthralin, or dithranol, is another old treatment of psoriasis, although its precise mechanism of action is not understood. It has potent anti-inflammatory and anti-proliferative activities.[49] Anthralin is best used as an adjunctive treatment especially on thick plaques or areas of large involvement. Concentrations of 0.1% up to 3% or higher are typically used; lower concentrations are used in more sensitive areas, whereas higher concentrations may be used to areas of thicker skin or thicker plaques, particularly as the skin becomes more tolerant. It is effective in the treatment of psoriasis in children[50,51] but irritation and transient staining of the skin may limit its use. Short-contact therapy with higher strength concentrations left on for short periods of time (10–30 minutes) before washing off can also be useful and may limit irritation and staining.
- The topical calcineurin inhibitors (tacrolimus, pimecrolimus) are nonsteroidal immunomodulators currently Food and Drug Administration–approved for use in atopic dermatitis. They are safe and effective in the treatment of psoriasis and are particularly good options in treating sensitive sites such as the face, flexures, and groin that are prone to adverse effects of long-term topical steroids.[52,53] Stinging, burning, and pruritus may sometimes be seen.
- Tazarotene is a topical retinoid that has been approved for the treatment of psoriasis in adults in the United States. Topical retinoids act by reducing inflammation and by restoring normal epidermal proliferation.[54] Tazarotene is available in gel and cream formulations and is best used on thick plaques not located in

sensitive areas. It has also been shown to be effective in the treatment of nail psoriasis.[55] The use of tazarotene may be limited by local skin irritation but limiting application to once daily or less can be helpful. It is a pregnancy category X medication.

- Keratolytics (salicylic acid, lactic acid, urea) can be useful as adjunctive treatments for psoriasis. They are helpful in removing layers of thick scale and should be used in combination with other treatment modalities. Salicylic acid is available as a shampoo or gel, whereas lactic acid and urea are available as lotions, creams, and ointments. Salicylic acid should not be used in infants because of the risk of salicylism.
- Antistreptococcal antibiotics should be used in patients found to have active streptococcal infection. When active infection is not found, antibiotics are not helpful in the treatment of psoriasis in children.[56]

Children with severe disease or disease refractory to topical measures may require further treatment. For these children, phototherapy and/or systemic treatment with medications such as methotrexate, cyclosporine, oral retinoids, and biologic medications may be warranted. The use of these treatments is individualized to each child and is beyond the scope of this review.

Nonpharmacologic Treatment

Bland moisturizers and emollients can be helpful in reducing itch and in removing some scale. Their use should be considered in all patients with psoriasis. Products are generally well-tolerated and easy to use and can be chosen by patient preference.

Surgical Treatment Options

Tonsillectomy is not proven to be beneficial and is not recommended as a treatment modality for children with psoriasis.[56]

Self-Management Strategies

Because of impact on QOL, psychosocial support is an important component of psoriasis treatment. Counseling may be helpful for some children and families. The National Psoriasis Foundation is a nonprofit patient advocacy group that can be a very useful resource for children and families. Their web site can be found at www.psoriasis.org.

COMPLICATIONS

Complications due to the skin disease itself are rare. Those with the rare forms of erythrodermic and generalized pustular psoriasis may have severe and life-threatening hypotension and hepatic or renal dysfunction. Other complications may be due to treatments for the disease itself, as discussed above.

Perhaps the most important and common complication of pediatric psoriasis is its psychosocial effects. Psoriasis is known to negatively impact the QOL of affected patients, children included. Children with psoriasis commonly endorse negative QOL because of itching, fatigue, and feelings of stigmatization, even those who have mild disease.[57,58] Affected children are also significantly more at risk than unaffected children of developing psychiatric disorders, especially depression and anxiety.[59,60] Thus, the profound physical and psychological effects of psoriasis on children cannot be underestimated.

SUMMARY

Pediatric psoriasis is a common inflammatory skin condition that is increasing in incidence and prevalence. Several triggers and comorbid conditions are associated. There is increasing prevalence of the metabolic syndrome even in the pediatric psoriasis population, an association that should be considered in all patients. Although topical treatment is indicated and effective for most affected children, treating the disease can be challenging. Psychosocial support should be given and attention paid to the QOL of children and their families.

REFERENCES

1. Lowes MA, Kikuchi T, Fuentes-Duculan J, et al. Psoriasis vulgaris lesions contain discrete populations of Th1 and Th17 T cells. J Invest Dermatol 2008;128(5): 1207–11.
2. Nograles KE, Zaba LC, Shemer A, et al. IL-22-producing "T22" T cells account for upregulated IL-22 in atopic dermatitis despite reduced IL-17-producing TH17 T cells. J Allergy Clin Immunol 2009;123(6):1244–52.e2.
3. Girolomoni G, Mrowietz U, Paul C. Psoriasis: rationale for targeting interleukin-17. Br J Dermatol 2012;167(4):717–24.
4. van Ruissen F, de Jongh GJ, van Erp PE, et al. Cell kinetic characterization of cultured human keratinocytes from normal and psoriatic individuals. J Cell Physiol 1996;168(3):684–94.
5. Roberson ED, Bowcock AM. Psoriasis genetics: breaking the barrier. Trends Genet 2010;26(9):415–23.
6. Mercy K, Kwasny M, Cordoro KM, et al. Clinical manifestations of pediatric psoriasis: results of a multicenter study in the United States. Pediatr Dermatol 2013; 30(4):424–8.
7. Morris A, Rogers M, Fischer G, et al. Childhood psoriasis: a clinical review of 1262 cases. Pediatr Dermatol 2001;18(3):188–98.
8. Brandrup F, Hauge M, Henningsen K, et al. Psoriasis in an unselected series of twins. Arch Dermatol 1978;114(6):874–8.
9. Nestle FO, Kaplan DH, Barker J. Psoriasis. N Engl J Med 2009;361(5):496–509.
10. Parisi R, Symmons DP, Griffiths CE, et al. Global epidemiology of psoriasis: a systematic review of incidence and prevalence. J Invest Dermatol 2013; 133(2):377–85.
11. Augustin M, Glaeske G, Radtke MA, et al. Epidemiology and comorbidity of psoriasis in children. Br J Dermatol 2010;162(3):633–6.
12. Tollefson MM, Crowson CS, McEvoy MT, et al. Incidence of psoriasis in children: a population-based study. J Am Acad Dermatol 2010;62(6):979–87.
13. Atherton DJ, Kahana M, Russell-Jones R. Naevoid psoriasis. Br J Dermatol 1989;120(6):837–41.
14. Honig PJ. Guttate psoriasis associated with perianal streptococcal disease. J Pediatr 1988;113(6):1037–9.
15. Farber EM, Carlsen RA. Psoriasis in childhood. Calif Med 1966;105(6):415–20.
16. Whyte HJ, Baughman RD. Acute guttate psoriasis and streptococcal infection. Arch Dermatol 1964;89:350–6.
17. Gupta MA, Gupta AK, Watteel GN. Early onset (< 40 years age) psoriasis is comorbid with greater psychopathology than late onset psoriasis: a study of 137 patients. Acta Derm Venereol 1996;76(6):464–6.
18. Abel EA, DiCicco LM, Orenberg EK, et al. Drugs in exacerbation of psoriasis. J Am Acad Dermatol 1986;15(5 Pt 1):1007–22.

19. Tsankov N, Angelova I, Kazandjieva J. Drug-induced psoriasis. Recognition and management. Am J Clin Dermatol 2000;1(3):159–65.
20. Koebnick C, Black MH, Smith N, et al. The association of psoriasis and elevated blood lipids in overweight and obese children. J Pediatr 2011;159(4):577–83.
21. Bernhard JD. Clinical pearl: Auspitz sign in psoriasis scale. J Am Acad Dermatol 1997;36(4):621.
22. Benoit S, Hamm H. Childhood psoriasis. Clin Dermatol 2007;25(6):555–62.
23. Howard R, Tsuchiya A. Adult skin disease in the pediatric patient. Dermatol Clin 1998;16(3):593–608.
24. Nanda A, Kaur S, Kaur I, et al. Childhood psoriasis: an epidemiologic survey of 112 patients. Pediatr Dermatol 1990;7(1):19–21.
25. Liao PB, Rubinson R, Howard R, et al. Annular pustular psoriasis–most common form of pustular psoriasis in children: report of three cases and review of the literature. Pediatr Dermatol 2002;19(1):19–25.
26. Hamminga EA, van der Lely AJ, Neumann HA, et al. Chronic inflammation in psoriasis and obesity: implications for therapy. Med Hypotheses 2006;67(4):768–73.
27. Zachariae H. Prevalence of joint disease in patients with psoriasis: implications for therapy. Am J Clin Dermatol 2003;4(7):441–7.
28. Gladman DD, Shuckett R, Russell ML, et al. Psoriatic arthritis (PSA)–an analysis of 220 patients. Q J Med 1987;62(238):127–41.
29. Shore A, Ansell BM. Juvenile psoriatic arthritis–an analysis of 60 cases. J Pediatr 1982;100(4):529–35.
30. Southwood TR, Petty RE, Malleson PN, et al. Psoriatic arthritis in children. Arthritis Rheum 1989;32(8):1007–13.
31. Boccardi D, Menni S, La Vecchia C, et al. Overweight and childhood psoriasis. Br J Dermatol 2009;161(2):484–6.
32. Wootton CI, Murphy R. Psoriasis in children: should we be worried about comorbidities? Br J Dermatol 2013;168(3):661–3.
33. Au SC, Goldminz AM, Loo DS, et al. Association between pediatric psoriasis and the metabolic syndrome. J Am Acad Dermatol 2012;66(6):1012–3.
34. Li WQ, Han JL, Manson JE, et al. Psoriasis and risk of nonfatal cardiovascular disease in U.S. women: a cohort study. Br J Dermatol 2012;166(4):811–8.
35. Lassus A, Mustakallio KK, Laine V. Psoriasis arthropathy and rheumatoid arthritis: a roentgenological comparison. Acta Rheumatol Scand 1964;10:62–8.
36. Mease PJ. Psoriatic arthritis: update on pathophysiology, assessment and management. Ann Rheum Dis 2011;70(Suppl 1):i77–84.
37. de Jager ME, de Jong EM, van de Kerkhof PC, et al. Efficacy and safety of treatments for childhood psoriasis: a systematic literature review. J Am Acad Dermatol 2010;62(6):1013–30.
38. Lara-Corrales I, Xi N, Pope E. Childhood psoriasis treatment: evidence published over the last 5 years. Rev Recent Clin Trials 2011;6(1):36–43.
39. Vogel SA, Yentzer B, Davis SA, et al. Trends in pediatric psoriasis outpatient health care delivery in the United States. Arch Dermatol 2012;148(1):66–71.
40. Herz G, Blum G, Yawalkar S. Halobetasol propionate cream by day and halobetasol propionate ointment at night for the treatment of pediatric patients with chronic, localized plaque psoriasis and atopic dermatitis. J Am Acad Dermatol 1991;25(6 Pt 2):1166–9.
41. Kimball AB, Gold MH, Zib B, et al. Clobetasol propionate emulsion formulation foam 0.05%: review of phase II open-label and phase III randomized controlled trials in steroid-responsive dermatoses in adults and adolescents. J Am Acad Dermatol 2008;59(3):448–54, 454.e1.

42. Darley CR, Cunliffe WJ, Green CM, et al. Safety and efficacy of calcipotriol ointment (Dovonex) in treating children with psoriasis vulgaris. Br J Dermatol 1996; 135(3):390–3.
43. van de Kerkhof PC, Hoffmann V, Anstey A, et al. A new scalp formulation of calcipotriol plus betamethasone dipropionate compared with each of its active ingredients in the same vehicle for the treatment of scalp psoriasis: a randomized, double-blind, controlled trial. Br J Dermatol 2009;160(1):170–6.
44. Lebwohl M, Siskin SB, Epinette W, et al. A multicenter trial of calcipotriene ointment and halobetasol ointment compared with either agent alone for the treatment of psoriasis. J Am Acad Dermatol 1996;35(2 Pt 1):268–9.
45. Brouda I, Edison B, Van Cott A, et al. Tolerability and cosmetic acceptability of liquor carbonis distillate (coal tar) solution 15% as topical therapy for plaque psoriasis. Cutis 2010;85(4):214–20.
46. Cram DL. Psoriasis: treatment with a tar gel. Cutis 1976;17(6):1197–8, 1202–3.
47. Pittelkow MR, Perry HO, Muller SA, et al. Skin cancer in patients with psoriasis treated with coal tar. A 25-year follow-up study. Arch Dermatol 1981;117(8): 465–8.
48. Roelofzen JH, Aben KK, Oldenhof UT, et al. No increased risk of cancer after coal tar treatment in patients with psoriasis or eczema. J Invest Dermatol 2010;130(4):953–61.
49. Reichert U, Jacques Y, Grangeret M, et al. Antirespiratory and antiproliferative activity of anthralin in cultured human keratinocytes. J Invest Dermatol 1985; 84(2):130–4.
50. Guerrier CJ, Porter DI. An open assessment of 0.1% dithranol in a 17% urea base ('Psoradrate' 0.1%) in the treatment of psoriasis of children. Curr Med Res Opin 1983;8(6):446–50.
51. Zvulunov A, Anisfeld A, Metzker A. Efficacy of short-contact therapy with dithranol in childhood psoriasis. Int J Dermatol 1994;33(11):808–10.
52. Brune A, Miller DW, Lin P, et al. Tacrolimus ointment is effective for psoriasis on the face and intertriginous areas in pediatric patients. Pediatr Dermatol 2007; 24(1):76–80.
53. Steele JA, Choi C, Kwong PC. Topical tacrolimus in the treatment of inverse psoriasis in children. J Am Acad Dermatol 2005;53(4):713–6.
54. Esgleyes-Ribot T, Chandraratna RA, Lew-Kaya DA, et al. Response of psoriasis to a new topical retinoid, AGN 190168. J Am Acad Dermatol 1994;30(4):581–90.
55. Bianchi L, Soda R, Diluvio L, et al. Tazarotene 0.1% gel for psoriasis of the fingernails and toenails: an open, prospective study. Br J Dermatol 2003;149(1):207–9.
56. Wilson JK, Al-Suwaidan SN, Krowchuk D, et al. Treatment of psoriasis in children: is there a role for antibiotic therapy and tonsillectomy? Pediatr Dermatol 2003;20(1):11–5.
57. de Jager ME, De Jong EM, Evers AW, et al. The burden of childhood psoriasis. Pediatr Dermatol 2011;28(6):736–7.
58. de Jager ME, van de Kerkhof PC, de Jong EM, et al. A cross-sectional study using the Children's Dermatology Life Quality Index (CDLQI) in childhood psoriasis: negative effect on quality of life and moderate correlation of CDLQI with severity scores. Br J Dermatol 2010;163(5):1099–101.
59. Bilgic A, Bilgic O, Akis HK, et al. Psychiatric symptoms and health-related quality of life in children and adolescents with psoriasis. Pediatr Dermatol 2010; 27(6):614–7.
60. Kimball AB, Wu EQ, Guerin A, et al. Risks of developing psychiatric disorders in pediatric patients with psoriasis. J Am Acad Dermatol 2012;67(4):651–7.e1–2.

Pediatric Melanoma, Moles, and Sun Safety

Elena B. Hawryluk, MD, PhD, Marilyn G. Liang, MD*

KEYWORDS

- Nevus • Congenital melanocytic nevus • Pediatric melanoma • Spitz nevus

KEY POINTS

- Melanoma is a rare but deadly disease among the pediatric population, and often has distinct clinical attributes compared with adult melanoma.
- Risk modification is important for pediatric patients at high risk for development of melanoma (eg, due to positive family history, skin phototype), and these patients should be counseled on features of concerning nevi, regular home skin examinations, and safe sun protection practices.
- Congenital nevi and atypical Spitz tumors are pediatric melanocytic lesions that can be challenging to manage and have increased risk for malignant potential.

INTRODUCTION

It is common for parents of pediatric patients to request evaluation of a "lesion" that is new, changing, or concerning in some way. The lesion may be plainly visible to a parent seeking more information, or concern may be related to a rising general overall awareness about melanoma and skin changes. Diagnosis and management of pigmented lesions, particularly pediatric dysplastic nevi and Spitz nevi, can be challenging. In this article, we provide an overview of pigmented lesions in the pediatric population, including melanoma, and management of melanoma risk factors and melanocytic nevi in children.

PEDIATRIC MELANOMA

Melanoma in children is rare. According to the Surveillance, Epidemiology, and End Results (SEER) program, which houses national cancer registry information that has been collected since the 1970s in several states and metropolitan areas, there were 1317 cases of childhood and adolescent melanoma diagnosed between 1973 and

Disclosure: No conflicts of interest relevant to this article were reported.
Dermatology Program, Boston Children's Hospital, 300 Longwood Avenue, Boston, MA 02115, USA
* Corresponding author.
E-mail address: Marilyn.Liang@childrens.harvard.edu

Pediatr Clin N Am 61 (2014) 279–291
http://dx.doi.org/10.1016/j.pcl.2013.11.004
0031-3955/14/$ – see front matter © 2014 Elsevier Inc. All rights reserved.

2009.[1] Only 104 cases were identified among children up to 9 years of age, and a large majority of pediatric cases (1230) were among white persons, corresponding to an incidence rate of 6 per 1,000,000 individuals. The analysis revealed an overall increase in pediatric melanoma by approximately 2% per year, with greatest increases among girls aged 15 to 19, and people with low ultraviolet (UV)-B exposure based on geographic locations, where those who live in these areas often get intermittently intense UV exposure.[1] Examination of all pediatric neoplasms among SEER data between 1992 and 2004 found an overall pediatric melanoma incidence of 4.9 per 1,000,000 individuals. Although this incidence is very low, the annual percentage change of 2.8% makes melanoma one of only a few pediatric neoplasms with significantly increased rates during this time period.[2]

Although a diagnosis of melanoma among pediatric patients is rare, it carries a similar prognosis and clinical course as adult melanoma. Histopathologic prognostic factors include Breslow depth of melanoma, ulceration, mitotic rate, and presence or absence of lymphovascular invasion.[3] It is especially important that the tissue is reviewed by a pathologist who is comfortable with the histopathology of skin from pediatric patients, as banal pediatric Spitz nevi and related tumors may harbor features concerning for melanoma, as discussed in this article.

Although melanoma disease course is similar between children and adults, clinical characteristics of pediatric melanomas do not always follow the typical "ABCDE" detection criteria of asymmetry, border irregularity, color variegation, diameter larger than 6 mm, and/or evolution (**Fig. 1**). Cordoro and colleagues[4] published a retrospective study of 70 cases of melanoma or ambiguous melanocytic tumors treated as melanoma from 1984 to 2009 and found that the most common pediatric melanoma characteristics are amelanosis, bleeding, "bumps," color uniformity, diameter variability, and de novo development. Among 10 pediatric patients who succumbed to disease in their series, 90% were aged 11 to 19 years, 70% had amelanotic lesions, and 60% had at least one risk factor for melanoma.[4] It is important to be cognizant of changing skin lesions and have a higher index of suspicion for patients with melanoma risk factors.

MELANOMA RISK FACTORS

Pediatric patients with inherent melanoma risk factors should be identified and counseled to minimize external factors that can further increase their risk of developing

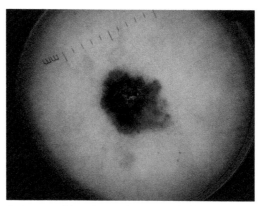

Fig. 1. Dermatoscopic image of invasive melanoma, which was detected by conventional ABCDE criteria.

melanoma. Examples of inherent risk factors that are nonmodifiable include age, pigmentation, nevi pattern, genetics and family history, and coincident medical conditions. Although risk of melanoma among pediatric patients is overall quite low, it increases with advancing age.[5] Patients with a pigmentation phenotype of Fitzpatrick I (fair skin with blonde or red hair) are at highest risk, followed by individuals who burn easily, tan poorly, and freckle.[6] A systematic meta-analysis of observational studies of melanoma risk factors identified an increased melanoma risk for physical attributes such as blue eye color (relative risk of 1.47 vs dark), fair skin color (2.06 vs dark), red hair color (3.64 vs dark), and high density of freckles (relative risk of 2.10).[7]

A 1997 case-control study by Tucker and colleagues[8] demonstrated the increased melanoma risk in adults with nevi. Risk is increased among patients with large numbers of banal nevi, such that having many small nevi increases risk approximately twofold, and having both small and large banal nevi imparts a fourfold increased risk. A personal history of having a single dysplastic nevus increases melanoma risk by twofold, whereas having 10 or more dysplastic nevi increases melanoma risk by a factor of 12.[8] Even the presence of a scar confers an independent increase in melanoma risk, as it suggests the possible prior removal of a nevus.[8] Melanoma enters the clinical differential when examining a pediatric patient who has clinically atypical or dysplastic nevi, a large congenital melanocytic nevus, or a Spitz nevus, which is discussed in further detail later in this article.

Having a primary family member with melanoma is associated with a relative risk of 1.74 of developing melanoma.[7] Fetal malignant melanoma is very rare and most often presents as melanoma from maternal metastasis.[9] Having a parent with multiple melanomas corresponds to a relative risk of 61.78.[10] Patients with 2 or more primary relatives with dysplastic nevi and a history of melanoma should prompt consideration of Familial Atypical Multiple Moles and Melanoma (FAMMM) syndrome, which often carries mutation in CDKN2A gene or the related signaling pathway, and is associated with increased rates of pancreatic and renal cell carcinoma. Both cutaneous and ocular melanomas are identified among kindreds with BAP1 genetic mutation.[11] Risk for development of melanoma is increased in patients with genetic diseases affecting photosensitivity or those affecting DNA repair mechanisms, such as xeroderma pigmentosum; these patients are diagnosed with melanomas at a 5% rate, with 65% of the melanomas distributed to photo-exposed areas.[12] Immunosuppression is another important consideration that increases melanoma risk among patients with AIDS, cancer, and transplantation.

It is important to identify patients with increased melanoma risk due to the intrinsic factors described previously, to counsel them to avoid extrinsic risk factors such as sunburns or exposures to medications or relevant activities (including photo exposure and tanning practice). Medications, such as psoralens, can artificially increase damage caused by UV rays, and a number of common phototoxic medications, including tetracycline antibiotics, cetirizine, propranolol, naproxen, and fluoxetine, lead to increased UV damage and sunburns. Long-term use of medications that cause immune system suppression can impact melanoma risk in a dose-dependent manner: among organ transplantation recipients, melanoma occurs in 14% of patients who received transplantation as a child, compared with 6% in adulthood.[13] Transplant patients may also take chronic systemic antifungal prophylaxis with voriconazole, which causes photosensitivity and is associated with melanoma.[14] Cutaneous surveillance is warranted, and the development of cutaneous neoplasms may prompt revision of the immunosuppression and prophylactic therapeutic regimens.

Excessive sun exposure and indoor tanning are exogenous risk factors for the development of melanoma. The World Health Organization's International Agency for Research on Cancer classified UV radiation as carcinogenic to humans in 2009.[15] An overall increased melanoma risk is associated with sporadic intermittent sun exposure, blistering sunburns, and self-reported sunburns.[6] All patients should be counseled to avoid sunburns through the use of sunscreen, sun-protective clothing, or sun-avoidance practice, as discussed further later in this article.

Indoor tanning is an extrinsic UV radiation exposure that contributes to increased melanoma risk, and is an important risk for adolescent patients. There are increasingly large studies and evidence shows more convincingly the link between indoor tanning and risk of melanoma. In 2012, Zhang and colleagues[16] used a large, well-characterized female nursing cohort to demonstrate a dose-response relationship between the use of tanning beds and melanoma risk (11% increased risk among participants who used tanning beds 4 times per year).

Despite increasing state legislation to prevent indoor tanning among minors (**Fig. 2**), Mayer and colleagues[17] reported that in the 100 most populated American cities, indoor tanning was used in the preceding year by 17.1% of adolescent girls and 3.2% of adolescent boys. Adolescent tanning was more common among white, older, and female adolescents, and those who have a parent who practices indoor tanning, a larger allowance, and live close to a tanning facility.[17] Among non-Hispanic white female high school students, 29.3% reported having tanned in the past, with 16.7% having tanned during the preceding year.[18] Counseling against indoor tanning is an important intervention to mitigate risk for skin cancer and melanoma.

CONGENITAL NEVI

Congenital nevi are traditionally defined as melanocytic nevi that are present at birth, and have historically been classified based on final, adult size (**Fig. 3**). In 2013, new recommendations were prepared for the categorization of cutaneous features of congenital melanocytic nevi with division of medium (M1: 1.5–10 cm, M2: >10–20 cm), large (L1: >20–30 cm, L2: >30–40 cm), and giant (G1: >40–60 cm, G2: >60 cm) sized nevi.[19] These investigators put forth additional descriptors with moderate to excellent expert interobserver agreement to describe the anatomic localization, color heterogeneity, surface rugosity, presence of hypertrichosis, presence of dermal or subcutaneous nodules, and number of satellite

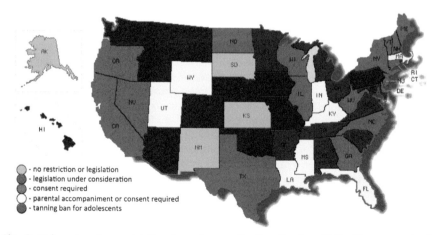

Fig. 2. Indoor tanning restriction for minors, effective October 2013. (*Courtesy of* John Adamson, diymaps.net.)

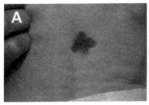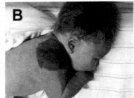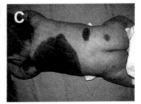

Fig. 3. Congenital nevi of medium (*A*), large (*B*), and giant (*C*) classification.

nevi (none, 1–20, >20–50, or >50). At the time of birth, one can expect a congenital nevus to reach at least large classification based on the growth of the nevus in proportion to the child's growth if its diameter is larger than 9 cm on the head, or larger than 6 cm on the body. Although small and medium-sized congenital nevi are skin-limited conditions, the presence of a large congenital nevus carries increased risk of both skin and systemic abnormalities.

Among all congenital nevi, the exact increase in melanoma risk is estimated at less than 1%, and among patients with small and medium-sized congenital nevi, this risk is virtually entirely after the patient reaches puberty. A number of studies have estimated the increase in melanoma risk associated with large congenital nevi, but given the rarity of these nevi and accumulation at referral centers, in addition to historic interpretation of proliferative nodules as melanomas, older estimates of melanoma risk may be artificially inflated. In 2013, Vourc'h-Jourdain and colleagues[20] performed a meta-analysis of studies published between 1966 and 2011 to examine melanoma risk for patients with congenital melanocytic nevi larger than 20 cm in size, and reported that 2% of 2578 patients developed melanomas, of which 74% had a nevus larger than 40 cm in size and 94% had satellite nevi.

The most prevalent systemic manifestation of large congenital nevi is neurocutaneous melanocytosis, in which melanocytes are present in the leptomeninges. This may be an asymptomatic or symptomatic phenomenon, and is not easily ascertained by available imaging studies. The risk for neurocutaneous melanocytosis is greatest among patients with congenital nevi larger than 40 cm in size and those with multiple satellite nevi; conflicting studies also implicate a posterior axial location of the congenital nevus. Among patients with large congenital nevi, additional abnormalities include complications attributed to nevus size and location, such as obstruction of orifices, urinary tract anomalies, musculoskeletal limitations, and neurologic sequelae of neurocutaneous melanocytosis.

Congenital nevi change over time, and some changes may prompt reevaluation. First and foremost, they are expected to grow in size in proportion to the patient's growth over time. Some may develop overlying hypertrichosis, which can be removed by clipping or shaving the hairs if desired. The surface of the congenital nevus may appear darker or lighter in color over time, undergo verrucous surface changes, or become overall thicker in depth. Nevi on the scalp are reported to spontaneously involute over time; it is advisable to monitor scalp nevi without intervention during a patient's first 2 years of life to allow for maximal improvement before any surgical manipulation.[21] Large and giant congenital nevi are also known to develop "proliferative nodules" within the nevus, which may reveal atypical histology but have reassuring genomic changes that are distinct from those of melanomas based on comparative genomic hybridization.[22] The decision to excise all or part of a congenital nevus is based on multiple factors, including personal and family history that may confer increased risk of melanoma, ease of monitoring, psychosocial factors, and risk of postoperative complications (such as scarring, contractures, and cosmesis), as excision of the nevus does not completely remove the risk of melanoma. Further, as many congenital nevi have large size and depth, ablative surgery or complete excision of deeper layers is often nearly impossible to achieve, and pigment recurrence in the setting of scarring poses great challenge to the pathologist reviewing reexcised tissue.

ACQUIRED BANAL AND DYSPLASTIC NEVI

Common acquired nevi appear after birth and increase in number over the first 2 decades of life. An Australian study of 2552 schoolchildren ages 5 to 14 tallied total-body nevus counts. At 5 years of age, median total-body nevus counts were 40 for girls and 51 for boys; the numbers of nevi increased over time with 14-year-old counts of 96 for girls and 120 for boys.[23] In 2009, Oliveria and colleagues[24] reported a population-based prospective study of nevi in a cohort of American children and identified predictors of nevus count, and found an association of nevus count with skin and hair color, and sun exposure, and sun protection behavior. There were increased nevi among males and children with freckling on their backs; fewer nevi were found among children with dark skin, dark hair, and no tendency to sunburn.[24] Sun exposure–related behaviors that were associated with increased number of nevi include hours spent in the sun, number of painful sunburns, and wearing a shirt or hat.[24]

Patients and parents should be counseled that the development of new nevi during childhood is normal and expected, and they should examine their full body for concerning changes in nevi over time. A nevus with unusual clinical features should be considered for biopsy, which may reveal features of a dysplastic nevus. This diagnosis is based on histopathologic criteria that were established by a panel of experts in 1991, including 2 major and 4 minor criteria, with a 92% mean concordance in diagnosis.[25] The presence of dysplastic nevi confers a slightly increased overall risk for melanoma.[8] That being said, the risk of any individual nevus turning into a melanoma is quite small: for a dysplastic nevus the lifetime transformation risk is approximately 1 in 10,000 (varying with grade of atypia),[26] such that most nevi (nondysplastic and clinically atypical nevi alike) are monitored clinically and biopsied only if concerning changes arise.

Many patients have a predominant nevus phenotype, such that many of their nevi have a similar clinical appearance, and they are regarded as "signature nevi."[27] Several signature nevi patterns have been described, including solid brown, solid pink, eclipse (tan with brown rim), pink eclipse (pink with brown rim), cockade (target), nevi with perifollicular hypopigmentation, multiple halo nevi, nonpigmented (white), fried-egg appearing, and lentiginous nevi.[27] Although some of these patterns individually appear unusual, the presence of several nevi of the same phenotypic pattern is reassuring. One approach to patients with numerous nevi is to identify their signature pattern by comparison, and examine for the presence of an "ugly duckling" outlier nevus that does not fit the signature pattern.

SPITZ NEVI

One particularly challenging pigmented lesion among the pediatric population is a Spitz nevus. The Spitz nevus, or spindle and epithelioid cell nevus, is a benign pigmented lesion that typically arises suddenly on the skin of children and young adults. This lesion differs from classic congenital and acquired benign nevi due to its far greater degrees of cytologic atypia and occasional association with locoregional recurrence and distant metastasis. Some of the histopathologic features are concerning for malignant melanoma, and there exists a "Spitzoid melanoma" variant that shares microscopic features with the benign Spitz nevus; the term "atypical Spitz tumor" describes the lesions of unknown malignant potential with greater atypia than a benign Spitz nevus. A 2011 study of long-term outcomes of patients with Spitz-type melanocytic tumors over 15 years found that among 157 patients, atypical Spitz tumors were associated with an increased risk of melanoma, minimal lethal potential, and moderate risk of regional lymph node metastasis.[28]

A classic Spitz nevus that appears in childhood, with typical history and clinical features, can be managed conservatively by clinical monitoring (**Fig. 4**). Those that are larger, nodular, changing, bleeding, ulcerated, or have other concerning features should be excised for pathologic review. Complete skin biopsy and histopathology review is the current gold standard for diagnosis of these entities, although among samples that do not clearly demonstrate classic features of Spitz nevi, there is often disagreement among expert dermatopathologists regarding diagnosis, with tremendous impact on clinical care. Given concern for melanoma, patients with unclear diagnoses often undergo conservative treatment with wide local excision. The true malignant potential of Spitzoid tumors is debated, as an overall positive rate of sentinel lymph node biopsy was found to be approximately 38%, whereas they only rarely result in negative clinical outcomes.[29] Among 24 patients with atypical Spitz tumors who were treated with excision alone, there were no reports of recurrence, additional lesions, or metastases identified during a follow-up duration of 8.4 years among 14 surveyed patients and 2.8 years among 10 patients followed by records alone.[30] Despite these positive outcomes, some patients undergo sentinel lymph node biopsy and potentially lymphadenectomy and chemotherapy because of the concern for metastasis.

Although many histologic and slide-based approaches have been attempted to differentiate Spitz nevi that will be cured by excision alone from the related tumors that are destined to behave more like malignant melanomas, no specific feature, test, or marker has proved successful. Molecular techniques including fluorescent in-situ hybridization (FISH) and array comparative genomic hybridization (aCGH) have not shown definitive diagnostic value. FISH has demonstrated cytogenetic alterations that are similar to melanoma, and a lack of clear distinction between the entities prompted Martin and colleagues[31] to advise cautious interpretation of FISH data, such that this approach may not be adding diagnostic value. Many of the studies are small because of the rarity of malignant Spitzoid tumors and lack of clinical follow-up to confirm patient outcomes. We recommend that concerning or atypical features on

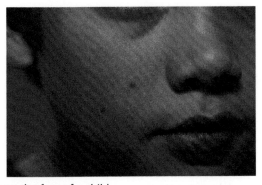

Fig. 4. Spitz nevus on the face of a child.

pathology should prompt complete excision, clear margins, and clinical follow-up, and we remain hopeful in the promise of future genomic tools to interpret histopathologic findings and better predict outcomes.

CHARACTERISTIC CHANGES IN NEVI

All nevi, including acquired banal nevi, have the capacity for subtle change over time, such as growth in proportion to the patient, appearing lighter or darker in color, or slowly becoming thicker in depth, over the course of years. Sometimes nevi undergo less-subtle changes, such as development of a halo or eczematous surface change.

Halo nevi are a result of the immunologic destruction of melanocytes and are considered an autoimmune phenomenon (**Fig. 5**). Although halo nevi may represent a signature pattern among a patient's nevi,[27] multiple halo nevi confer a higher risk of vitiligo and other autoimmune diseases.[32] The halo, which forms a hypopigmented or depigmented circular macule centered on a nevus, can persist an average of 7.8 years, with eventual involution and return to normal-appearing skin.[33] When halo nevi are identified, it is important to closely examine the entire skin's surface, as the immunologic targeting of melanocytes may be a response to a melanocyte abnormality, such as melanoma; however this phenomenon is rare among pediatric patients.[34] A halo may also represent the immune system's response to a traumatized nevus or may be an idiopathic phenomenon.

The Meyerson phenomenon describes an eczematous change over a nevus,[35] which is occasionally associated with atopic dermatitis. Eczematous surface changes can be treated with topical corticosteroids. The Meyerson phenomenon can also be associated with nonpigmented lesions, including capillary malformations, hemangiomas, nevus sebaceous, and others.

EVALUATION, TREATMENT, AND COUNSELING

A nevus is typically evaluated by examination of clinical features, including the classic "ABCDE" criteria (asymmetry, border irregularity, color variegation, diameter >6 mm, and/or evolution) and pediatric-specific melanoma criteria of amelanosis, bleeding, "bumps," color uniformity, diameter variability, and de novo development.[4] If a patient has a "signature nevus" pattern,[27] it is important also to consider a comparative approach of the patient's nevi to identify any nevi outside the common pattern in that patient (the so called "ugly duckling sign"), for close evaluation and consideration for biopsy.

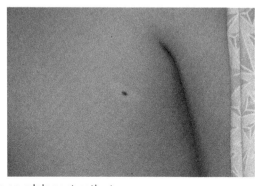

Fig. 5. Halo nevi in an adolescent patient.

One useful tool to closely examine nevi of concern is dermatoscopy, also known as dermoscopy or surface microscopy, which uses a handheld magnification device to visualize key morphologic structures of pigmented and nonpigmented lesions. Two meta-analyses demonstrated that use of dermatoscopy has improved sensitivity over naked-eye examination for melanoma detection, when performed by trained, experienced examiners.[36] Increased dermatoscopy use may yield an improved recognition of early nevus changes, in addition to improved close patient monitoring and tendency to check banal-appearing nevi more closely.[37] Among adult patients with many clinically atypical nevi, a combination of dermatoscopy, total-body photography, and digital dermatoscopy may help to improve early detection of melanomas,[38] although these approaches can be costly in terms of time and resources. Additional diagnostic aids are in development, including techniques of confocal scanning laser microscopy, MelaFind (MELA Sciences, Inc, Irvington, NY, USA), SIAscopy (MedX Health Corp, Ontario, Canada), and noninvasive genomic detection.[39] Although MelaFind has received US Food and Drug Administration premarket approval, it is expected to be made available for use exclusively by dermatologists who receive training and lease the device, and its cost is not intended to be covered by health insurance.[39] Although initial results have shown promise,[40] the studies are limited by evaluation of pigmented lesions that were pre-selected for biopsy by dermatologists, and MelaFind did not significantly outperform dermatologists in detection of melanoma.[41] Such tools may provide reassurance in deciding to follow a specific lesion clinically, versus making the decision that excisional biopsy is clinically indicated.

Among pediatric patients, there are a number of considerations that factor into a decision to biopsy or excise a pigmented lesion of concern. First and foremost, one should consider the clinical necessity, based on the lesion's history, clinical, or dermatoscopic features. Additional reasons to consider removing a pigmented lesion include location in a difficult-to-monitor site (from the patient's or parent's perspective), cosmesis, or ongoing concern regarding a specific lesion. The lesion's location should be considered for ease of removal in terms of both surgical approach and healing, as scars on sites such as the chest or face may not heal with desired cosmetic outcomes, and scars overlying joints may have functional limitations for the patient. A pediatric patient's self-image should be considered, as young children tend to develop an awareness of physical features around the time they enter school, such that elective procedures during infancy and early childhood can be delayed until age 4 to 5. Some patients and parents pursue removal of nevi because of anxiety regarding the nevus; in such cases one should be mindful of providing the best treatment possible for the patient, and to avoid creation of unnecessary permanent scars. The anxiety regarding a concerning nevus should be balanced against the patient's anxiety about the excision procedure in determining the ideal timing for removal. Pediatric patients will often require general anesthesia for a excision of a nevus, whereas local anesthesia may be more appropriate for a quick biopsy or an excision on an adolescent patient.

All removed tissue should be sent for histopathologic review, as even banal-appearing amelanotic growths may yield notable histopathology. Although banal nevi are readily diagnosed, and dysplastic nevi have set criteria with high expert interobserver concordance,[25] severely dysplastic nevi, melanomas, and atypical Spitz tumors can cause significant challenge for diagnosticians. A retrospective review of 478 cutaneous melanocytic tumors sent to a tertiary-care melanoma center (in both historic and contemporary cohorts) demonstrated that approximately 13% of referred melanocytic tumors defied definitive diagnosis (without consensus regarding benign vs malignant classification), independent of the subspecialty training of the initial pathologist, thereby impacting patient management.[42] A number of ancillary tissue and molecular-based tests are in development and are increasingly available to help identify tissue-based attributes that are concerning for melanoma, including aCGH and FISH techniques; however, at this time none have proven diagnostic for mainstream use, and such tests are not considered as standard of care.

Occasionally patients inquire about alternatives to surgical approaches to remove nevi. Despite the availability of over-the-counter creams and products claiming to "remove moles," no topical product has been shown to safely treat or remove melanocytic nevi, and available products carry risk of local destruction, contact or irritant dermatitis, and/or scarring.[43] Further, topical treatment of a nevus may alter the histopathology, causing confusion and potential concern for malignancy if the lesion is later biopsied. Laser for the treatment of pigmented lesions is not recommended because of the unknown effects and potential activation of dysplastic changes, and similar disruption of histopathology.

For patients who have Fitzpatrick I skin phenotype, many nevi, clinically atypical nevi, or a personal or family history of dysplastic nevi or melanoma, it is helpful to monitor their skin and changes over time. Patients and parents often request periodic examinations or "full skin checks" to monitor their nevi, which should be met with a complete skin examination and histopathologic evaluation of concerning nevi (**Fig. 6**). Photo-documentation provides an excellent resource for both office follow-up and home self-monitoring. Pediatric patients and their parents should be educated to examine their skin periodically and take note of their nevi; concerning changes including bleeding, new symptoms, or visible change should prompt evaluation by their pediatrician or dermatologist, and possible consideration for biopsy or excision. The differential diagnosis of a rapidly changing lesion in a pediatric patient can include both pigmented and nonpigmented diagnoses, such as a tick bite, pyogenic granuloma, or even playstation purpura.[44]

Daily sunscreen use has been shown to reduce both the rate of total melanomas and the rate of invasive melanomas, in a 10-year follow-up of a randomized prospective study.[45] The Food and Drug Administration announced new requirements for sunscreen marketing in 2011, providing definition for Broad Spectrum designation (protecting against UV-A and UV-B), restricting use of claims to prevent skin cancer and early skin aging to Broad Spectrum sunscreen with SPF of at least 15, and definition of water resistance claims. The American Academy of Dermatology has provided recommendations on the selection of a sunscreen (**Box 1**). Sun protection

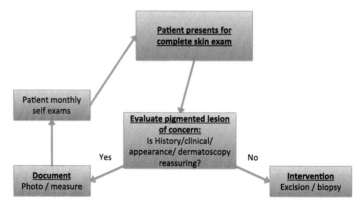

Fig. 6. Clinical management of a concerning pigmented lesion.

Box 1
American Academy of Dermatology sunscreen recommendations

SPF 30 or higher

Broad spectrum

Water resistant

Data from American Academy of Dermatology. Available at: http://www.aad.org/media-resources/stats-and-facts/prevention-and-care/sunscreens.

---

with physical sunscreens (containing ingredients such as zinc oxide and titanium dioxide) are generally regarded as safer among pediatric patients as they provide a barrier against both UV-A and UV-B radiation and are not absorbed by the skin. Patients are encouraged to reapply sunscreens when spending time in the water or extended durations outdoors, as a single application is not sufficient for prolonged protection. In general, one can minimize exposure to the most intense UV rays by planning outdoor activities before 10 AM or after 2 PM, and by wearing hats and clothing (fabric that is engineered to protect from the sun's rays is designated with a UV protection factor rating). All pediatric patients should be counseled to not engage in an indoor tanning practice, as even a single exposure will increase overall melanoma risk.[46]

SUMMARY

Although melanoma remains rare among pediatric patients, there is an overall increase in incidence, possibly attributed to exogenous factors such as indoor tanning exposure. A general increase in population awareness in melanoma may contribute to a parent's desire to seek evaluation or treatment of nevi. It is important to educate parents and patients regarding safe sun practices and self-examinations to recognize concerning changes to their skin.

REFERENCES

1. Wong JR, Harris JK, Rodriguez-Galindo C, et al. Incidence of childhood and adolescent melanoma in the United States: 1973–2009. Pediatrics 2013;131: 846–54.
2. Linabery AM, Ross JA. Trends in childhood cancer incidence in the U.S. (1992–2004). Cancer 2008;112:416–32.
3. Balch CM, Gershenwald JE, Soong SJ, et al. Final version of 2009 AJCC melanoma staging and classification. J Clin Oncol 2009;27:6199–206.
4. Cordoro KM, Gupta D, Frieden IJ, et al. Pediatric melanoma: results of a large cohort study and proposal for modified ABCD detection criteria for children. J Am Acad Dermatol 2013;68:913–25.
5. Psaty EL, Scope A, Halpern AC, et al. Defining the patient at high risk for melanoma. Int J Dermatol 2010;49:362–76.
6. Rigel DS. Epidemiology of melanoma. Semin Cutan Med Surg 2010;29:204–9.
7. Gandini S, Sera F, Cattaruzza MS, et al. Meta-analysis of risk factors for cutaneous melanoma: III. Family history, actinic damage and phenotypic factors. Eur J Cancer 2005;41:2040–59.
8. Tucker MA, Halpern A, Holly EA, et al. Clinically recognized dysplastic nevi. A central risk factor for cutaneous melanoma. JAMA 1997;277:1439–44.

9. Campbell WA, Storlazzi E, Vintzileos AM, et al. Fetal malignant melanoma: ultrasound presentation and review of the literature. Obstet Gynecol 1987;70: 434–9.

10. Hemminki K, Zhang H, Czene K. Familial and attributable risks in cutaneous melanoma: effects of proband and age. J Invest Dermatol 2003;120:217–23.

11. Njauw CN, Kim I, Piris A, et al. Germline BAP1 inactivation is preferentially associated with metastatic ocular melanoma and cutaneous-ocular melanoma families. PLoS One 2012;7:e35295.

12. Kraemer KH, Lee MM, Scotto J. Xeroderma pigmentosum. Cutaneous, ocular, and neurologic abnormalities in 830 published cases. Arch Dermatol 1987;123: 241–50.

13. Penn I. Malignant melanoma in organ allograft recipients. Transplantation 1996; 61:274–8.

14. Miller DD, Cowen EW, Nguyen JC, et al. Melanoma associated with long-term voriconazole therapy: a new manifestation of chronic photosensitivity. Arch Dermatol 2010;146:300–4.

15. El Ghissassi F, Baan R, Straif K, et al, WHO International Agency for Research on Cancer Monograph Working Group. A review of human carcinogens—part D: radiation. Lancet Oncol 2009;10:751–2.

16. Zhang M, Qureshi AA, Geller AC, et al. Use of tanning beds and incidence of skin cancer. J Clin Oncol 2012;30:1588–93.

17. Mayer JA, Woodruff SI, Slymen DJ, et al. Adolescents' use of indoor tanning: a large-scale evaluation of psychosocial, environmental, and policy-level correlates. Am J Public Health 2011;101:930–8.

18. Guy GP, Berkowitz Z, Watson M, et al. Indoor tanning among young non-Hispanic white females. JAMA Intern Med 2013;173(20):1920–2.

19. Krengel S, Scope A, Dusza SW, et al. New recommendations for the categorization of cutaneous features of congenital melanocytic nevi. J Am Acad Dermatol 2013;68:441–51.

20. Vourc'h-Jourdain M, Martin L, Barbarot S, aRED. Large congenital melanocytic nevi: therapeutic management and melanoma risk: a systematic review. J Am Acad Dermatol 2013;68:493–8.e1–14.

21. Strauss RM, Newton Bishop JA. Spontaneous involution of congenital melanocytic nevi of the scalp. J Am Acad Dermatol 2008;58:508–11.

22. Phadke PA, Rakheja D, Le LP, et al. Proliferative nodules arising within congenital melanocytic nevi: a histologic, immunohistochemical, and molecular analyses of 43 cases. Am J Surg Pathol 2011;35:656–69.

23. English DR, Armstrong BK. Melanocytic nevi in children. I. Anatomic sites and demographic and host factors. Am J Epidemiol 1994;139:390–401.

24. Oliveria SA, Satagopan JM, Geller AC, et al. Study of Nevi in Children (SONIC): baseline findings and predictors of nevus count. Am J Epidemiol 2009;169: 41–53.

25. Clemente C, Cochran AJ, Elder DE, et al. Histopathologic diagnosis of dysplastic nevi: concordance among pathologists convened by the World Health Organization Melanoma Programme. Hum Pathol 1991;22:313–9.

26. Tsao H, Bevona C, Goggins W, et al. The transformation rate of moles (melanocytic nevi) into cutaneous melanoma: a population-based estimate. Arch Dermatol 2003;139:282–8.

27. Suh KY, Bolognia JL. Signature nevi. J Am Acad Dermatol 2009;60:508–14.

28. Sepehr A, Chao E, Trefrey B, et al. Long-term outcome of Spitz-type melanocytic tumors. Arch Dermatol 2011;147:1173–9.

29. Luo S, Sepehr A, Tsao H. Spitz nevi and other Spitzoid lesions part II. Natural history and management. J Am Acad Dermatol 2011;65:1087–92.
30. Cerrato F, Wallins JS, Webb ML, et al. Outcomes in pediatric atypical Spitz tumors treated without sentinel lymph node biopsy. Pediatr Dermatol 2012;29:448–53.
31. Martin V, Banfi S, Bordoni A, et al. Presence of cytogenetic abnormalities in Spitz naevi: a diagnostic challenge for fluorescence in-situ hybridization analysis. Histopathology 2012;60:336–46.
32. Patrizi A, Bentivogli M, Raone B, et al. Association of halo nevus/i and vitiligo in childhood: a retrospective observational study. J Eur Acad Dermatol Venereol 2013;27:e148–52.
33. Aouthmany M, Weinstein M, Zirwas MJ, et al. The natural history of halo nevi: a retrospective case series. J Am Acad Dermatol 2012;67:582–6.
34. Lai C, Lockhart S, Mallory SB. Typical halo nevi in childhood: is a biopsy necessary? J Pediatr 2001;138:283–4.
35. Tauscher A, Burch JM. Picture of the month–quiz case. Diagnosis: Meyerson phenomenon within a congenital melanocytic nevus. Arch Pediatr Adolesc Med 2007;161:471–2.
36. Kittler H, Pehamberger H, Wolff K, et al. Diagnostic accuracy of dermoscopy. Lancet Oncol 2002;3:159–65.
37. Argenziano G, Albertini G, Castagnetti F, et al. Early diagnosis of melanoma: what is the impact of dermoscopy? Dermatol Ther 2012;25:403–9.
38. Puig S, Malvehy J. Monitoring patients with multiple nevi. Dermatol Clin 2013;31:565–77.
39. Ferris LK, Harris RJ. New diagnostic aids for melanoma. Dermatol Clin 2012;30:535–45.
40. Monheit G, Cognetta AB, Ferris L, et al. The performance of MelaFind: a prospective multicenter study. Arch Dermatol 2011;147:188–94.
41. Wells R, Gutkowicz-Krusin D, Veledar E, et al. Comparison of diagnostic and management sensitivity to melanoma between dermatologists and MelaFind: a pilot study. Arch Dermatol 2012;148:1083–4.
42. Hawryluk EB, Sober AJ, Piris A, et al. Histologically challenging melanocytic tumors referred to a tertiary care pigmented lesion clinic. J Am Acad Dermatol 2012;67:727–35.
43. McAllister JC, Petzold CR, Lio PA. Adverse effects of a mole removal cream. Pediatr Dermatol 2009;26:628–9.
44. Robertson SJ, Leonard J, Chamberlain AJ. PlayStation purpura. Australas J Dermatol 2010;51:220–2.
45. Green AC, Williams GM, Logan V, et al. Reduced melanoma after regular sunscreen use: randomized trial follow-up. J Clin Oncol 2011;29:257–63.
46. Boniol M, Autier P, Boyle P, et al. Cutaneous melanoma attributable to sunbed use: systematic review and meta-analysis. BMJ 2012;345:e4757.

Diagnosis and Management of Nail Disorders in Children

Derek H. Chu, MD, Adam I. Rubin, MD*

KEYWORDS

- Nail unit • Onychomycosis • Melanonychia • Trachyonychia • Onychomadesis
- Nail pitting

KEY POINTS

- Before initiating treatment of onychomycosis, it is important to establish the diagnosis with confirmatory testing.
- Most cases of longitudinal melanonychia in children are benign; rare cases of melanoma in situ have been reported.
- Trachyonychia is most commonly associated with lichen planus, psoriasis, and alopecia areata.
- The onset of onychomadesis is delayed and often appears subsequent to a systemic illness causing transient arrest of the nail matrix.
- Nail pitting is a nonspecific sign that may not require therapy.

INTRODUCTION

Although pediatric nail disorders are a limited part of a general pediatric practice, it is important for practitioners to be able to recognize and treat common nail pathology and determine when referral to a dermatologist is indicated. There is a wide spectrum of congenital, inflammatory, infectious, and neoplastic conditions that may affect the nail unit in children. Some of these conditions are isolated to the nail unit, whereas others have associated mucocutaneous or systemic manifestations. Herein, we describe several frequently encountered pediatric nail changes and disorders, as well as diagnostic considerations and treatment options.

NORMAL NAIL ANATOMY

To understand the pathologic processes affecting the nail unit, it is important to first recognize normal anatomy. The nail unit is composed of a variety of structures,

Disclosure: The authors have no conflicts of interest to report.
Department of Dermatology, Hospital of the University of Pennsylvania, 2 Maloney Building, 3600 Spruce Street, Philadelphia, PA 19104, USA
* Corresponding author.
E-mail address: Adam.rubin@uphs.upenn.edu

Pediatr Clin N Am 61 (2014) 293–308
http://dx.doi.org/10.1016/j.pcl.2013.11.005
0031-3955/14/$ – see front matter © 2014 Elsevier Inc. All rights reserved.

including the nail plate, nail bed, nail matrix, proximal and lateral nail folds, and hyponychium (**Fig. 1**).

The nail plate is the hard and translucent portion of the nail unit, composed of onychocytes, which we normally clip at its free edge. It is bounded on 3 sides by the proximal and lateral nail folds. The cuticle seals the nail plate from the outside environment at the proximal nail fold. The nail matrix is located beneath the proximal nail fold and is the germinative epithelium that creates the nail plate. The nail bed represents the epithelium and connective tissue on which the nail plate rests. The hyponychium is the distal aspect of the nail unit, at the junction of the free edge of the nail plate and the nail bed.

ONYCHOMYCOSIS

Onychomycosis is defined as a fungal infection of the nail plate. Although it is a nail problem that dermatologists frequently encounter, it is relatively uncommon in children less than 18 years of age, with an estimated prevalence of 0.3% worldwide.[1] The number of cases in children seems to be increasing each year. This increase is perhaps related to increased use of occlusive foot wear, communal locker rooms, public swimming pools, and inoculation from affected family members. Adolescents may develop onychomycosis more commonly than younger children, and toenails are more often affected than fingernails. Immunocompromised individuals (ie, HIV, transplant recipients) and children with Down syndrome are more likely to acquire fungal infections of the nail.[2,3]

Onychomycosis can be caused by dermatophytes (Trichophyton species, Microsporum species, Epidermophyton species), as well as nondermatophyte molds and Candida. *Trichophyton rubrum* is the most common cause of onychomycosis. There are several types of onychomycosis described in the literature:

- Distal lateral subungual onychomycosis
- Proximal subungual onychomycosis
- Superficial white onychomycosis
- Candida onychomycosis
- Endonyx onychomycosis
- Total dystrophic onychomycosis

The most common type of onychomycosis seen in children is distal lateral subungual onychomycosis,[4–6] characterized by yellow discoloration of the nail plate,

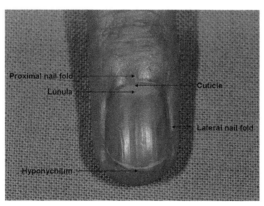

Fig. 1. Normal nail unit. Specific anatomic areas are highlighted.

subungual debris, onycholysis (separation of the nail plate from the nail bed), and thickening of the distal and lateral aspects of the nail plate (**Fig. 2**). The fungus typically derives from the plantar skin and infects the nail via the hyponychium and nail bed. Proximal subungual onychomycosis and superficial white onychomycosis are observed much less frequently.[7] Both can present with leukonychia (white discoloration of the nail). Superficial white onychomycosis results from infection of the dorsal nail plate, whereas the proximal subungual variant is secondary to fungal penetration from the proximal nail fold into the deep proximal aspect of the nail plate and has also been postulated to be caused by systemic spread.[8] Candida onychomycosis is rare, classically occurs in patients with chronic mucocutaneous candidiasis, and often presents in association with a paronychia.[9] Endonyx onychomycosis is characterized by nail plate pigmentation, pitting, milky-white patches, and transverse indentations.[10] Total dystrophic onychomycosis, resulting from infection of the entire nail plate, is the most severe variant and is extremely rare in children.[11]

It is essential to remember that fungal infections of the nail can be pigmented and can mimic melanocytic lesions. Furthermore, several conditions other than onychomycosis may lead to dystrophy of the nails, including trauma, psoriasis, lichen planus, alopecia areata, atopic dermatitis or eczema, and congenital nail dystrophies. Consequently, a complete physical examination of the skin and oral mucosa should be performed to evaluate for associated cutaneous findings.

Establishing the diagnosis of onychomycosis before initiation of treatment is of paramount importance. Systemic antifungal medications have the potential for serious adverse effects. There exists a variety of methods to obtain laboratory confirmation of onychomycosis, including histologic examination of nail clippings (fixed in formalin) stained with periodic acid-Schiff or Grocott methenamine silver (**Fig. 3**), mycologic culture, and direct microscopy with potassium hydroxide preparation. PCR is a method to diagnose onychomycosis, which may have a greater role in the future, but is currently not widely available. Before submitting a specimen for fungal culture, the target nail should be cleansed with an alcohol swab or with soap and water. The nail is then clipped back to the mycelial front (the most active area of infection), which lies at the most proximal aspect of the junction between the nail bed and nail plate that remains intact. Hyperkeratotic material can be removed from this exposed area for culture and/or microscopy. Submitting small nail clippings from the distal free edge of the nail plate are of low yield and often contain contaminants. There are several

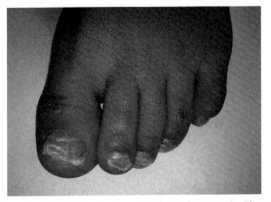

Fig. 2. A 3-year-old girl with histologically proved onychomycosis. The toenails are thickened and yellow at the distal and lateral aspects. (*Courtesy of* Dr Patrick McMahon.)

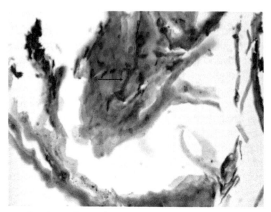

Fig. 3. Histologic examination of onychomycosis. Hyphal fungal elements are seen within the nail plate. The arrow highlights one of the multiple fungi seen in this image. (Periodic Acid Schiff; ×400).

advantages and disadvantages to each diagnostic method (**Table 1**). A negative test result does not necessarily rule out onychomycosis and may be the result of sampling error.

The management of onychomycosis should take into consideration patient age, the causative pathogen, cost-effectiveness, and drug-drug interactions. To date, no medication is approved by the Food and Drug Administration for the treatment of onychomycosis in children (**Table 2**). The gold standard treatment of onychomycosis is

Table 1
Diagnostic testing for onychomycosis

Diagnostic Test	Advantage	Disadvantage	Technique
Histology (PAS)	• Confirmation of fungi in parenchyma of nail plate • Permanent record of specimen • High sensitivity	• Cost • Inability to confirm fungal species and whether fungus is alive	Perform nail clipping and place specimen in formalin
Fungal culture	• Fungal speciation to guide therapy	• Lengthy time for culture to grow (weeks) • Interpretation of results can be complex if potential contaminants are recovered	Clean the nail, clip back free edge of nail plate, collect hyperkeratotic material and submit for fungal culture
KOH prep	• Convenience (in office procedure) • Cost • Rapid results	• Inability to confirm fungal species and whether fungus is alive • Can be time consuming during a busy clinic	Clip back free edge of nail plate, collect hyperkeratotic material and place it on glass slide, add KOH, and interpret with microscope

Abbreviations: KOH, potassium hydroxide; PAS, periodic acid-Schiff.

Table 2
Medical treatment of pediatric onychomycosis

Antifungal	Dosage		Duration of Therapy
Oral terbinafine[1,13–15]	Continuous therapy		
	<20 kg	62.5 mg/d	Toenails: 12 wk
	20–40 kg	125 mg/d	Fingernails: 6 wk
	>40 kg	250 mg/d	
Oral itraconazole[1,12–14]	Pulse therapy[a]		
	<20 kg	5 mg/kg/d	Toenails: 3 pulses
	20–40 kg	100 mg/d	Fingernails: 2 pulses
	40–50 kg	200 mg/d	
	>50 kg	200 mg twice daily	
	Continuous therapy		
	<50 kg	5 mg/kg/d	Toenails: 12 wk
	>50 kg	200 mg/d	Fingernails: 6 wk
Oral fluconazole[1,13,14]	Intermittent therapy		
	3–6 mg/kg once per wk		Toenails: 18–26 wk
			Fingernails: 12–16 wk
Topical ciclopirox 8% nail lacquer[17,19,b]	Apply once daily to all affected nails		Toenails: 12 mo Fingernails: 6 mo
Topical amorolfine 5% nail lacquer[17,18,b,c]	Apply once or twice weekly to all affected nails		Toenails: 9–12 mo Fingernails: 6 mo

Note: No oral antifungals are approved by the Food and Drug Administration for the treatment of onychomycosis in children.
[a] 1 pulse = 1 week on treatment, 3 weeks off treatment.
[b] Duration of therapy is based on adult data. Duration may be shorter for infants and young children.
[c] Not available in the United States.

oral antifungal therapy, with the literature supporting the use of oral itraconazole[1,12–14] or terbinafine[1,13–15] in children with similar efficacy and safety as adults.[16] Oral fluconazole[1,13,14] and griseofulvin[1] do not appear to be as effective.[16] Under certain circumstances, topical therapy can be used as an alternative, particularly in the setting of superficial white onychomycosis or mild to moderate subungual onychomycosis without onycholysis or matrix involvement.[17–19] A recent study by Friedlander and colleagues[19] demonstrated the efficacy of topical ciclopirox in the pediatric age group for onychomycosis.

MELANONYCHIA

Melanonychia refers to brown or black pigmentation of the nail caused by melanin deposition (**Fig. 4**). It most commonly presents as a longitudinal streak (longitudinal melanonychia), but can also present as a transverse band (transverse melanonychia) or involve the entire nail plate (total melanonychia). Increased melanin production within the nail matrix will result in subsequent incorporation of melanin into the nail plate. Melanonychia can involve a single nail or multiple nails. When multiple nails are involved, one should consider the possibility that it is a normal variant, particularly in the setting of dark-skinned patients, or that it represents a manifestation of an underlying syndrome (ie, Peutz-Jeghers syndrome, Laugier-Hunziker syndrome) or medication-induced pigmentation (ie, hydroxyurea, minocycline, zidovudine, antimalarials, cancer chemotherapeutics). In contrast, when an isolated nail is involved, a neoplastic process is suspected. Typically, a pediatrician is confronted with the

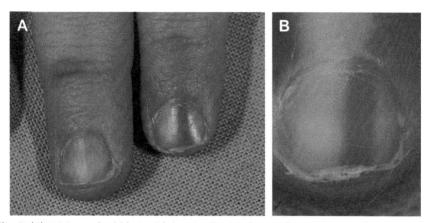

Fig. 4. (A) A 26-month-old boy with longitudinal melanonychia. Nail matrix biopsy showed histologic features favoring a melanocytic nevus. (B) Dermoscopy of longitudinal melanonychia seen in (A). The image clarifies the multiple pigmented bands that are present.

scenario of evaluating a single nail with pigmentation. As such, this will be the focus of discussion.

Parental anxiety around pigmentation of the nail is a reflection of their concern for possible melanoma. Melanoma of the nail unit is exceedingly rare in children.[20] Of the cases documented in the literature, most have occurred in dark-skinned patients, with only 2 cases described in fair-skinned children.[21] To date, all cases of melanoma presenting initially as longitudinal melanonychia in children have been pathologically determined to be melanoma in-situ.[20,21]

Overwhelmingly, longitudinal melanonychia signifies a benign process in the pediatric population. In a study of 40 children with melanonychia aged less than 16 years, no malignant lesions were identified on histologic examination. The final diagnosis was benign nevus in 19 cases, lentigo in 12 cases, and melanocytic activation in 9 cases.[22] Additional reports support these findings.[23–25] Also unique to children is the concept of spontaneous regression of melanonychia.[26,27] This fading of pigmentation may indicate decreased melanocyte activity.

The differential diagnosis of melanonychia includes exogenous pigment deposition (ie, topical agents or systemic medications), trauma or subungual hematoma, and pigmented bacterial or fungal infections of the nail. These conditions should be considered and ruled out in the assessment of melanonychia.

The evaluation and management of childhood melanonychia can be challenging. The practitioner must weigh the remote risk of discovering a melanoma against the risks of sedation and the potential for permanent nail dystrophy related to nail matrix biopsy. The practitioner must also consider patient and family preference. Excision would avoid long-term follow-up, which can often be anxiety provoking. As such, melanonychia should be assessed on a case by case basis. Generally, melanonychia of a single nail will require referral to a dermatologist or nail specialist.

Helpful tools for evaluation of melanonychia include nail clippings to rule out a pigmented onychomycosis, dermoscopy,[27–32] and serial photographs. There are several classically concerning features to bear in mind, which if present in adults, should raise suspicion for melanoma (**Box 1**).[21,33,34] However, these rules do not always apply to the pediatric population, as many of these characteristics can be observed with benign melanocytic proliferations in children.[21] For example, pediatric nail unit nevi can have associated periungual pigmentation (pseudo-Hutchinson sign), heterogeneity of

---

Box 1
Concerning features for melanoma of the nail unit

1. Pigment develops abruptly in previously normal nail or changes over time
2. Rapid darkening or widening of band
3. Lack of pigmentary homogeneity
4. Blurred lateral borders of a band
5. Associated nail dystrophy with pigmentation
6. Triangular shaped band
7. Periungual pigmentation (Hutchinson sign)
8. Occurs in patient with history of melanoma
9. Develops after history of trauma (subungual hematoma ruled out)
10. Involves thumb, index finger, or great toe

Data from Refs.[21,33,34]

---

pigmentation, and variation in width of the pigmented band (triangular shape of pigmentation). Unfortunately, there are no absolute criteria established to help definitively differentiate benign and malignant lesions in children on clinical grounds alone.[35] If concerning or changing features are observed, prompt referral is warranted. Excision should be considered for histologic examination (**Fig. 5**). There are multiple biopsy methods, depending on the origin of the pigmentation, including a nail matrix shave biopsy, lateral longitudinal excision, or a punch excision. Incisional or partial biopsies are not recommended as this negatively affects the accuracy of diagnosis and clinical follow-up of the remaining lesion.

TRACHYONYCHIA

Trachyonychia is a common diagnosis referred to nail specialty clinics. Trachyonychia is defined as roughness of the nails (**Fig. 6**). Usually multiple nails are affected, and sometimes all 20 nails can be involved. When all 20 nails show characteristic changes, the term twenty-nail dystrophy has been used as a descriptor. Trachyonychia has

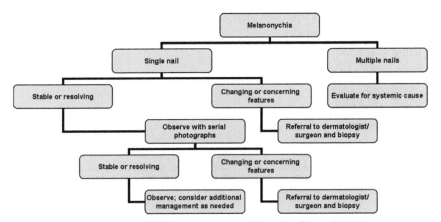

Fig. 5. Recommended melanonychia management algorithm for pediatricians.

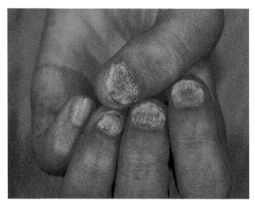

Fig. 6. An 11-year-old girl with trachyonychia. The fingernails are rough and have a sandpa-perlike appearance.

been grouped into 2 types: shiny trachyonychia and opaque trachyonychia; this likely represents the spectrum of disease severity.[36] In our experience, opaque trachyony-chia is more commonly seen. Trachyonychia can present at any age. The incidence of trachyonychia in the pediatric population is not known.

The clinical features of trachyonychia include a sandpaperlike appearance of the nails, longitudinal ridging, brittleness, and nail pitting. Koilonychia (spoon nails) can be seen in association with trachyonychia as well.[37] Trachyonychia has been corre-lated with various general cutaneous disorders, having been predominantly described in the setting of alopecia areata,[38,39] lichen planus,[40–42] and psoriasis.[36,43] There are other less common associations (**Box 2**),[43,44] as well as idiopathic trachyonychia,[45] defined as isolated nail involvement in the absence of other cutaneous disease.

Trachyonychia is often misdiagnosed as onychomycosis. Therefore, it is essential to perform laboratory studies before initiation of antifungal therapy. Evaluation should also include a comprehensive skin examination to look for characteristic fea-tures of an associated dermatosis and/or hair loss. Nail unit biopsies are generally not recommended to diagnose trachyonychia primarily because it is a benign,

---

Box 2
Other select conditions associated with trachyonychia

1. Atopic dermatitis/eczema

2. Ichthyosis vulgaris

3. Vitiligo

4. Incontinentia pigmenti

5. Primary biliary cirrhosis

6. Immunoglobulin A deficiency

7. Pemphigus vulgaris

Adapted from Grover C, Khandpur S, Nagi Reddy BS, et al. Longitudinal nail biopsy: utility in 20-nail dystrophy. Dermatol Surg 2003;29(11):1125–9. http://dx.doi.org/10.1046/j.1524-4725. 2003.29351.x, with permission; and Gordon K, Tosti A, Vega J. Trachyonychia: a comprehensive review. Indian J Dermatol Venereol Leprol 2011;77(6):640. http://dx.doi.org/10.4103/0378-6323. 86470, with permission.

nonscarring process and can remit spontaneously. When biopsies have been performed, histology has demonstrated changes representative of the underlying associated dermatosis.[39,43,45]

Patients and families are often disturbed by the appearance of the nails and seek treatment. There is a paucity of literature on the treatment of trachyonychia, with no evidence-based treatment guidelines. Case reports and small case series have cited various treatment strategies, including topical/intralesional/systemic corticosteroids, topical/systemic retinoids, phototherapy, or other immunomodulating agents.[44] In general, topical medications have poor penetration through the proximal nail fold and are normally ineffective. In our experience, we have achieved good results with nail unit triamcinolone injections. Pursuing this form of treatment requires motivation from the patient and family, because response to treatment can be slow. In most cases, watchful waiting and observation is reasonable. In about half of patients, nail changes will resolve or show significant improvement within 5 to 6 years.[36] Referral to a dermatologist for evaluation of trachyonychia can be helpful to confirm the diagnosis and/or attempt therapies.

ONYCHOMADESIS

Onychomadesis is defined as separation of the proximal nail plate from the nail bed (**Fig. 7**), which may ultimately result in shedding of the entire nail plate.[46] It is believed that both onychomadesis and Beau's lines (transverse ridging of the nail plate) fall along a spectrum of nail dystrophies that occur secondary to temporary nail matrix arrest, with onychomadesis representing the more severe form. Events that may contribute to nail matrix arrest include

- Severe systemic illness
- Infection
- High fever
- Medications
- Nutritional deficiency
- Periungual inflammation
- Trauma[47]

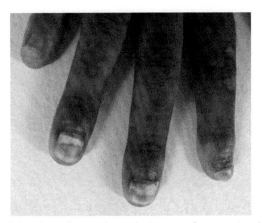

Fig. 7. A 14-year-old girl with onychomadesis secondary to Lamictal-induced toxic epidermal necrolysis. Note the separation of the nail plate from the nail bed proximally. (*Courtesy of* Dr Patrick McMahon.)

The exact mechanism by which these entities inhibit nail matrix activity is unclear. It is conceivable that periungual inflammation and trauma could cause direct damage to the nail matrix, whereas antimitotic agents such as chemotherapeutics inhibit matrix proliferation.[48]

Onychomadesis is likely an underreported phenomenon. It has been observed in children of all ages, including neonates.[49] Depending on the underlying cause, there may be involvement of a single nail or multiple nails. Various systemic and dermatologic conditions have been reported in association with onychomadesis (**Box 3**).[38,50–53] Systemic medications such as anticonvulsants,[54] antibiotics,[55] chemotherapy agents,[56] and retinoids have also been reported as inciting factors. In fact, drug eruptions can trigger the onset of onychomadesis, as evident in the case of a child with penicillin allergy.[57] Neonatal onychomadesis is thought to be related to perinatal stressors and birth trauma, with possible exacerbation by superimposed candidiasis.[58] Idiopathic onychomadesis occurring in a familial pattern has been described.[59]

In recent years, the relationship between hand foot and mouth disease (HFMD) and onychomadesis has been a frequent topic of discussion. HFMD is a common and highly contagious enteroviral infection that primarily affects young children and is characterized by an erosive stomatitis, vesicles on the palms and soles, and a generalized macular and papular eruption. Onychomadesis occurs as a delayed phenomenon, usually 3 to 8 weeks following the acute illness. Numerous outbreaks of HFMD and onychomadesis have been observed in Spain, Finland, Taiwan, and North America.[60–63] To date, HFMD-related onychomadesis has been attributed to multiple viral serotypes, including Coxsackie virus A6, A10, A16, B1, and B2.[47] Experts hypothesize that inflammation created around the nail matrix may be the root cause of nail shedding. Alternatively, viral replication itself may directly damage the nail matrix, as suggested by the detection of Coxsackie virus A6 in shedding nail particles.[61] There does not appear to be a relationship between the severity of HFMD and onychomadesis.

Onychomadesis is a clinical diagnosis. The presence of distinct nail changes and a probable exposure help to confirm the diagnosis. There is no specific treatment. Onychomadesis is generally self-limited and reversible on removal or resolution of the inciting cause. It is important to counsel families and provide reassurance.

Box 3
Systemic and dermatologic conditions associated with onychomadesis

1. Kawasaki disease[50]

2. Stevens-Johnson syndrome

3. Systemic lupus erythematosus

4. Alopecia areata[38]

5. Pemphigus vulgaris[51]

6. Epidermolysis bullosa

7. Scarlet fever

8. Hand foot and mouth disease[52]

9. Varicella infection[53]

10. Paronychia

Data from Refs.[38,50–53]

NAIL PITTING

Nail pits are superficial punctate depressions of the dorsal nail plate (**Fig. 8**). Multiple nails may have pitting, with fingernails more commonly affected. The proximal nail matrix gives rise to the dorsal nail plate and is therefore primarily affected by a causative dermatosis. The ventral aspect of the proximal nail fold closely approximates the nail plate and may also play a role in pathogenesis. It is believed that clusters of cells with retained nuclei develop in the superficial layers of the developing nail plate, and as the nail grows outward, these cells are sloughed off leaving pits in the nail plate.[64] Deeper depressions suggest involvement of the intermediate and distal portions of the nail matrix, in addition to the proximal portion. The amount of time in which the matrix is free of disease correlates directly with the length of normal nail plate growth observed.[64]

It is important to understand that nail pitting is not specific for any one disease (**Box 4**).[65] Perhaps the most common associated condition is psoriasis. Few studies have assessed the prevalence of nail psoriasis in the pediatric population. It is estimated that between 7% and 39.4% of children with psoriasis have nail disease,[66] which can consist of nail pitting, as well as onycholysis, subungual hyperkeratosis, longitudinal ridging, oil spots, splinter hemorrhages, discoloration, and/or trachyonychia. In one study, 61.8% of children with nail psoriasis had evidence of pitting.[67] Psoriatic nail pitting has been described in infancy as well.[68] Although data in adults have correlated psoriasis severity and psoriatic arthritis with nail disease, the same relationships so far have not been established in the pediatric literature.[69]

The number of pits and the type of pitting may occasionally be suggestive of the associated disease. It has been proposed that having less than 20 nail pits is nonspecific and can be present in nonpsoriatic conditions, whereas 20 to 60 pits is suggestive of psoriasis and greater than 60 pits is unlikely to be found in the absence of psoriasis.[70] Irregular pits and deeper pits are often seen with psoriasis. In contrast, fine geometric pitting (longitudinal or transverse lines) is more characteristic of alopecia areata, and coarse pitting may indicate eczematous dermatitis. Rarely, uniform pitting over the entire nail plate can be a developmental anomaly.[65]

The evaluation of nail pitting should include a thorough history and physical examination, assessing for concomitant psoriatic skin lesions, joint symptoms, atopy, hair loss, and additional nail changes suggestive of an inflammatory dermatosis. Nail

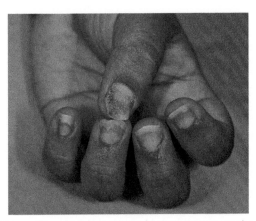

Fig. 8. A 6-year-old boy with nail pitting. Multiple pits are seen on the thumbnail and the fourth fingernail.

Box 4
Causes of nail pitting

1. Psoriasis
2. Alopecia areata
3. Lichen planus
4. Eczema
5. Vitiligo
6. Reactive arthritis
7. Chronic renal failure

Adapted from Jadhav V, Mahajan P, Mhaske C. Nail pitting and onycholysis. Indian J Dermatol Venereol Leprol 2009;75(6):631. http://dx.doi.org/10.4103/0378-6323.57740; with permission.

---

pitting in isolation is benign and does not require treatment. However, the use of intra-lesional triamcinolone for pitted nails in children has been effective, although only tran-siently.[71] If psoriasis is suspected and nail disease is severe, referral to a specialist for management may be necessary. Topical tazarotene[72] and indigo naturalis oil extract[73] have been reported to be useful in pediatric nail psoriasis. Other traditionally used top-icals, radiation therapies, and systemic agents for nail psoriasis have been studied predominantly in adults.[64]

SUMMARY

Nail disorders in the pediatric population are unusual. However, among the nail abnor-malities encountered in children, onychomycosis, melanonychia, trachyonychia, ony-chomadesis, and nail pitting represent relatively common diagnoses. Certainly, these entities do not encompass all diagnostic possibilities, and one should consider other possible conditions when evaluating a child with onychodystrophy. Nevertheless, it is important for general practitioners to be able to diagnose and manage these nail dis-orders and to refer to specialists when appropriate.

REFERENCES

1. Gupta AK, Sibbald RG, Lynde CW, et al. Onychomycosis in children: prevalence and treatment strategies. J Am Acad Dermatol 1997;36(3 Pt 1):395–402.
2. Prose NS. HIV infection in children. J Am Acad Dermatol 1990;22(6 Pt 2): 1223–31.
3. Barankin B, Guenther L. Dermatological manifestations of Down's syndrome. J Cutan Med Surg 2001;5(4):289–93. http://dx.doi.org/10.1007/s102270000021.
4. Gupta AK, Chang P, Del Rosso JQ, et al. Onychomycosis in children: preva-lence and management. Pediatr Dermatol 1998;15(6):464–71.
5. Rodríguez-Pazos L, Pereiro-Ferreirós MM, Pereiro M, et al. Onychomycosis observed in children over a 20-year period: onychomycosis in children over a 20-year period. Mycoses 2011;54(5):450–3. http://dx.doi.org/10.1111/j.1439-0507.2010.01878.x.
6. Lange M, Roszkiewicz J, Szczerkowska-Dobosz A, et al. Onychomycosis is no longer a rare finding in children. Mycoses 2006;49(1):55–9. http://dx.doi.org/10.1111/j.1439-0507.2005.01186.x.

7. Ploysangam T, Lucky AW. Childhood white superficial onychomycosis caused by Trichophyton rubrum: report of seven cases and review of the literature. J Am Acad Dermatol 1997;36(1):29–32. http://dx.doi.org/10.1016/S0190-9622(97)70321-9.

8. Baran R, McLoone N, Hay RJ. Could proximal white subungual onychomycosis be a complication of systemic spread? The lessons to be learned from Maladie Dermatophytique and other deep infections. Br J Dermatol 2005;153(5):1023–5. http://dx.doi.org/10.1111/j.1365-2133.2005.06838.x.

9. Tosti A, Piraccini BM, Vincenzi C, et al. Itraconazole in the treatment of two young brothers with chronic mucocutaneous candidiasis. Pediatr Dermatol 1997;14(2):146–8. http://dx.doi.org/10.1111/j.1525-1470.1997.tb00223.x.

10. Fletcher CL, Moore MK, Hay RJ. Endonyx onychomycosis due to Trichophyton soudanense in two Somalian siblings. Br J Dermatol 2001;145(4):687–8. http://dx.doi.org/10.1046/j.1365-2133.2001.04452.x.

11. Gupta AK, Skinner AR, Baran R. Onychomycosis in children: an overview. J Drugs Dermatol 2003;2(1):31–4.

12. Gupta AK, Cooper EA, Ginter G. Efficacy and safety of itraconazole use in children. Dermatol Clin 2003;21(3):521–35.

13. Gupta AK, Skinner AR. Onychomycosis in children: a brief overview with treatment strategies. Pediatr Dermatol 2004;21(1):74–9. http://dx.doi.org/10.1111/j.0736-8046.2004.21117.x.

14. De Berker D. Childhood nail diseases. Dermatol Clin 2006;24(3):355–63. http://dx.doi.org/10.1016/j.det.2006.03.003.

15. Gupta AK, Cooper EA, Lynde CW. The efficacy and safety of terbinafine in children. Dermatol Clin 2003;21(3):511–20.

16. Gupta AK, Paquet M. Systemic antifungals to treat onychomycosis in children: a systematic review. Pediatr Dermatol 2013;30(3):294–302. http://dx.doi.org/10.1111/pde.12048.

17. Gupta AK, Paquet M, Simpson FC. Therapies for the treatment of onychomycosis. Clin Dermatol 2013;31(5):544–54. http://dx.doi.org/10.1016/j.clindermatol.2013.06.011.

18. Hsu MM. Rapid response of distal subungual onychomycosis to 5% amorolfine nail lacquer in a 20-month-old healthy infant. Pediatr Dermatol 2006;23(4):410–1. http://dx.doi.org/10.1111/j.1525-1470.2006.00272.x.

19. Friedlander SF, Chan YC, Chan YH, et al. Onychomycosis does not always require systemic treatment for cure: a trial using topical therapy. Pediatr Dermatol 2013;30(3):316–22. http://dx.doi.org/10.1111/pde.12064.

20. Iorizzo M, Tosti A, Di Chiacchio N, et al. Nail melanoma in children: differential diagnosis and management. Dermatol Surg 2008;34(7):974–8. http://dx.doi.org/10.1111/j.1524-4725.2008.34191.x.

21. Tosti A, Piraccini BM, Cagalli A, et al. In situ melanoma of the nail unit in children: report of two cases in fair-skinned caucasian children: nail melanoma in two caucasian children. Pediatr Dermatol 2012;29(1):79–83. http://dx.doi.org/10.1111/j.1525-1470.2011.01481.x.

22. Goettmann-Bonvallot S, André J, Belaich S. Longitudinal melanonychia in children: a clinical and histopathologic study of 40 cases. J Am Acad Dermatol 1999;41(1):17–22. http://dx.doi.org/10.1016/S0190-9622(99)70399-3.

23. Tosti A, Baran R, Piraccini BM, et al. Nail matrix nevi: a clinical and histopathologic study of twenty-two patients. J Am Acad Dermatol 1996;34(5 Pt 1):765–71.

24. Léauté-Labrèze C, Bioulac-Sage P, Taïeb A. Longitudinal melanonychia in children. A study of eight cases. Arch Dermatol 1996;132(2):167–9.

25. Buka R, Friedman KA, Phelps RG, et al. Childhood longitudinal melanonychia: case reports and review of the literature. Mt Sinai J Med 2001;68(4–5):331–5.

26. Tosti A, Baran R, Morelli R, et al. Progressive fading of longitudinal melanonychia due to a nail matrix melanocytic nevus in a child. Arch Dermatol 1994; 130(8):1076–7.

27. Murata Y, Kumano K. Dots and lines: a dermoscopic sign of regression of longitudinal melanonychia in children. Cutis 2012;90(6):293–6, 301.

28. Lazaridou E, Giannopoulou C, Fotiadou C, et al. Congenital nevus of the nail apparatus-diagnostic approach of a case through dermoscopy. Pediatr Dermatol 2012. http://dx.doi.org/10.1111/j.1525-1470.2012.01813.x.

29. Chiacchio ND, de Farias DC, Piraccini BM, et al. Consensus on melanonychia nail plate dermoscopy. An Bras Dermatol 2013;88(2):309–13. http://dx.doi.org/10.1590/S0365-05962013000200029.

30. Thomas L, Dalle S. Dermoscopy provides useful information for the management of melanonychia striata. Dermatol Ther 2007;20(1):3–10. http://dx.doi.org/10.1111/j.1529-8019.2007.00106.x.

31. Ronger S, Touzet S, Ligeron C, et al. Dermoscopic examination of nail pigmentation. Arch Dermatol 2002;138(10):1327–33.

32. Bilemjian AP, Piñeiro-Maceira J, Barcaui CB, et al. Melanonychia: the importance of dermatoscopic examination and of nail matrix/bed observation. An Bras Dermatol 2009;84(2):185–9. http://dx.doi.org/10.1590/S0365-05962009000200013.

33. Braun RP, Baran R, Le Gal FA, et al. Diagnosis and management of nail pigmentations. J Am Acad Dermatol 2007;56(5):835–47. http://dx.doi.org/10.1016/j.jaad.2006.12.021.

34. Adigun CG, Scher RK. Longitudinal melanonychia: when to biopsy and is dermoscopy helpful? Dermatol Ther 2012;25(6):491–7. http://dx.doi.org/10.1111/j.1529-8019.2012.01554.x.

35. Tosti A, Piraccini BM, de Farias DC. Dealing with melanonychia. Semin Cutan Med Surg 2009;28(1):49–54. http://dx.doi.org/10.1016/j.sder.2008.12.004.

36. Sakata S, Howard A, Tosti A, et al. Follow up of 12 patients with trachyonychia. Australas J Dermatol 2006;47(3):166–8. http://dx.doi.org/10.1111/j.1440-0960.2006.00264.x.

37. Richert B, André J. Nail disorders in children: diagnosis and management. Am J Clin Dermatol 2011;12(2):101–12. http://dx.doi.org/10.2165/11537110-000000000-00000.

38. Tosti A, Morelli R, Bardazzi F, et al. Prevalence of nail abnormalities in children with alopecia areata. Pediatr Dermatol 1994;11(2):112–5.

39. Tosti A, Fanti PA, Morelli R, et al. Trachyonychia associated with alopecia areata: a clinical and pathologic study. J Am Acad Dermatol 1991;25(2 Pt 1):266–70.

40. Joshi RK, Abanmi A, Ohman SG, et al. Lichen planus of the nails presenting as trachyonychia. Int J Dermatol 1993;32(1):54–5.

41. Taniguchi S, Kutsuna H, Tani Y, et al. Twenty-nail dystrophy (trachyonychia) caused by lichen planus in a patient with alopecia universalis and ichthyosis vulgaris. J Am Acad Dermatol 1995;33(5 Pt 2):903–5.

42. Tosti A, Piraccini BM, Cambiaghi S, et al. Nail lichen planus in children: clinical features, response to treatment, and long-term follow-up. Arch Dermatol 2001; 137(8):1027–32.

43. Grover C, Khandpur S, Nagi Reddy BS, et al. Longitudinal nail biopsy: utility in 20-nail dystrophy. Dermatol Surg 2003;29(11):1125–9. http://dx.doi.org/10.1046/j.1524-4725.2003.29351.x.

44. Gordon K, Tosti A, Vega J. Trachyonychia: a comprehensive review. Indian J Dermatol Venereol Leprol 2011;77(6):640. http://dx.doi.org/10.4103/0378-6323.86470.
45. Tosti A, Bardazzi F, Piraccini BM, et al. Idiopathic trachyonychia (twenty-nail dystrophy): a pathological study of 23 patients. Br J Dermatol 1994;131(6): 866-72.
46. Shah KN, Rubin AI. Nail disorders as signs of pediatric systemic disease. Curr Probl Pediatr Adolesc Health Care 2012;42(8):204-11. http://dx.doi.org/10.1016/j.cppeds.2012.02.004.
47. Bettoli V, Zauli S, Toni G, et al. Onychomadesis following hand, foot, and mouth disease: a case report from Italy and review of the literature. Int J Dermatol 2013; 52(6):728-30. http://dx.doi.org/10.1111/j.1365-4632.2011.05287.x.
48. Clementz GC, Mancini AJ. Nail matrix arrest following hand-foot-mouth disease: a report of five children. Pediatr Dermatol 2000;17(1):7-11.
49. Parmar B, Lyon C. Neonatal onychomadesis. Pediatr Dermatol 2010;27(1):115. http://dx.doi.org/10.1111/j.1525-1470.2009.01075.x.
50. Ciastko AR. Onychomadesis and Kawasaki disease. CMAJ 2002;166(8): 1069.
51. Tosti A, André M, Murrell DF. Nail involvement in autoimmune bullous disorders. Dermatol Clin 2011;29(3):511-3. http://dx.doi.org/10.1016/j.det.2011.03.006, xi.
52. Haneke E. Onychomadesis and hand, foot and mouth disease–is there a connection? Euro Surveill 2010;15(37).
53. Kocak AY, Koçak O. Onychomadesis in two sisters induced by varicella infection. Pediatr Dermatol 2013;30(5):e108-9. http://dx.doi.org/10.1111/pde.12038.
54. Poretti A, Lips U, Belvedere M, et al. Onychomadesis: a rare side-effect of valproic acid medication? Pediatr Dermatol 2009;26(6):749-50. http://dx.doi.org/10.1111/j.1525-1470.2009.00867.x.
55. Aksoy B, Aksoy HM, Civas E, et al. Azithromycin-induced onychomadesis. Eur J Dermatol 2008;18(3):362-3. http://dx.doi.org/10.1684/ejd.2008.0423.
56. Cetin M, Utas S, Unal A, et al. Shedding of the nails due to chemotherapy (onychomadesis). J Eur Acad Dermatol Venereol 1998;11(2):193-4.
57. Shah RK, Uddin M, Fatunde OJ. Onychomadesis secondary to penicillin allergy in a child. J Pediatr 2012;161(1):166. http://dx.doi.org/10.1016/j.jpeds.2012.01.073.
58. Patel NC, Silverman RA. Neonatal onychomadesis with candidiasis limited to affected nails. Pediatr Dermatol 2008;25(6):641-2. http://dx.doi.org/10.1111/j.1525-1470.2008.00792.x.
59. Mehra A, Murphy RJ, Wilson BB. Idiopathic familial onychomadesis. J Am Acad Dermatol 2000;43(2 Pt 2):349-50.
60. Davia JL, Bel PH, Ninet VZ, et al. Onychomadesis outbreak in Valencia, Spain associated with hand, foot, and mouth disease caused by enteroviruses. Pediatr Dermatol 2011;28(1):1-5. http://dx.doi.org/10.1111/j.1525-1470.2010.01161.x.
61. Osterback R, Vuorinen T, Linna M, et al. Coxsackievirus A6 and hand, foot, and mouth disease, Finland. Emerg Infect Dis 2009;15(9):1485-8. http://dx.doi.org/10.3201/eid1509.090438.
62. Wei SH, Huang YP, Liu MC, et al. An outbreak of coxsackievirus A6 hand, foot, and mouth disease associated with onychomadesis in Taiwan, 2010. BMC Infect Dis 2011;11:346. http://dx.doi.org/10.1186/1471-2334-11-346.
63. Mathes EF, Oza V, Frieden IJ, et al. "Eczema coxsackium" and unusual cutaneous findings in an enterovirus outbreak. Pediatrics 2013;132(1):e149-57. http://dx.doi.org/10.1542/peds.2012-3175.

64. Jiaravuthisan MM, Sasseville D, Vender RB, et al. Psoriasis of the nail: anatomy, pathology, clinical presentation, and a review of the literature on therapy. J Am Acad Dermatol 2007;57(1):1–27. http://dx.doi.org/10.1016/j.jaad.2005.07.073.

65. Jadhav V, Mahajan P, Mhaske C. Nail pitting and onycholysis. Indian J Dermatol Venereol Leprol 2009;75(6):631. http://dx.doi.org/10.4103/0378-6323.57740.

66. Klaassen KM, van de Kerkhof PC, Pasch MC. Nail psoriasis: a questionnaire-based survey. Br J Dermatol 2013;169(2):314–9. http://dx.doi.org/10.1111/bjd.12354.

67. Al-Mutairi N, Manchanda Y, Nour-Eldin O. Nail changes in childhood psoriasis: a study from Kuwait. Pediatr Dermatol 2007;24(1):7–10. http://dx.doi.org/10.1111/j.1525-1470.2007.00324.x.

68. Akinduro OM, Venning VA, Burge SM. Psoriatic nail pitting in infancy. Br J Dermatol 1994;130(6):800–1.

69. Mercy K, Kwasny M, Cordoro KM, et al. Clinical manifestations of pediatric psoriasis: results of a multicenter study in the United States. Pediatr Dermatol 2013;30(4):424–8. http://dx.doi.org/10.1111/pde.12072.

70. Singh SK. Finger nail pitting in psoriasis and its relation with different variables. Indian J Dermatol 2013;58(4):310–2. http://dx.doi.org/10.4103/0019-5154.113955.

71. Khoo BP, Giam YC. A pilot study on the role of intralesional triamcinolone acetonide in the treatment of pitted nails in children. Singapore Med J 2000;41(2):66–8.

72. Diluvio L, Campione E, Paternò EJ, et al. Childhood nail psoriasis: a useful treatment with tazarotene 0.05%. Pediatr Dermatol 2007;24(3):332–3. http://dx.doi.org/10.1111/j.1525-1470.2007.00421.x.

73. Liang CY, Lin TY, Lin YK. Successful treatment of pediatric nail psoriasis with periodic pustular eruption using topical indigo naturalis oil extract. Pediatr Dermatol 2013;30(1):117–9. http://dx.doi.org/10.1111/j.1525-1470.2012.01721.x.

Diagnosis and Management of Morphea and Lichen Sclerosus and Atrophicus in Children

Elena Pope, MD, MSc[a],*, Ronald M. Laxer, MDCM[b]

KEYWORDS

- Morphea • Localized scleroderma • En coup de sabre • Parry-Romberg syndrome
- Lichen sclerosus et atrophicus • Atrophoderma of Pasini and Pierini

KEY POINTS

- Early recognition may facilitate early intervention and decrease chances of residual cosmetic and functional problems.
- A team approach is beneficial in management of patients with morphea.
- Treatment of morphea depends on the extent, level of activity, and potential for cosmetic and functional disability.
- Treatment of lichen sclerosus et atrophicus alleviates symptoms.

INTRODUCTION
Overview

Morphea or localized scleroderma is a rare fibrosing disorder of the skin and underlying tissues. It is an inflammatory disorder characterized by skin hardening caused by increased collagen density resulting from a complex interplay of immune, genetic, and environmental factors. Morphea should be differentiated from systemic sclerosis (SSc) based on the appearance and distribution of the cutaneous manifestations and absence of severe internal organ involvement. Lichen sclerosus et atrophicus is a rare chronic inflammatory dermatosis that tends to affect primarily prepubertal girls. Both genital and extragenital involvement may occur. It can be coexistent with morphea, hence the inclusion of the entity in the morphea classification, or on its own with no evidence of other skin findings.

Disclosure: None to declare.
[a] Section of Dermatology, Department of Paediatrics, The Hospital for Sick Children, University of Toronto, 555 University Avenue, Toronto, ON M5G 1X8, Canada; [b] Departments of Paediatrics and Medicine, The Hospital for Sick Children, University of Toronto, 555 University Avenue, Toronto, ON M5G 1X8, Canada
* Corresponding author.
E-mail address: elena.pope@sickkids.ca

Pediatr Clin N Am 61 (2014) 309–319
http://dx.doi.org/10.1016/j.pcl.2013.11.006 **pediatric.theclinics.com**

Epidemiology

Epidemiologic studies have reported incidence rates for morphea of up to 2.7 cases per 100, 000 population.[1] A female predominance of 2.4:1 has been noted.[2,3] Although morphea affects all races, it is more prevalent in Caucasians.[1–3] It usually starts in childhood, especially the linear subtypes, with nearly 90% of children presenting at a mean age of 7 years. There is another peak between 40 and 50 years of age for circumscribed or plaque morphea.[4]

The exact incidence of lichen sclerosus et atrophicus in childhood is not known, as most data on its frequency come from the specialized vulvar clinics that follow both adults and children. A prevalence of 1 in 900 cases has been reported.[5] Anogenital lichen sclerosus et atrophicus is primarily recognized in prepubertal girls.

Pathophysiology

The etiology and pathogenesis of morphea are not completely understood. A complex interplay of autoimmunity and environmental factors including possibly infection and/ or trauma leads to local inflammation and ultimately increased collagen synthesis and deposition in the skin. This process is believed to occur due to increased fibroblast proliferation and extracellular matrix deposition through activation and release of transforming growth factor (TGF) α and β; platelet-derived growth factor (PDGF); connective tissue growth factor (CTGF); and interleukin (IL) 4, 6 and 8, among others; and a decrease in the collagen degradation through a decrease in the matrix metalloproteinases (MMPs).[6] A family history of autoimmune conditions is present in 12% to 24% of cases or morphea.[2,7] Moreover, 5% of children have other autoimmune diseases, and up to 69% of them have antinuclear antibodies.[7,8] Among infectious agents, *Borrelia* species organisms have been extensively studied, but their pathogenic role, particularly outside Europe, remains unclear.[6,9] Lichen sclerosus et atrophicus has a strong autoimmune association; 65% of a cohort of pediatric patients were homozygous for HLA-DQ7, as opposed to 5% of controls.[10]

HISTORY

Lesions of morphea occur insidiously. As they are largely asymptomatic, and the early stages of the disease are nonspecific, seeking medical attention is often delayed. Moreover, lack of familiarity with this condition further adds to delay in diagnosis and treatment. Significant delay has been described ranging from 6 months up to years.[11–13] Anogenital lichen sclerosus et atrophicus seems to be diagnosed within 1 year from onset, likely due to its symptomatic nature.[5] Extragenital lichen sclerosus et atrophicus is likely underdiagnosed, as it is generally asymptomatic.

CLINICAL FEATURES

The clinical picture of morphea depends on the stage (**Fig. 1**).[2,3,14,15] The inflammatory phase presents with local redness or violaceous discoloration. When the discoloration is at the periphery of the lesion, it creates the classical lilac ring appearance. It is often mistaken for other entities (see differential diagnosis) or overlooked. Color changes are accompanied by increased local temperature. Local edema and increased collagen deposition will ensue, particularly in the middle part of the lesion, often with waxy, shiny, white discoloration (porcelain-like). As the disease progresses toward more collagen synthesis, the skin becomes indurated and bound down. Burnt-out lesions are characterized by dyspigmentation (often hyperpigmentation), epidermal atrophy (shiny skin with visible venous pattern), dermal atrophy (cliff drop appearance), and

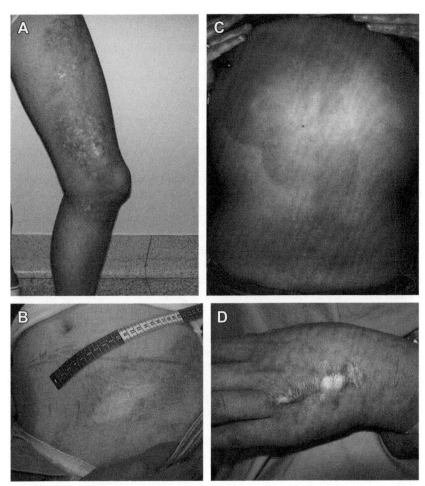

Fig. 1. (*A*) Linear morphea of the limb. (*B*) Plaque morphea with active violaceous border and central waxy infiltration. (*C*) Burnt-out plaque morphea. (*D*) Linear morphea with residual thickening and sclerosis.

subcutaneous atrophy (lipoatrophy to the fascia). Recognition of the level of activity of the lesion is very important in the therapeutic decision algorithm. The extent and location of morphea are also important. Various classification schemes have been proposed; however, the most clinically applicable one includes 5 morphea variants: circumscribed (with superficial and deep variants), generalized, linear (with trunk/limb variant and head variant), pansclerotic and mixed.[9] Other described variants such as guttate or bullous morphea are considered variants of these 5 subtypes, and other conditions such as atrophoderma of Pasini and Pierini, eosinophilic fasciitis, and lichen sclerosus et atrophicus are considered to be part of the spectrum of localised scleroderma (LSc).[2,3,14,16,17]

The most common presentation in children is linear morphea, either on the extremities or the head (en coup de sabre [ECS] or Parry-Romberg syndrome [PRS]/progressive hemifacial atrophy).[4,9]

Plaque or circumscribed morphea usually presents on the trunk, as an oval-shaped plaque, with a waxy, ivory sclerotic center, and an erythematous or violaceous border.

Linear morphea is characterized by longitudinally arranged, band-like lesions located predominantly on the extremities, sometimes following the Blaschko lines (demarcation lines, not normally visible, that follow migration patterns of the embryologic skin cells).[6] Deep involvement in a growing child may lead to impaired growth with a limb length discrepancy, muscle atrophy (rarely myositis and myalgia), weakness, flexion contractures, and significant disability. The ECS subtype of linear morphea occurs on the frontoparietal region of the head, usually ranging from the hair-bearing scalp, where it causes alopecia, to the forehead or even to the mandible. Progressive facial hemiatrophy (Parry-Romberg syndrome) is considered a variant of linear morphea. This condition is characterized by primary atrophy of subcutaneous tissue, muscle, and bone with little or no skin involvement. This often results in severe facial asymmetry.[4,6,9] The deep type of morphea (morphea profunda) is extremely rare; the fibrotic process affects the deeper layers of connective tissue (fat, fascia, and muscle), resulting in firm and bound down skin. It may manifest without any clinical signs of inflammation.[4,6,9] Generalized morphea presents as 4 or more indurated plaques of more than 3 cm of diameter involving 2 or more anatomic sites. These can coalesce into larger lesions. A rare variant of the generalized type is disabling pansclerotic morphea, which predominantly occurs in childhood, and leads to extensive involvement of the skin, fat, fascia, muscle, and bone, resulting in severe contractures and disability.[4,6,9] Mixed forms, seen in 15% of cases, are characterized by different types of lesions occurring simultaneously.[9] Guttate morphea is a rare subtype that presents with multiple yellowish or whitish small sclerotic lesions with a shiny surface, primarily on the trunk. Atrophoderma of Pasini and Pierini is possibly an abortive type of morphea, in which there is deeper atrophy, and the lesions have a distinct cliff-border depression compared with the rest of the skin.[4] Eosinophilic fasciitis is considered by some authors to be a subtype of generalized morphea, which exclusively affects extremities and presents with a rapid onset of symmetric swelling of the skin, progressively becoming indurated and fibrotic with a typical peau d'orange-like appearance.[4]

Lichen sclerosus et atrophicus is a condition in which patients develop characteristic pale, shiny, atrophic plaques (**Fig. 2**). It predominantly affects the anogenital area (with an hour-glass appearance), but it also can present in any other part of the body. Patients with anogenital involvement are often symptomatic with significant pruritus and/or burning sensation. Fissuring may occur, causing further discomfort. Occasionally hemorrhagic blistering may develop, raising concern about child abuse. There is a high prevalence of lichen sclerosus et atrophicus in patients with circumscribed and generalized morphea. Lichen sclerosus et atrophicus coexists with other autoimmune diseases, suggesting a common pathogenic background.[17]

PHYSICAL EXAMINATION

The physical examination should focus on establishing the extent of the skin involvement, the signs suggestive of disease activity, and the potential cosmetic and functional impact. Extracutaneous involvement should also be sought. Proper documentation (with the advent of photography) is important, as the body asymmetry may progress even in the absence of ongoing disease activity.

COMORBIDITIES

Approximately 40% of children with morphea have extracutaneous manifestations such as arthritis, neurologic symptoms (headache, seizures), vascular abnormalities (Raynaud phenomenon), ocular involvement, and gastrointestinal and respiratory

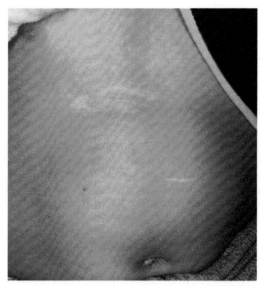

Fig. 2. Lichen sclerosis et atrophicus with hypopigmentation and atrophic changes.

symptoms.[3,4,18] In linear scleroderma involving the face, neurologic involvement such as seizures or brain calcifications, and ocular changes such as uveitis or episcleritis have also been described and require screening even in the absence of symptoms.[4,6]

DIFFERENTIAL DIAGNOSIS

Differential diagnosis depends on the stage of presentation (**Tables 1** and **2**).

DIAGNOSTIC RECOMMENDATIONS

Diagnosis of morphea and lichen sclerosus et atrophicus is largely clinical with pathology confirmation when in doubt. To date, there is no diagnostic test that is helpful in deciding if therapeutic intervention is warranted based on the degree of disease activity.

HISTOLOGY

Early inflammatory stages of morphea are characterized by a mixed perivascular infiltrate of predominantly lymphocytes with rare plasma cells and eosinophils in the reticular dermis. In the later stages, there is excessive deposition of dense collagen. The

Table 1 Differential diagnosis of morphea		
Inflammatory Phase	**Infiltrative (Indurated) Phase**	**Burnt-Out Phase**
Port-wine stain	Lipodermatosclerosis	Postinflammatory hyperpigmentation
Bruising	Pretibial myxedema	Vitiligo
Erythema migrans	Panniculitis	Trauma-induced fat necrosis/lipoatrophy
	Chronic graft vs host disease	Porphyria cutanea tarda

Table 2	
Differential diagnosis of lichen sclerosus et atrophicus	
Common Entities	**Rare Entities**
Postinflammatory hypopigmentation	Nevus depigmentosus
Vitiligo	Child abuse
	Idiopathic guttate hypomelanosis

eccrine glands become atrophied, and the subcutaneous fat appears trapped in the dermis because of the extension of collagen into the subcutaneous tissues. The characteristic histologic findings of lichen sclerosus et atrophicus are an atrophic epidermis and edematous homogenized hyalinized collagen in the papillary dermis. These changes can be found in combination with deeper alterations when the plaques of morphea are both superficial and deep.[1–3,19]

LABORATORY STUDIES

Most patients with morphea have laboratory testing done, although positive findings are not indicative of disease activity. Positive antinuclear antibodies (ANA) are found in 23% to 73% of patients.[6,8,9] Less frequently, antihistone antibodies (AHA) and antisingle-stranded DNA (ssDNA) serology may be seen.[11] Anticardiolipin antibodies have been found in 46% adult and 12.6% pediatric patients.[20] Patients with active morphea may also present positive rheumatoid factor,[9] hypergammaglobulinemia, and eosinophilia.[6] None of these markers are indicative of active disease, but seem to correlate with disease extent, presence of functional limitations, and severity of the skin score.[8] Elevation of the s-IL-2 receptor, a marker of T-cell activation, correlated with active disease in 1 study.[21] Elevation of various cytokines and chemokines, including tumor necrosis factor (TNF) α and IL-13 has been reported.[22]

RADIOLOGY

Routine imaging has limited utility in most patients with morphea. Evaluation is largely directed by symptoms and signs of extracutaneous involvement. Most practitioners will evaluate joints that are crossed over by a lesion of morphea. Deep involvement of a limb may require magnetic resonance imaging (MRI) examination to rule out fascial and muscle involvement. Increasingly, patients with linear morphea of the face (ECS or PRS) will have MRI examinations of the brain to rule out calcifications and central nervous system (CNS) vasculitis. However, clinical and imaging findings do not necessarily correlate, perhaps limiting the utility of brain imaging. However, it can serve as an important baseline in patients who may develop neurologic disease later in the course.

THERAPEUTIC RECOMMENDATIONS

Treatment of morphea is challenging. To date, there is limited evidence for each therapy used, largely hampered by the small number of patients and lack of objective outcome measures. The choice of treatment will depend on the extent, location, disease activity, and potential for functional or cosmetic deformity (**Table 3**).

Table 3
Morphea treatment algorithm

	Plaque	Linear Limb	Linear Face	Generalized
Active	• Topical corticosteroids[a] • Topical tacrolimus • Topical calcipotriene +/− betamethasone	• Methotrexate +/− corticosteroids[b] • Mycophenolate mofetil	• Methotrexate +/− corticosteroids • Mycophenolate mofetil	• Methotrexate • Mycophenolate mofetil • Phototherapy[c]
Residual sclerosis	• Topical imiquimod	• Topical imiquimod • Physiotherapy	• Topical imiquimod	
Burnt-out	• Cosmetic camouflage	• Physiotherapy	• Surgical reconstruction[d] • Cosmetic camouflage	• Cosmetic camouflage

[a] Mid- to high-potency steroids are more effective; discontinue use if no signs of improvement in 2–3 months.
[b] Corticosteroids could be administered as oral prednisone (1–2 mg/kg/d) or intravenous methylprednisolone (30 mg/kg/d for 3 days, monthly for 3 months).
[c] Narrow band ultraviolet radiation could be used; ultraviolet A1 phototherapy has also been reported.
[d] Fat injection, bone paste, fat transplant, maxillofacial reconstruction, tendon lengthening.

Pharmacologic Treatment

For patients with localized plaques of morphea without any restriction in movement or growth or development, topical treatment is an excellent option. There are many options available such as topical corticosteroids alone or in combinations with vitamin D3 analogues such as calcipotriene.[23] Topical tacrolimus has also been found to improve localized plaques.[24] Imiquimod is an immunomodulator that upregulates interferon-α and -γ and inhibits the collagen production by fibroblasts, likely by down-regulating TGF-β. It is particularly effective in more indurated lesions.[25,26] Local phototherapy with ultraviolet A1 radiation (UVA1), with or without psoralen, and narrow band ultraviolet B (NB UVB) is another possible choice, especially for super-ficial lesions, but true evidence of efficacy is lacking, particularly in the pediatric population.[27–29]

Treatment of lichen sclerosus et atrophicus affecting the body is treated similarly to the plaque morphea. Lichen sclerosus et atrophicus of the genital area responds well to either topical pimecrolimus, tacrolimus, or mid- to high-potency corticosteroids.[30]

Systemic treatment is recommended for morphea lesions that have potential for causing functional or cosmetic disfigurement. These include linear lesions of the ex-tremity crossing over a joint, linear lesions on the face, or generalized forms.[6,12,16,31]

Early recognition and prompt referral for appropriate therapy are recommended for these locations.

The combination of low-dose methotrexate (MTX), administered orally or subctaneosuly in doses of 15 mg/m^2/wk (maximum 25 mg/kg/wk) and systemic corticosteroids (CS), either given as pulses with intravenous methylprednisolone (30 mg/kg/d, for 3 days a month, monthly for 3 months, maximum 1 g/d) or oral pred-nisone (1–2 mg/kg/d, maximum 60 mg/d), has shown good response rates and excellent tolerability.[31–33] Other treatments that have been used with variable suc-cess rates are phototherapy,[26–28] antimalarials,[34] cyclosporine,[35] mycophenolate mofetil (MMF).[36]

The ideal combination, dosage, and duration are not currently known. The Child-hood Arthritis and Rheumatic Diseases Research Alliance (CARRA), Scleroderma Chapter, decided on 3 prospective protocols for moderately or highly severe localized scleroderma requiring systemic treatment: MTX alone, MTX plus CS (intravenous methylprednisolone or oral prednisone), or MMF for patients who did not tolerate or did not respond to treatment with MTX.[37]

There is also limited information regarding the length of treatment needed. The authors' practice is to treat, on average, for at least 2 to 3 years, allowing for a minimum 1 year of disease inactivity before treatment discontinuation. Even with this regimen, 15% to 28% of patients will experience disease recurrence after treatment discontin-uation, especially patients with the linear limb subtype and older age of onset.[33,38]

Nonpharmacologic Treatment

Physiotherapy is important for patients who have joint involvement to improve their functionality. Cosmetic cover-up is a suitable option for residual hyperpigmentation.

Surgical treatment options

Damage can be corrected, if desired, once the disease has been inactive for at least 2 years and the patient has reached full growth. Joint contractures may be surgically corrected with tendon-lengthening procedures. Dental abnormalities benefit from orthodontic treatment or more advanced maxillofacial surgery. Facial deformities have been successfully corrected with a range of plastic surgery procedures, such as injectable fillers or fat, autologous fat transplantation, or bone implants.[12,39]

PROGNOSIS

Typically, clinical activity in morphea persists for 3 to 4 years, but new lesions can develop even after longer periods. Overall, the prognosis of plaque morphea is good, especially in patients with limited involvement. At the most severe spectrum, patients with extensive linear morphea, morphea profunda, or pansclerotic morphea may develop growth retardation, irreversible structural deformities, joint contractures, and residual skin and subcutaneous changes that may lead to functional impairment and psychological distress.

SUMMARY

Despite its rarity, morphea requires early recognition and intervention to control the disease activity and prevent permanent sequelae. Investigations for possible extracutaneous involvement are warranted. Patients and families require education about their disease and psychological support to deal with some of the visible, irreversible changes or body asymmetry. A team approach (dermatologist, rheumatologist, physiotherapist, psychologist/social worker, ophthalmologist, plastic and reconstructive surgeon, and orthopedic surgeon) is recommended whenever possible, particularly for severe disease.

REFERENCES

1. Peterson LS, Nelson AM, Su WP, et al. The epidemiology of morphea (localized scleroderma) in Olmsted County 1960–1993. J Rheumatol 1997;24:73–80.
2. Zulian F, Athreya BH, Laxer R, et al. Juvenile localized scleroderma: clinical and epidemiological features in 750 children. An international study. Rheumatology (Oxford) 2006;45:614–20.
3. Christen-Zaech S, Hakim MD, Afsar FS, et al. Pediatric morphea (localized scleroderma): review of 136 patients. J Am Acad Dermatol 2008;59:385–96.
4. Atzeni F, Bardoni A, Cutolo M, et al. Localized and systemic forms of scleroderma in adults and children. Clin Exp Rheumatol 2006;24:S36–45.
5. Powell J, Wojnarowska F. Childhood vulvar lichen sclerosus: an increasingly common problem. J Am Acad Dermatol 2001;44(5):803–6.
6. Kreuter A. Localized scleroderma. Dermatol Ther 2012;25:135–47.
7. Leitenberger JJ, Cayce RL, Haley RW, et al. Distinct autoimmune syndromes in morphea: a review of 245 adult and pediatric cases. Arch Dermatol 2009;145: 545–50.
8. Warner Dharamsi J, Victor S, Aguwa N, et al. Morphea in adults and children cohort III: nested case–control study—the clinical significance of autoantibodies in morphea. JAMA Dermatol 2013;149(10):1159–65.
9. Laxer RM, Zulian F. Localized scleroderma. Curr Opin Rheumatol 2006;18: 606–13.
10. Powell J, Wojnarowska F, Winsey S, et al. Lichen sclerosus premenarche: autoimmunity and immunogenetics. Br J Dermatol 2000;142:481–4.
11. Nouri S, Jacobe H. Recent developments in diagnosis and assessment of morphea. Curr Rheumatol Rep 2013;15:308.
12. Zwischenberger BA, Jacobe HT. A systematic review of morphea treatments and therapeutic algorithm. J Am Acad Dermatol 2011;65:925–41.
13. Johnson W, Jacobe H. Morphea in adults and children cohort II: patients with morphea experience delay in diagnosis and large variation in treatment. J Am Acad Dermatol 2012;67:881–9.

14. Peterson LS, Nelson AM, Su WP. Classification of morphea (localized scleroderma). Mayo Clin Proc 1995;70:1068–76.
15. Fett NM. Morphea (localized scleroderma). JAMA Dermatol 2013;149:1124.
16. Uziel Y, Krafchik BR, Silverman ED, et al. Localized scleroderma in childhood: a report of 30 cases. Semin Arthritis Rheum 1994;23:328–40.
17. Kreuter A, Wischnewski J, Terras S, et al. Coexistence of lichen sclerosus and morphea: a retrospective analysis of 472 patients with localized scleroderma from a German tertiary referral center. J Am Acad Dermatol 2012;67:1157–62.
18. Zulian F, Vallongo C, Woo P, et al. Localized scleroderma in childhood is not just a skin disease. Arthritis Rheum 2005;52:2873–81.
19. Succaria F, Kurban M, Kibbi AG, et al. Clinicopathological study of 81 cases of localized and systemic scleroderma. J Eur Acad Dermatol Venereol 2013;27: e191–6.
20. Sato S, Fujimoto M, Hasegawa M, et al. Antiphospholipid antibody in localised scleroderma. Ann Rheum Dis 2003;62:771–4.
21. Uziel Y, Krafchik BR, Feldman B, et al. Serum levels of soluble interleukin-2 receptor. A marker of disease activity in localized scleroderma. Arthritis Rheum 1994; 37:898–901.
22. Hasegawa M, Sato S, Nagaoka T, et al. Serum levels of tumor necrosis factor and interleukin-13 are elevated in patients with localized scleroderma. Dermatology 2003;207:141–7.
23. Cunningham BB, Landells ID, Langman C, et al. Topical calcipotriene for morphea/linear scleroderma. J Am Acad Dermatol 1998;39:211–5.
24. Cantisani C, Miraglia E, Richetta AG, et al. Generalized morphea successfully treated with tacrolimus 0.1% ointment. J Drugs Dermatol 2013;12:14–5.
25. Gupta AK, Browne M, Bluhm R. Imiquimod: a review. J Cutan Med Surg 2002;6: 554–60.
26. Pope E, Doria AS, Theriault M, et al. Topical imiquimod 5% cream for pediatric plaque morphea: a prospective, multiple-baseline, open-label pilot study. Dermatology 2011;223:363–9.
27. Andres C, Kollmar A, Mempel M, et al. Successful ultraviolet A1 phototherapy in the treatment of localized scleroderma: a retrospective and prospective study. Br J Dermatol 2010;162:445–7.
28. Uchiyama M, Okubo Y, Kawashima H, et al. Case of localized scleroderma successfully treated with bath psoralen and ultraviolet A therapy. J Dermatol 2010; 37:75–80.
29. Pavlotsky F, Sakka N, Lozinski A, et al. Bath psoralen-UVA photochemotherapy for localized scleroderma: experience from a single institute. Photodermatol Photoimmunol Photomed 2013;29:247–52.
30. Chi CC, Kirtschig G, Baldo M, et al. Systematic review and meta-analysis of randomized controlled trials on topical interventions for genital lichen sclerosus. J Am Acad Dermatol 2012;67:305–12.
31. Uziel Y, Feldman BM, Krafchik BR, et al. Methotrexate and corticosteroid therapy for pediatric localized scleroderma. J Pediatr 2000;136:91–5.
32. Zulian F, Martini G, Vallongo C, et al. Methotrexate treatment in juvenile localized scleroderma: a randomized, double-blind, placebo-controlled trial. Arthritis Rheum 2011;63:1998–2006.
33. Zulian F, Vallongo C, Patrizi A, et al. A long-term follow-up study of methotrexate in juvenile localized scleroderma (morphea). J Am Acad Dermatol 2012;67: 1151–6.

34. Brownell I, Soter NA, Franks AG Jr. Familial linear scleroderma (en coup de sabre) responsive to antimalarials and narrowband ultraviolet B therapy. Dermatol Online J 2007;13:11.

35. Perez Crespo M, Betlloch Mas I, Mataix Diaz J, et al. Rapid response to cyclosporine and maintenance with methotrexate in linear scleroderma in a young girl. Pediatr Dermatol 2009;26:118–20.

36. Martini G, Ramanan AV, Falcini F, et al. Successful treatment of severe or methotrexate-resistant juvenile localized scleroderma with mycophenolate mofetil. Rheumatology (Oxford) 2009;48:1410–3.

37. Li SC, Torok KS, Pope E, et al. Development of consensus treatment plans for juvenile localized scleroderma: a roadmap toward comparative effectiveness studies in juvenile localized scleroderma. Arthritis Care Res (Hoboken) 2012; 64:1175–85.

38. Mirsky L, Chakkittakandiyil A, Laxer RM, et al. Relapse after systemic treatment in paediatric morphoea. Br J Dermatol 2012;166:443–5.

39. Palmero ML, Uziel Y, Laxer RM, et al. En coup de sabre scleroderma and Parry-Romberg syndrome in adolescents: surgical options and patient-related outcomes. J Rheumatol 2010;37:2174–9.

Diagnosis and Management of Cutaneous Vasculitis in Children

Tracy V. Ting, MD, MS

KEYWORDS

- Cutaneous vasculitis • Leukocytoclastic vasculitis • HSP • Palpable purpura
- Cutaneous polyarteritis nodosa • Pediatric

KEY POINTS

- Cutaneous vasculitis is rare in children.
- Henoch-Schönlein purpura is the most common vasculitis in childhood.
- Leukocytoclastic vasculitis describes the typical histopathologic findings on skin biopsy of most childhood cutaneous vasculitic lesions: small vessel wall inflammation with fibrinoid necrosis and immune complex deposition.
- Differential diagnosis of cutaneous vasculitis includes infectious causes, systemic forms of vasculitis, and other connective tissue diseases.
- Referral to a dermatologist and/or rheumatologist is warranted, particularly when the rash and/or presentation is atypical.

INTRODUCTION

Vasculitis is an inflammatory cell-mediated process involving cellular infiltration, necrosis, and destruction of blood vessels. Cutaneous vasculitis (CV) can be seen among a spectrum of heterogeneous conditions. Although it can be limited to cutaneous deposition only, it can also be associated with other inflammatory and autoimmune conditions such as systemic vasculitides and connective tissue diseases, and has also been associated with certain medications, infections, and malignancy (although malignancy is more commonly seen among adults). This article focuses on the childhood conditions most commonly associated with CV and the varying histopathology, clinical presentation, and treatment, including leukocytoclastic vasculitis (Henoch-Schönlein purpura [HSP], urticarial vasculitis [UV], acute hemorrhagic edema of infancy [AHEI]) and cutaneous polyarteritis nodosa (cPAN). There is also a brief discussion of systemic conditions and other causes or mimickers of CV.

The author has nothing to disclose.
Division of Pediatric Rheumatology, Cincinnati Children's Hospital Medical Center, 3333 Burnet Avenue, MLC 4010, Cincinnati, OH 45229, USA
E-mail address: tracy.ting@cchmc.org

Pediatr Clin N Am 61 (2014) 321–346
http://dx.doi.org/10.1016/j.pcl.2013.11.007 **pediatric.theclinics.com**

PATHOPHYSIOLOGY

The exact mechanism leading to vasculitis remains uncertain. It is presumed that CV is an immune complex–mediated condition with the majority of lesions having immunoglobulin and/or complement deposition on direct immunofluorescence. For example, in leukocytoclastic vasculitis (LCV), immunoglobulin (Ig) A, IgG, IgM, fibrin, and activated third component of complement (C3) deposition is noted.[1,2] Endothelial cell factors, inflammatory mediators, and adhesion molecules are also presumed to play a role in the damage seen in vasculitis. Following immune complex deposition, complement (C3a, C5a) is activated triggering the recruitment of inflammatory cells including neutrophils and mast cells.[3] Adhesion molecules, including intracellular adhesion molecule-1, P-selectin, and E-selectin, have been found to be expressed within vasculitic lesions.[4–6] Activated lymphocytes and macrophages trigger further complement activation and cytokine production, including production of tumor necrosis factor (TNF) alpha and interferon gamma, which serve to induce and upregulate adhesion molecules, thus perpetuating the vascular destruction.[7,8] Other autoantibodies, including antineutrophil cytoplasmic antibodies (ANCA), may play a role in some cases of CV, particularly those cases seen in certain systemic vasculitides.

EPIDEMIOLOGY

Given the rarity of childhood cases of CV, limited information is available for incidence and prevalence. HSP is the most common systemic vasculitis in children, occurring in 1 in 5000 children annually in the United States,[9] with Kawasaki disease being the second most common vasculitis. Although not specific to the pediatric population, causes of CV in adults are typically idiopathic (45%–55%) but can be associated with infection (15%–20%), autoimmune conditions (15%–20%), medications (10%–15%), and malignancy (<5%).[5,10] Other inflammatory conditions like systemic lupus erythematosus (SLE), rheumatoid arthritis (RA), Sjögren syndrome (SS), Behçet disease (BD), and inflammatory bowel disease can have cutaneous findings of CV as part of the clinical manifestation of disease. Medications associated with CV in children include penicillins, paracetamol, and/or nonsteroidal antiinflammatory drugs (NSAIDs).[11] Multiple infections, primarily upper respiratory infections (viral, bacterial, mycobacterial),[12–15] and vaccinations including hepatitis A, hepatitis B, influenza, and H1N1[15–19] have also been implicated. Other potential triggers seen more frequently in adults include chemical exposures, foods, and illicit drugs.[20,21] Diagnosing drug-induced vasculitis is difficult given the lack of diagnostic tests; however, eosinophilia has been found in some cases.[22] Therefore, other causes must first be excluded. Some clues to drug-induced vasculitis include the temporal relationship of skin findings to the drug (typically 5–7 days after exposure, although it can be years), effect of withdrawal of the drug, effects of rechallenge with the drug, dose exposure, and the type of drug.[10]

CLINICAL FEATURES
History

To date, classification criteria have been controversial for vasculitic syndromes, in part because of the heterogeneity of the different diseases. Nonetheless, in pediatrics, a revised classification criteria was proposed in 2008 via a consensus panel by the European League against Rheumatism (EULAR), the Pediatric Rheumatology International Trials Organisation (PRINTO), and the Paediatric Rheumatology European Society (PRES)[23] to better define childhood vasculitic syndromes. Additional criteria for systemic disease has been suggested by both the American College of Rheumatology (ACR)[24] and the North Carolina Chapel Hill Consensus Congress,[25] but these have limitations and are unique to the adult population.

At present, when evaluating a child with suspected CV, key criteria to consider include the size of the vessel(s) involved, histopathologic features, as well as extent of disease with or without additional systemic symptoms (limited cutaneous vs systemic). Skin is composed of both small and medium-sized vessels. Small-vessel disease involves inflammation within the superficial dermis of capillaries, postcapillary venules, and nonmuscular arterioles and presents clinically as palpable purpura, petechiae, vesicles, pustules, and/or urticaria. Medium-sized vessels of the skin are arterioles located deep in the junction of dermis and subcutis with medium-vessel vasculitis presenting clinically as subcutaneous nodules, livedo reticularis, cutaneous ulcers or infarcts, and/or necrotic lesions.

DIAGNOSTIC RECOMMENDATIONS

A thorough history and physical examination helps to guide the need for laboratory and imaging studies. The history should focus on recent illnesses, drug or vaccination exposure, family history, and medical history. Constitutional symptoms including fever, weight loss, anorexia, malaise, arthralgias, and myalgias are helpful to elicit. Additional organ-specific symptoms should be reviewed to evaluate for possible systemic disease.

Laboratory Studies

In general, laboratory studies may not be helpful in making the diagnosis of CV limited only to skin. However, they may be helpful when differentiating isolated cutaneous versus systemic disease. In all cases, there may be evidence of mild to moderate systemic inflammation (increased white blood cell [WBC] count, erythrocyte sedimentation rate [ESR], or c-reactive protein [CRP]); however, in systemic disease, there may be greater increases of inflammatory markers. Additional screening should include a complete metabolic panel (CMP), urinalysis (UA), urine protein/creatinine ratio (an indirect measure of proteinuria), antinuclear antibody (ANA), complement levels (C3, C4, CH50), ANCA, antistreptolysin-O (ASO) antibodies, anti-DNase antibodies, and other bacterial or viral studies as appropriate. Rheumatoid factor (RF), anti-SSA, anti-SSB, cryoglobulins, and hepatitis B/C titers may be considered but are less commonly seen among children.

Histology

A skin biopsy is helpful when performed correctly. It is important to consider both location and timing of the biopsy for optimal diagnostic yield.[26,27] The type of biopsy (punch of 3–4 mm vs incisional/excisional >6 mm) should be chosen based on vessel size of interest, with larger vessels present in deeper tissue. Lesions of choice should be active (appearing no more than 48 hours before biopsy) and ideally include a tender, reddish, purpuric lesion.[27] In small-vessel (diameter<50 μm) vasculitis, a punch biopsy should be sufficient; however, for cPAN, a deeper biopsy including subcutaneous fat is needed for adequate evaluation of medium-sized (diameter 50–150 μm) vessels, and therefore an incisional or excisional biopsy may be more appropriate.

Timing of the skin biopsy is also critical. Classic lesions less than 24 hours old typically reveal fibrin deposits and neutrophilic infiltration with hemorrhage (caused by extravasation of erythrocytes) and nuclear debris. However, soon thereafter, neutrophils are replaced with infiltration of lymphocytes and macrophages and, by 48 hours, lymphocytes predominate.[28] Thus, it is strongly recommended that the lesion be less than 48 hours old. Furthermore, immunofluorescence deposition declines with time.[5,29,30]

In addition to standard hematoxylin and eosin staining, all skin biopsies should undergo direct immunofluorescence (DIF), particularly given the hallmark finding of IgA deposition in HSP. In immune complex–mediated vasculitis, all biopsies should stain for immunoglobulins within the first 48 hours. However, only 70% are present at 48 to 72 hours, and none are detected after 72 hours.[5] In contrast, complement may still be seen in most lesions of vasculitis even after 72 hours.[5] A lesional biopsy is also preferred for DIF, although perilesional (2–3 mm from active lesion) biopsies may reveal positive immunoglobulin deposition.[31] A diagnosis of LCV-type vasculitis was associated with IgA deposition within lesional (sensitivity 87%, specificity 73%) and perilesional (sensitivity 68%, specificity 66.7%) biopsies.[31] Likewise, in LCV, IgM and IgG were also more commonly seen in lesional (56%, 20% respectively) than perilesional (34%, 8%) skin biopsies.[31]

THERAPEUTIC RECOMMENDATIONS
Pharmacologic Treatment

Because most isolated cutaneous lesions have a benign course, treatment is mainly supportive with rest, elevation, and NSAIDs. Avoidance or removal of potential triggers (ie, medications) should also occur and appropriate treatment of identified infections should be implemented. Patients who do not respond readily to these supportive measures, or in whom there is significant pain or involvement, may benefit from dapsone, colchicine, or hydroxychloroquine. There is anecdotal evidence that a short course of oral (and possibly topical) steroids may provide rapid relief but should be reserved for severe cases of cutaneous disease and should likely be tapered slowly to prevent rebound. Those cases of CV associated with systemic conditions require more specific immune suppressants including systemic corticosteroids; a discussion of this is beyond the scope of this article.

PROGNOSIS

CV of the skin only is typically benign and self-limited with a good prognosis. Those skin lesions associated with systemic conditions are at risk of greater organ involvement and, therefore, greater morbidity.

LEUKOCYTOCLASTIC VASCULITIS
HSP

Introduction/overview
HSP is the most common small vessel vasculitis of childhood with a classic presentation of palpable purpura. HSP is typically a benign, self-limited condition, although some patients have a protracted course with relapses and renal complications. Skin findings are the absolute criteria for diagnosis; therefore, awareness of the variations of cutaneous presentation can be helpful. Most cases of HSP are diagnosed and managed by the general pediatrician; however, at times, with atypical presentations or unusual skin findings, a dermatologist's evaluation can be helpful. Additional consultants may include a rheumatologist if there is consideration for an alternate systemic vasculitis or treatment recommendations, a nephrologist for renal disease, and a gastroenterologist or urologist if necessary.

PATHOPHYSIOLOGY

HSP is an immune complex–mediated leukocytoclastic vasculitis affecting small blood vessels including arterioles, venules, and capillaries. Polymorphonuclear infiltration of vascular and perivascular tissue is frequently seen. It is an IgA-mediated disease with deposition noted on histopathology. Direct immunofluorescence may further reveal additional IgM and C3 deposition.[1] Other autoantibodies including ANCA, endothelial cell factors like vascular endothelial growth factor (VEGF[32]), inflammatory mediators, and adhesion molecules are also presumed to play a role in the damage seen in vasculitis. In a 2004 study evaluating the presence of ANCA in HSP, blood samples of IgA ANCA were found with greater prevalence (82.3%) among patients with HSP in the acute stages compared with IgG ANCA (2.8%) and in comparison with healthy controls (0%) and patients without LCV vasculitis (38%). In the resolution phase, IgA ANCA was seen in only 12% of patients with HSP, indicating that ANCA testing could be a useful biomarker of disease, although further studies have yet to be reported. This finding further indicates the potential pathogenic involvement of ANCA.[33]

EPIDEMIOLOGY

The annual incidence of HSP in children has been reported at 14 to 20.4 per 100,000.[9,34,35] As one of the most common vasculitides in childhood, it accounts for more than half of all cases of pediatric vasculitis.[26,34,36] There may be a slight gender predilection affecting male rather than female patients at a 2:1 ratio.[9,37–39] Average age of onset is approximately 2 to 11 years.[9,38–40] Although skin disease is always present, vasculitis can also involve the gastrointestinal tract, kidneys, scrotum, and joints. Frequent association with a preceding illness has been reported, in particular with beta-hemolytic streptococcus (20%–50%), parvovirus B19, *Bartonella henselae*, *Staphylococcus aureus*, *Helicobacter pylori*, *Haemophilus parainfluenza*, Coxsackie virus, mycobacteria, *Salmonella*, other viral illnesses, immunizations, and medications.[39,41–44] The seasonal predilection (primarily fall and winter) for HSP provides further evidence of a strong association with infectious triggers.[35,37,39,45]

PROGNOSIS

In most classic cases of HSP, patients have a short-lived (<1 month), benign course and require little to no treatment (other than supportive care). About one-third of patients tend to have a remitting and relapsing course, particularly with skin findings.[37,43] Nevertheless, each subsequent episode is less severe and shorter in duration than the one before. Approximately 2% to 20% of all patients with HSP develop permanent renal disease.[46,47]

CLINICAL FEATURES
History

In children with HSP, classic symptoms of palpable purpura typically occur 5 to 7 days following an upper respiratory infection or other trigger noted earlier.[41] The rash is the presenting symptom in nearly three-quarters of cases.[37,48,49]

Physical Examination

Children with HSP classically present with palpable purpura (**Fig. 1**) located in areas of dependency, including the buttock and lower extremities. A rash can also appear on

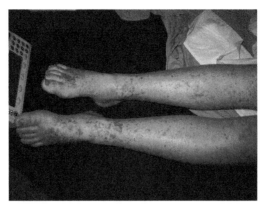

Fig. 1. Typical HSP skin rash (palpable purpura) of the lower limb.

other sites, including the arms and trunk. Lesions may occur following trauma or under pressure (eg, sites such as the waistband). There can also be mucosal involvement. In addition to classic purpura, papules, vesicles, and urticaria-like lesions can occur. Less common findings include petechiae and necrotic, ulcerated, hemorrhagic, or bullous lesions (**Fig. 2**).[1] More atypical skin lesions (necrotic, ulcerative) seem to be associated with a longer duration to presentation (2–3 weeks) and worse gastrointestinal (upper gastrointestinal bleed, abdominal pain, or gastritis) and renal (oliguria, hypertension, hematuria) symptoms.[1] However, several case reports of bullous lesions in children with HSP do not seem to be associated with worse prognosis or renal outcomes.[50,51]

Systemic symptoms may include peripheral edema or periarticular swelling and corresponding arthralgias. True arthritis, typically symmetric involvement of large joints (hips, knees, ankles) may be apparent (66% of patients).[37,39,48,52] Some patients also have gastrointestinal symptoms (56%) of sharp, colicky pain; gastritis; bleeding; and/or intussusception (0.7%–13.6%).[52,53] Male patients can have scrotal edema. Renal findings (30%) can vary from hypertension, hematuria, oliguria, nephritis/nephrotic range proteinuria, to end-stage renal disease (end-stage renal disease is

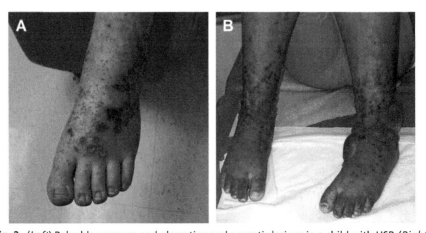

Fig. 2. (*Left*) Palpable purpura and ulcerative and necrotic lesions in a child with HSP. (*Right*) Palpable purpura with bullous lesions on the lower limb in a different child with HSP.

a late complication).[39,52,54] If renal disease is present and severe, consultation with nephrology is appropriate. Typical onset is 4 weeks from initial symptom onset and risk of serious, long-standing renal disease may be related to severity of disease at presentation, with greater risk (19%) associated with nephritic or nephrotic syndromes.[47] Other rare manifestations include serositis, ascites, pancreatitis, cerebral vasculitis, orchitis, and pulmonary hemorrhage.[55,56]

Differential Diagnosis

Possible differential diagnoses include idiopathic thrombocytopenic purpura, thrombotic thrombocytopenic purpura, disseminated intravascular coagulation, sepsis, scurvy, other systemic vasculitis, and connective tissue diseases like juvenile idiopathic arthritis or SLE. A thorough history, physical examination, and additional laboratory testing should help identify these conditions.

DIAGNOSTIC RECOMMENDATIONS

A revised childhood classification criteria for HSP was proposed in 2008 (**Table 1**),[23] with a sensitivity of 100% and specificity of 87%. Laboratory and radiology recommendations are generally nonspecific in HSP and imaging is not always necessary (**Table 2**). On histology, the classic leukocytoclastic vasculitis appearance includes disruption of the vasculature with segmental regions of transmural inflammatory infiltration (primarily neutrophils) and fibrinoid necrosis (**Fig. 3**). Leukocytoclasis, or granulocyte debris, is frequently noted, as is hemorrhage from extravasated erythrocytes. Direct immunofluorescence reveals deposition primarily of IgA (**Fig. 4**) but also C3 and IgM.

Table 1
Classification criteria for HSP

Criteria	Definition
Purpura or petechiae must be present Plus at least one of the following:	Palpable purpura or petechiae[a] predominantly located on the lower extremities[b]
Abdominal pain	Pain is of acute onset, diffuse, colicky, or GI bleeding, or intussusception
Histopathology Skin	Leukocytoclastic vasculitis with IgA deposition
Renal	Proliferative glomerulonephritis with IgA deposition
Arthritis or arthralgias	Acute-onset joint swelling or pain with limitation of motion
Renal involvement	Proteinuria: >0.3 g/24 h or >30 mmol (urine protein/creatinine ratio[c]), or Hematuria: >5 RBC/HPF or RBC casts or ≥2+ on dipstick

Abbreviations: GI, gastrointestinal; HPF, high power field; RBC, red blood cells.
 [a] Not caused by thrombocytopenia.
 [b] If distribution of lesions is atypical, then biopsy must show IgA deposition.
 [c] First morning void.
 Adapted from Ozen S, Pistorio A, Iusan SM, et al. EULAR/PRINTO/PRES criteria for Henoch-Schonlein purpura, childhood polyarteritis nodosa, childhood Wegener granulomatosis and childhood Takayasu arteritis: Ankara 2008. Part II: Final classification criteria. Ann Rheum Dis 2010;69(5):798–806.

Table 2
Diagnostic recommendations for HSP

Laboratory Studies	Laboratory Findings in HSP
CBC and differential	Normal to increased platelet count Normal to increased WBC Otherwise normal CBC
Inflammatory markers ESR, CRP	Normal to increased
Complete metabolic profile	Normal
Lipase or amylase (if abdominal pain present)	Normal
PT, PTT, INR	Normal
UA, urine protein, urine creatinine	Normal or proteinuria, hematuria, RBC casts
BUN, creatinine	Normal to mildly increased BUN
Imaging Studies Indication	Imaging Modality
Suspect intussusception	Abdominal ultrasound, ±barium enema
Scrotal edema, concern for torsion	Testicular ultrasound

Abbreviations: CBC, complete blood count; CRP, c-reactive protein; ESR, erythrocyte sedimentation rate; INR, international normalized ratio; PT, prothrombin time; PTT, partial thromboplastin time.

THERAPEUTIC RECOMMENDATIONS
Pharmacologic Treatment

For most cases of HSP, only supportive care is necessary. NSAIDs are often provided for mild to moderate pain (abdominal, joint, edema). However, there may be instances when more aggressive immune suppression is required. Potential indications for advanced immunotherapy (ie, oral or parenteral corticosteroids) include severe abdominal pain, gastrointestinal bleeding, severe renal disease (proteinuria, hematuria), and/or serious scrotal edema.[57–60] The use of corticosteroids, the dose, and timing for their use remain controversial. A recent multisite randomized placebo-controlled trial was performed in the United Kingdom assessing potential benefits of early corticosteroid therapy in preventing long-term renal morbidity. The results of this large cohort (180 treatment and 170 controls) did not show benefit in reducing

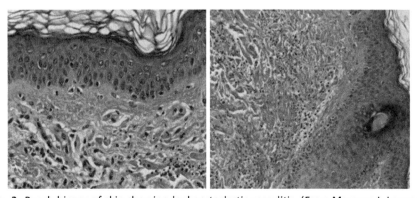

Fig. 3. Punch biopsy of skin showing leukocytoclastic vasculitis. (*From* Marques I, Lagos A, Reis J, et al. Reversible Henoch-Schölein purpura complicating adalimumab therapy. J Crohns Colitis 2012;6(7):796–9; with permission.)

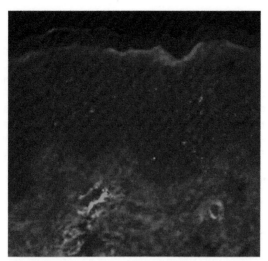

Fig. 4. IgA immunofluorescence showing perivascular IgA deposition. (*Courtesy of* Amy W. Davis, MD, Pittsburgh, PA.)

proteinuria 1 year after diagnosis following implementation of oral corticosteroids within 1 week of onset of symptoms.[61] The literature on the benefits of corticosteroids on both renal and gastrointestinal disease remains contradictory.[60,62,63] Nonetheless, there seems to be some benefit to corticosteroid use for hospitalized patients with respect to duration of hospitalization, need for abdominal surgery, and hospital readmission.[64] Routine steroid use cannot be recommended based on the evidence to date.

COMPLICATIONS

Morbidity associated with HSP is primarily caused by gastrointestinal (intussusception, bleeding, pancreatitis) and/or renal involvement. Of the ~2% to 20% of all patients with HSP who develop permanent renal disease,[46,47] nearly 97% of patients do so by 6 months following disease onset.[47] Therefore, routine blood pressure and urinalysis are recommended for 6–12 months.

AHEI

AHEI is a benign LCV condition affecting children aged 4 months to 2 years with a slight male predilection.[65,66] There have been approximately 300 cases reported in the literature.[65] It is surmised to be a variant of HSP; however, unlike HSP, the location and histology of skin lesions differ.[65]

CLINICAL FEATURES
History

There is a classic triad of symptoms in AHEI. This triad includes fever (low grade) in an otherwise well-appearing infant; edema; and a classic purpuric rash involving the face, ears, and extremities. There is almost always a preceding trigger or prodrome (60%–75%), frequently an upper respiratory tract infection of viral or bacterial cause (group A streptococcus, *Mycoplasma pneumoniae*), certain medications (paracetamol, antibiotics, NSAIDs), or immunizations.[65,66]

Physical Examination

The classic rash of AHEI includes 1-cm to 5-cm iris-like or targetoid red or purple purpuric lesions with surrounding indurated edema scattered symmetrically in a cockade pattern (**Fig. 5**). Lesions are located on the face, ears, and eyelids as well as lower and upper extremities and perianal region. Although the rash can be significant in appearance and infants may have a low-grade fever, children appear well. The edema can be painful and nonpitting in extremities, face, and ears. There can be scrotal swelling in boys.[65,66] There are a few case reports of additional systemic symptoms including transient arthralgias, arthritis, and renal symptoms (glomerulonephritis, hematuria, proteinuria); abdominal pain; gastrointestinal bleeding; and/or intussusception.[66]

Differential Diagnosis

Table 3 presents a list of differentials for AHEI.

DIAGNOSTIC RECOMMENDATIONS
Laboratory Studies

Although generally nonspecific, there may be slight leukocytosis or thrombocytosis along with mildly increased inflammatory markers (ESR, CRP). Additional laboratory testing is normal; however, there have been a few case reports of increased immunoglobulins[67] but normal complement levels.[68] In 2007, Watanabe and Sato[69] reported a case of transiently low C1q, C4, and CH50 with renal involvement in a patient with AHEI.

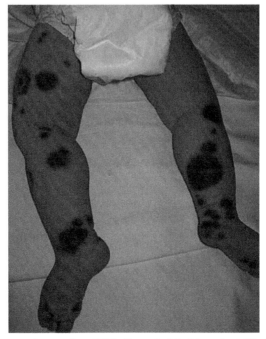

Fig. 5. Bruiselike purpuric macules: AHEI. (*From* Pulido-Pérez A, Avilés-Izquierdo, Suárez-Fernández R. Cutaneous vasculitis. Actas Dermo-Sifiliográficas (English Edition) 2012;103(3):179–91; with permission.)

Table 3 Differential diagnoses for AHEI	
Diagnoses	**Clinical or Laboratory Findings**
Nonaccidental trauma (abuse)	History of trauma; other indicators for trauma may be apparent on examination or imaging
Purpura fulminans	Fever, toxic appearing, rapidly spreading petechiae/purpura/edema
Other rashes	Urticaria, erythema multiforme, erythema nodosum
Gianotti-Crosti syndrome	Infantile papular acrodermatitis: papular or pustulovesicular (not purpuric) lesions on face and distal extremities
Neonatal-onset Sweet syndrome	Fever, painful erythematous plaques, associated immunodeficiency
Neonatal lupus	Maternal history of anti-Ro or anti-La antibodies Annular, erythematous plaques, slightly scaly on face, neck, or scalp May have congenital heart block, cytopenias, increased transaminases

Histology

Like all leukocytoclastic vasculitides, AHEI lesions show a perivascular neutrophilic infiltration with leukocytoclasia (fragmentation of nuclei) of small vessels. Direct immunofluorescence shows a predominance of IgM (80%), IgA (30%), IgE (30%), and IgG (20%).[66,70] This distribution of immunoglobulin deposition is in contrast with that of HSP, in which IgA predominates. Furthermore, there has been evidence for C1q deposition in AHEI but not in HSP.[71] For these reasons, controversy remains surrounding the notion that AHEI is merely an HSP condition of early childhood.

THERAPEUTIC RECOMMENDATIONS
Pharmacologic Treatment

In general, given the self-limited nature of the disease, systemic medication therapy is unnecessary. Treatment is generally directed at symptom management.

PROGNOSIS

AIHE has a good prognosis, with most cases being self-limited and resolving within 1 to 3 weeks without long-term complications or progression to chronic systemic disease.

UV

Clinical features

UV is a rare LCV condition among children.[72,73] Among adults, UV makes up 5% to 10% of cases of chronic urticaria.[74,75] In classic UV, 2 types have been described: normocomplementemic (NUV) and hypocomplementemic (HUV). Patients presenting with mild to moderate forms of UV typically experience pruritus but no pain. In contrast, patients with true UV (NUV, HUV) primarily have a painful, burning wheal-like lesion that persists for longer than 24 hours and results in hyperpigmentation during the healing process (**Fig. 6**). This is thought to occur because of the extravasation of red blood cells in LCV. Lesions can occur anywhere on the body but are most common on the lower extremities.

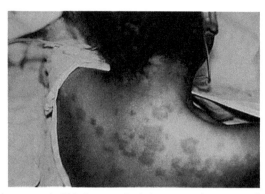

Fig. 6. Hypocomplementemic UV. Scattered, violaceous, edematous plaques on the back. (*From* DeAmicis T, Mofid MZ, Cohen B, et al. Hypocomplementemic urticarial vasculitis: report of a 12-year-old girl with systemic lupus erythematosus. J Am Acad Dermatol 2002;47(Suppl 5):S273–4; with permission.)

Associated systemic findings may be more common and more severe in HUV but can be seen in all types. These symptoms include fever, edema or angioedema, renal involvement (hematuria, proteinuria), nonspecific gastrointestinal findings (abdominal pain, diarrhea, nausea, vomiting, hepatosplenomegaly), arthralgias/arthritis, Raynaud phenomenon, and inflammatory eye disease (uveitis, episcleritis).[72,75,76]

Most cases of UV are idiopathic. Symptoms may be triggered by exposure to certain medications or illnesses.[77] A moderate form of UV has been associated with certain syndromes (eg, AHA [arthritis, hives, angioedema], Schnitzler syndrome, Muckle-Wells syndrome, and Cogan syndrome).[75] HUV, and infrequently NUV, can be associated with other conditions, including connective tissue diseases like SLE, SS, RA, and mixed cryoglobulinemia.[73,78–80]

DIAGNOSTIC RECOMMENDATIONS
Laboratory Studies

Complement levels (C1q, C3, C4, CH50) should be evaluated and are low in HUV. C1q antibodies are present in HUV,[81,82] unlike in SLE. Inflammatory markers (ESR, CRP) may be increased. ANA testing is frequently positive; however, additional screening tests for SLE (eg, anti–double-stranded DNA, anti-Smith antibodies) tend to be negative, unless there is concern for overlap or diagnosis of SLE.

Histology

A skin biopsy is necessary to make the diagnosis of UV. Although lesions clinically appear urticaria-like, histopathology should reveal the classic LCV appearance with immunoglobulin (IgG) and complement (C3, C1q) deposition on DIF. Like other LCV conditions, it is presumed that UV is a type III hypersensitivity reaction associated with antigen-antibody complex deposition. Following immune complex deposition, complement activation occurs, as does neutrophil chemotaxis and subsequent mast cell activation. Mast cells further recruit eosinophils, leading to increased vascular permeability and release of basic proteins that contribute to cellular necrosis. Adhesion molecules expressed on endothelial cells further act to recruit neutrophils, lymphocytes, monocytes, and eosinophils.[83]

THERAPEUTIC RECOMMENDATIONS
Pharmacologic Treatment

If localized to the skin, supportive care with antihistamines and NSAIDs may be sufficient. Other first-line (for mild disease) immune-suppressant medications include dapsone, colchicine, and hydroxychloroquine.[84] For more severe systemic symptoms, treatment may include systemic corticosteroids, methotrexate, azathioprine, cyclosporine, cyclophosphamide, and mycophenolate mofetil.[84,85] Rituximab and intravenous immunoglobulin (IVIG) have proved beneficial in separate cases of HUV with SLE.[86,87] To date, there is limited evidence to offer specific guidance for therapy, particularly in children.

PROGNOSIS

Depending on the type of UV, prognosis can be good, although all forms are generally chronic. Most idiopathic UV is isolated to the skin with resolution over time. However, HUV syndrome is more severe and systemic complications can occur. Among pediatric cases of idiopathic HUV reported in the literature, the prognosis has been good.[72,88–90] Close assessment and follow-up for association with SLE is warranted.

cPAN

Epidemiology/pathophysiology

Classic polyarteritis nodosa (PAN) is a necrotizing vasculitis of small and medium-sized arteries resulting in tissue necrosis that can affect multiple organ systems. Cutaneous PAN (cPAN) was first described in 1931 as a form of systemic PAN that was limited only to the skin. Unlike the systemic form, cPAN is a rare, benign condition. The rarity of this condition does not allow prevalence or incidence rates to be determined; however, a review of the current literature indicates fewer than 100 reported cases among children. cPAN affects children of all ages without a clear gender predilection.[91–93] There has been a case report of a 3-day-old infant with peripheral gangrene born to a mother diagnosed with cPAN in her second trimester.[94] Although the exact cause of cPAN is unknown, it is presumed that the cause is an immune complex–mediated reaction with deposition of IgM and C3 visualized on histopathology.[95]

PROGNOSIS

cPAN is a benign condition, although it often has a relapsing, remitting chronic course. Nevertheless, the term benign may be a misnomer for those few children who have digital autoamputation, which is an infrequent but serious complication. These cases are also rare, but seem to occur with higher frequency among children diagnosed at less than 10 years of age.[93,96] Unlike its systemic counterpart, cPAN does not affect major organs and does not evolve into other systemic conditions over time. The most likely cause of morbidity is associated with treatment; if more aggressive, prolonged therapy is needed.

CLINICAL FEATURES
History

Children may have a preceding illness, most commonly group A streptococcal pharyngitis.[91,93] Other reported triggers have included immunizations (diphtheria-pertussis-tetanus), wasp stings, antibiotics (penicillin, tetracycline), and viral illnesses.[93] In the adult form of cPAN, there have been associations with an active hepatitis B infection; however, this is rarely seen in children, although a case report of cPAN following hepatitis B vaccination has been reported.[18]

Physical Examination

The typical presentation includes painful, subcutaneous nodules located primarily in the lower extremities but these lesions can also appear on the trunk and upper extremities (**Fig. 7**).[97] Nodules tend to be less than 0.5 cm in size and can be erythematous to violaceous in color. Other skin findings include livedo reticularis and, much less commonly, ulcerations, gangrene, or necrotic patches (ie, autoamputation). Associated systemic symptoms include high-grade fever (often >39°C), malaise, arthralgias, and/or arthritis. Patients may appear ill with pallor. If present, arthritis of the large joints (eg, knees, ankles) may be palpated. Because this condition does not affect major organ systems, the physical examination is otherwise normal.

COMORBIDITIES

There are typically no associated comorbidities with cPAN because progression to systemic disease does not occur. There have been few case reports of associated Crohn's disease, ulcerative colitis,[98,99] and antiphospholipid antibodies but, in general, no clear indications for systemic disease.[100]

DIFFERENTIAL DIAGNOSIS

Possible differential diagnoses for cPAN include systemic PAN, erythema nodosum (histology typically reveals a septal panniculitis and involves small vessels including venules), other systemic vasculitides (granulomatosis with polyangiitis, Churg-Strauss, microscopic polyangiitis), and other connective tissue diseases (SLE, sarcoidosis).

DIAGNOSTIC RECOMMENDATIONS
Laboratory Studies

It is important to rule out systemic PAN and other conditions with initial screening laboratory studies. A basic complete blood count and differential, ESR, and/or CRP may show signs of inflammation, with most patients presenting with increased inflammatory markers. Additional recommendations include a CMP, streptococcal titers (ASO and anti-DNase B) and/or throat culture, urinalysis, ANA, ANCA, and antiphospholipid antibodies. When appropriate (ie, in the event of gangrene or autoamputation), additional hypercoagulable work-up may be warranted but should be normal.[96]

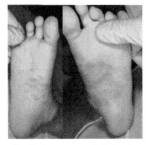
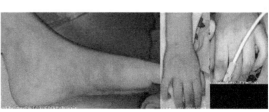

Fig. 7. Violaceous painful subcutaneous nodules in a child with cPAN.

Histology

Depending on the presence of ulcerations, a full-thickness biopsy may be preferred. However, a wedge or excisional biopsy may be sufficient to reveal any small to medium arteriole and artery involvement. Histology reveals a necrotizing vasculitis with variable mononuclear cells, neutrophils, and eosinophils (**Fig. 8**).[91–93,95] Fibrinoid necrosis and leukocytoclasia may be present, as may periarteriolar panniculitis.[95] Direct immunofluorescence may reveal IgM and C3 deposits.[95]

THERAPEUTIC RECOMMENDATIONS
Pharmacologic Treatment

In mild cases, NSAIDs may be sufficient treatment; however, most cases require systemic corticosteroids (1 mg/kg/d of oral prednisone or greater depending on severity of disease). There are some case reports of patients treated with steroid-sparing agents for refractory cases including colchicine, dapsone, cyclophosphamide, methotrexate, anti-TNF agents, IVIG, and mycophenolate mofetil[91,93,96,101–105] with varying degrees of efficacy. Also, given the association with antecedent streptococcal infection, patients with evidence for preceding infection are frequently initiated on long-term penicillin (or similar) prophylaxis; however, evidence is limited and efficacy remains unclear.[91,93,106] Patients with extreme necrosis/gangrene may require more aggressive vasodilatory therapy, including aspirin and/or other anticoagulant, calcium channel blockers, topical nitroglycerin paste, systemic vasodilators,[96] or pentoxifylline.[105,107]

Surgical Treatment Options

Surgical interventions are typically unnecessary unless there is severe autoamputation with secondary infection requiring debridement.[93,96]

COMPLICATIONS

cPAN is generally benign and self-limited with relapsing, remitting course. Most patients do well without significant complication. There are rare reports, particularly

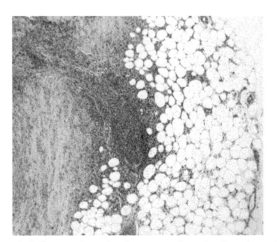

Fig. 8. cPAN. There is inflammation of a large vessel at the junction of the dermis and subcutaneous fat. (*From* Leonard N. Panniculitis. Curr Diagn Pathol 2005;11(4):236–44; with permission.)

Table 4
Differential diagnoses and mimickers of CV

Differential Diagnoses	Clinical Manifestations	Laboratory Findings	Histopathology (skin biopsy)	Imaging Findings
		Systemic Vasculitides		
Medium Vessel				
Kawasaki disease	Maculopapular rash, conjunctival injection, strawberry red tongue, lymphadenopathy, desquamation of fingertips and toes	Increased WBC/platelets/ESR/CRP, sterile pyuria	Necrotizing medium-vessel vasculitis	Aneurysms on echocardiogram
Polyarteritis nodosa	Palpable purpura, painful subcutaneous nodules, livedo reticularis, hypertension, abdominal pain, renal failure, neuropathy	ANCA−, increased ESR/CRP/WBC/platelets	Medium-sized arterial vasculitis	Vasculopathy, microaneurysms on angiography
Cutaneous polyarteritis nodosa	Painful subcutaneous nodules, livedo reticularis with burst like appearance	ANCA−, increased ESR/CRP	Medium-sized arterial vasculitis	N/A
Small Vessel				
Granulomatosis with polyangiitis	Palpable purpura, livedo reticularis, urticaria, mucosal/cutaneous ulcerations, upper respiratory involvement (sinusitis, saddle nose, pulmonary hemorrhage), renal disease (proteinuria, hematuria, hypertension, glomerulonephritis)	cANCA+ (PR3), increased ESR/CRP/WBC/platelets, anemia	Necrotizing small vessel vasculitis with granulomas (skin and renal), LCV, pauci-immune	Ground-glass, nodules, cavitary lesions on chest CT

	Clinical features	Laboratory	Vasculitis type	Imaging/other
HSP	Palpable purpura, petechiae, bullae, necrotic lesions, pustular lesions, gastrointestinal, renal, scrotal edema, arthralgias/arthritis	Increased ESR/CRP, ANCA–	LCV IgA deposition	Possible intussusception
Microscopic polyangiitis	Palpable purpura, renal disease (glomerulonephritis), alveolar hemorrhage	pANCA+ (MPO) > cANCA (PR3), increased ESR/CRP	Small and medium-sized vessel vasculitis (skin and renal), pauci-immune	Ground-glass, patchy opacifications on chest imaging
Churg-Strauss	Palpable purpura, painful subcutaneous nodules, asthma, allergy symptoms	pANCA+ (MPO), eosinophilia, increased IgE	Small and medium-vessel LCV vasculitis with granulomas and eosinophils	Ground-glass, patchy opacifications on chest imaging
Connective Tissue Diseases				
SLE	Palpable purpura, digital ulcerations, subcutaneous nodules, livedo reticularis, urticaria malar rash, photosensitivity, mucosal ulcerations, arthritis, hematuria/proteinuria, hypertension, Raynaud	ANA+, dsDNA+, anti-Sm+, low C3/C4	Small vessel vasculitis (more common in drug-induced SLE)	Serositis on chest radiograph or echocardiogram, renal biopsy suggesting lupus nephritis
Sjögren's	Palpable purpura, livedo reticularis, dry eyes, dry mouth, arthralgias, malaise	ANA+, Anti-Ro+, Anti-La+	Small vessel vasculitis	Abnormal sialogram or salivary scintigraphy
Mixed connective tissue disease	Palpable purpura, digital ulcerations, subcutaneous nodules, livedo reticularis, urticarial malar rash, photosensitivity, mucosal ulcerations, arthritis, myositis, hematuria/proteinuria, hypertension, Raynaud	ANA+, anti-RNP+, anti-Sm−	Small vessel vasculitis	Serositis on chest radiograph or echocardiogram, myositis on MRI, diminished DLco on pulmonary function tests

(continued on next page)

Table 4
(continued)

Differential Diagnoses	Clinical Manifestations	Laboratory Findings	Histopathology (skin biopsy)	Imaging Findings
Scleroderma	Livedo reticularis, Raynaud with ulceration, livedo reticularis, gastroesophageal reflux/dysmotility, skin tightening/sclerodactyly	ANA+, anti–Scl-70+ > anticentromere, anemia	Small vessel vasculitis	GERD on barium swallow, pulmonary hypertension, diminished DLco on pulmonary function tests
Juvenile idiopathic arthritis	Arthritis, uveitis	±ANA, ±RF	Small vessel vasculitis	Slit-lamp eye examination with anterior chamber inflammation
Other: Behçet, inflammatory bowel disease, sarcoidosis	Erythema nodosum	Variable	Septal panniculitis	Variable
Other Causes				
Antiphospholipid antibody syndrome	Clotting (deep venous thrombosis, pulmonary embolus), recurrent miscarriage, livedo reticularis	APA +	Microthrombi	DVT on ultrasound, pulmonary embolus on spiral chest CT
Idiopathic thrombocytopenic purpura	Petechiae, bleeding gums	Low platelets	N/A	N/A
Thrombotic thrombocytopenic purpura	Petechiae, bleeding gums, mental status changes	Low platelets, hemolytic anemia, acute renal abnormalities	N/A	N/A

				Vegetations on echocardiogram
Infective endocarditis	Fever, malaise, splinter hemorrhages, purpura or petechiae	+ Blood cultures, anemia, increased ESR/CRP	N/A	Vegetations on echocardiogram
Scurvy	Petechiae, ecchymoses, perifollicular hemorrhage, bleeding gums, diet low in vitamin C, poor wound healing	Anemia (macrocytic), leukopenia, low ascorbic acid levels	Perivascular and perifollicular hemorrhage	N/A
Purpura fulminans/disseminated coagulation/sepsis	Purpura/petechiae with edema and necrosis ± bullae, vesicles (hemorrhagic infarction), fever, toxic appearing, diffuse, rapidly progressing, multiorgan dysfunction	Anemia, thrombocytopenia, coagulopathy, increased D-dimer	Microvascular thrombosis ± acute vasculitis	N/A
Drug induced	Drug exposure	± ANCA, APA, antihistone antibodies, anemia, increased ESR/CRP	Small vessel LCV, ± eosinophilia	N/A

Abbreviations: ANA, antinuclear antibody; APA, antiphospholipid antibodies; cANCA, cytoplasmic ANCA; CRP, c-reactive protein; CT, computed tomography; DLco, carbon monoxide diffusion in the lung; dsDNA, double-stranded DNA; DVT, deep vein thrombosis; ESR, erythrocyte sedimentation rate; GERD, gastroesophageal reflux disease; INR, international normalized ratio; MPO, myeloperoxidase; N/A, not applicable; pANCA, perinuclear ANCA; PT, prothrombin time; PTT, partial thromboplastin time; PR3, proteinase-3; RF, rheumatoid factor; Sm, Smith.

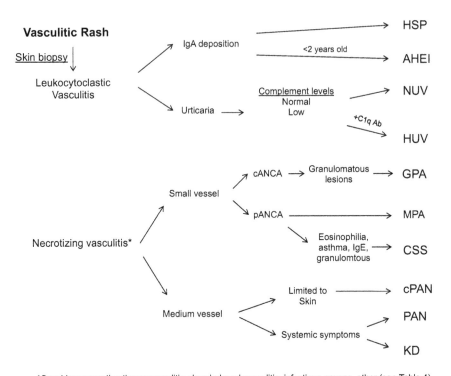

*Consider connective tissue vasculitis, drug induced vasculitis, infectious causes, other (see Table 4)

Fig. 9. Algorithm for approaching a child with CV.

in children diagnosed before the age of 10 years, of autoamputation/digital necrosis, as discussed earlier.

Differential Diagnoses and Mimickers of CV in Childhood

Purpuric lesions and painful nodules are common in other conditions. Mimickers may include infectious causes and autoimmune-mediated conditions like idiopathic thrombocytopenia or antiphospholipid antibody syndrome, which can present with purpura, petechiae, or other vasculitic rashes. It is also important to consider other systemic forms of vasculitis, including Kawasaki disease, systemic PAN, granulomatous polyangiitis (formerly Wegener granulomatosis), microscopic polyangiitis, and Churg-Strauss. Other inflammatory conditions, including BD and inflammatory bowel disease, may present with similar skin lesions, although they more frequently involve erythema nodosum. In many of these conditions, skin findings occur with other clinical manifestations; thus, close evaluation for additional organ involvement is critical. **Table 4** presents a list of conditions that should be considered in the differential when evaluating a child with CV.

Fig. 9 provides an algorithm for approaching a child with CV. If there is concern for these conditions, consultation with a rheumatologist and dermatologist would be helpful for both diagnostic and treatment purposes.

SUMMARY

CV can occur among a wide range of heterogeneous conditions. The most common vasculitis in childhood is HSP, a leukocytoclastic vasculitis of small vessels. Most cases of CV in childhood are benign; however, there is a potential for more systemic, complicated disease. Infants, albeit rarely, can have a similar HSP-like condition with good prognosis. Limited cPAN affects medium-sized arterial vessels and generally has a good prognosis. At times, CV can be associated with systemic conditions with greater potential for complications. A skin biopsy can help to make the diagnosis of CV, and both dermatology and rheumatology should be consulted in complex cases.

REFERENCES

1. Murgu A, Mihaila D, Cozma L, et al. Indications and limitations of histopathological skin investigation of Henoch-Schonlein purpura in children. Rom J Morphol Embryol 2012;53(Suppl 3):769–73.
2. Faille-Kuyber EH, Kater L, Kooiker CJ, et al. IgA-deposits in cutaneous blood-vessel walls and mesangium in Henoch-Schonlein syndrome. Lancet 1973; 1(7808):892–3.
3. Baumann U, Chouchakova N, Gewecke B, et al. Distinct tissue site-specific requirements of mast cells and complement components C3/C5a receptor in IgG immune complex-induced injury of skin and lung. J Immunol 2001;167(2): 1022–7.
4. Bielsa I, Carrascosa JM, Hausmann G, et al. An immunohistopathologic study in cutaneous necrotizing vasculitis. J Cutan Pathol 2000;27(3):130–5.
5. Sais G, Vidaller A, Jucgla A, et al. Adhesion molecule expression and endothelial cell activation in cutaneous leukocytoclastic vasculitis. An immunohistologic and clinical study in 42 patients. Arch Dermatol 1997;133(4):443–50.
6. Burrows NP, Molina FA, Terenghi G, et al. Comparison of cell adhesion molecule expression in cutaneous leucocytoclastic and lymphocytic vasculitis. J Clin Pathol 1994;47(10):939–44.
7. Cid MC. Endothelial cell biology, perivascular inflammation, and vasculitis. Cleve Clin J Med 2002;69(Suppl 2):SII45–9.
8. Hernandez-Rodriguez J, Segarra M, Vilardell C, et al. Tissue production of pro-inflammatory cytokines (IL-1beta, TNFalpha and IL-6) correlates with the intensity of the systemic inflammatory response and with corticosteroid requirements in giant-cell arteritis. Rheumatology (Oxford) 2004;43(3):294–301.
9. Gardner-Medwin JM, Dolezalova P, Cummins C, et al. Incidence of Henoch-Schonlein purpura, Kawasaki disease, and rare vasculitides in children of different ethnic origins. Lancet 2002;360(9341):1197–202.
10. Fiorentino DF. Cutaneous vasculitis. J Am Acad Dermatol 2003;48(3):311–40.
11. Sanchez-Borges M, Capriles-Hulett A, Caballero-Fonseca F. Risk of skin reactions when using ibuprofen-based medicines. Expert Opin Drug Saf 2005; 4(5):837–48.
12. Edwards MS, Baker CJ. Complications and sequelae of meningococcal infections in children. J Pediatr 1981;99(4):540–5.
13. Coppo R, Amore A, Gianoglio B. Clinical features of Henoch-Schonlein purpura. Italian Group of Renal Immunopathology. Ann Med Interne (Paris) 1999;150(2): 143–50.
14. Nong BR, Huang YF, Chuang CM, et al. Fifteen-year experience of children with Henoch-Schonlein purpura in southern Taiwan, 1991–2005. J Microbiol Immunol Infect 2007;40(4):371–6.
15. Rigante D, Castellazzi L, Bosco A, et al. Is there a crossroad between infections, genetics, and Henoch-Schonlein purpura? Autoimmun Rev 2013;12(10): 1016–21.

16. Jariwala S, Vernon N, Shliozberg J. Henoch-Schonlein purpura after hepatitis A vaccination. Ann Allergy Asthma Immunol 2011;107(2):180–1.
17. Hughes R, Lacour JP, Baldin B, et al. Urticarial vasculitis secondary to H1N1 vaccination. Acta Derm Venereol 2010;90(6):651–2.
18. Ventura F, Antunes H, Brito C, et al. Cutaneous polyarteritis nodosa in a child following hepatitis B vaccination. Eur J Dermatol 2009;19(4):400–1.
19. Famularo G, Nicotra GC, Minisola G, et al. Leukocytoclastic vasculitis after influenza vaccination. J Clin Rheumatol 2006;12(1):48–50.
20. Calabrese LH, Duna GF. Drug-induced vasculitis. Curr Opin Rheumatol 1996; 8(1):34–40.
21. Merkel PA. Drug-induced vasculitis. Rheum Dis Clin North Am 2001;27(4): 849–62.
22. Bahrami S, Malone JC, Webb KG, et al. Tissue eosinophilia as an indicator of drug-induced cutaneous small-vessel vasculitis. Arch Dermatol 2006;142(2):155–61.
23. Ozen S, Pistorio A, Iusan SM, et al. EULAR/PRINTO/PRES criteria for Henoch-Schonlein purpura, childhood polyarteritis nodosa, childhood Wegener granulomatosis and childhood Takayasu arteritis: Ankara 2008. Part II: final classification criteria. Ann Rheum Dis 2010;69(5):798–806.
24. Hunder GG, Arend WP, Bloch DA, et al. The American College of Rheumatology 1990 criteria for the classification of vasculitis. Introduction. Arthritis Rheum 1990;33(8):1065–7.
25. Jennette JC, Falk RJ, Bacon PA, et al. 2012 revised International Chapel Hill Consensus Conference Nomenclature of Vasculitides. Arthritis Rheum 2013; 65(1):1–11.
26. Carlson JA, Ng BT, Chen KR. Cutaneous vasculitis update: diagnostic criteria, classification, epidemiology, etiology, pathogenesis, evaluation and prognosis. Am J Dermatopathol 2005;27(6):504–28.
27. Chen KR, Carlson JA. Clinical approach to cutaneous vasculitis. Am J Clin Dermatol 2008;9(2):71–92.
28. Carlson JA, Cavaliere LF, Grant-Kels JM. Cutaneous vasculitis: diagnosis and management. Clin Dermatol 2006;24(5):414–29.
29. Cochrane CG, Weigle WO. The cutaneous reaction to soluble antigen-antibody complexes; a comparison with the Arthus phenomenon. J Exp Med 1958; 108(5):591–604.
30. Stone JH, Nousari HC. "Essential" cutaneous vasculitis: what every rheumatologist should know about vasculitis of the skin. Curr Opin Rheumatol 2001;13(1):23–34.
31. Barnadas MA, Perez E, Gich I, et al. Diagnostic, prognostic and pathogenic value of the direct immunofluorescence test in cutaneous leukocytoclastic vasculitis. Int J Dermatol 2004;43(1):19–26.
32. Topaloglu R, Sungur A, Baskin E, et al. Vascular endothelial growth factor in Henoch-Schonlein purpura. J Rheumatol 2001;28(10):2269–73.
33. Ozaltin F, Bakkaloglu A, Ozen S, et al. The significance of IgA class of antineutrophil cytoplasmic antibodies (ANCA) in childhood Henoch-Schonlein purpura. Clin Rheumatol 2004;23(5):426–9.
34. Rostoker G. Schonlein-Henoch purpura in children and adults: diagnosis, pathophysiology and management. BioDrugs 2001;15(2):99–138.
35. Piram M, Mahr A. Epidemiology of immunoglobulin A vasculitis (Henoch-Schonlein): current state of knowledge. Curr Opin Rheumatol 2013;25(2):171–8.
36. Bowyer S, Roettcher P. Pediatric rheumatology clinic populations in the United States: results of a 3 year survey. Pediatric Rheumatology Database Research Group. J Rheumatol 1996;23(11):1968–74.

37. Trapani S, Micheli A, Grisolia F, et al. Henoch Schonlein purpura in childhood: epidemiological and clinical analysis of 150 cases over a 5-year period and review of literature. Semin Arthritis Rheum 2005;35(3):143–53.
38. Yang YH, Hung CF, Hsu CR, et al. A nationwide survey on epidemiological characteristics of childhood Henoch-Schonlein purpura in Taiwan. Rheumatology (Oxford) 2005;44(5):618–22.
39. Chen O, Zhu XB, Ren P, et al. Henoch Schonlein Purpura in children: clinical analysis of 120 cases. Afr Health Sci 2013;13(1):94–9.
40. Dolezalova P, Telekesova P, Nemcova D, et al. Incidence of vasculitis in children in the Czech Republic: 2-year prospective epidemiology survey. J Rheumatol 2004;31(11):2295–9.
41. Yang YH, Chuang YH, Wang LC, et al. The immunobiology of Henoch-Schonlein purpura. Autoimmun Rev 2008;7(3):179–84.
42. Levy M, Broyer M, Arsan A, et al. Anaphylactoid purpura nephritis in childhood: natural history and immunopathology. Adv Nephrol Necker Hosp 1976;6: 183–228.
43. Saulsbury FT. Epidemiology of Henoch-Schonlein purpura. Cleve Clin J Med 2002;69(Suppl 2):SII87–9.
44. Al-Mayouf SM, Bahabri S, Majeed M. Cutaneous leukocytoclastic vasculitis associated with mycobacterial and salmonella infection. Clin Rheumatol 2007; 26(9):1563–4.
45. Atkinson SR, Barker DJ. Seasonal distribution of Henoch-Schonlein purpura. Br J Prev Soc Med 1976;30(1):22–5.
46. Ronkainen J, Ala-Houhala M, Huttunen NP, et al. Outcome of Henoch-Schoenlein nephritis with nephrotic-range proteinuria. Clin Nephrol 2003;60(2):80–4.
47. Narchi H. Risk of long term renal impairment and duration of follow up recommended for Henoch-Schonlein purpura with normal or minimal urinary findings: a systematic review. Arch Dis Child 2005;90(9):916–20.
48. Calvino MC, Llorca J, Garcia-Porrua C, et al. Henoch-Schonlein purpura in children from northwestern Spain: a 20-year epidemiologic and clinical study. Medicine 2001;80(5):279–90.
49. Jauhola O, Ronkainen J, Koskimies O, et al. Clinical course of extrarenal symptoms in Henoch-Schonlein purpura: a 6-month prospective study. Arch Dis Child 2010;95(11):871–6.
50. Park SE, Lee JH. Haemorrhagic bullous lesions in a 3-year-old girl with Henoch-Scholein purpura. Acta Paediatr 2011;100(12):e283–4.
51. Trapani S, Mariotti P, Resti M, et al. Severe hemorrhagic bullous lesions in Henoch Schonlein purpura: three pediatric cases and review of the literature. Rheumatol Int 2010;30(10):1355–9.
52. Peru H, Soylemezoglu O, Bakkaloglu SA, et al. Henoch Schonlein purpura in childhood: clinical analysis of 254 cases over a 3-year period. Clin Rheumatol 2008;27(9):1087–92.
53. Chang WL, Yang YH, Lin YT, et al. Gastrointestinal manifestations in Henoch-Schonlein purpura: a review of 261 patients. Acta Paediatr 2004;93(11): 1427–31.
54. Chang WL, Yang YH, Wang LC, et al. Renal manifestations in Henoch-Schonlein purpura: a 10-year clinical study. Pediatr Nephrol 2005;20(9):1269–72.
55. Ebert EC. Gastrointestinal manifestations of Henoch-Schonlein Purpura. Dig Dis Sci 2008;53(8):2011–9.
56. Roberts PF, Waller TA, Brinker TM, et al. Henoch-Schonlein purpura: a review article. South Med J 2007;100(8):821–4.

57. Szer IS. Gastrointestinal and renal involvement in vasculitis: management strategies in Henoch-Schonlein purpura. Cleve Clin J Med 1999;66(5):312–7.
58. Leung SP. Use of intravenous hydrocortisone in Henoch-Schonlein purpura. J Paediatr Child Health 2001;37(3):309–10.
59. Rosenblum ND, Winter HS. Steroid effects on the course of abdominal pain in children with Henoch-Schonlein purpura. Pediatrics 1987;79(6):1018–21.
60. Weiss PF, Feinstein JA, Luan X, et al. Effects of corticosteroid on Henoch-Schonlein purpura: a systematic review. Pediatrics 2007;120(5):1079–87.
61. Dudley J, Smith G, Llewelyn-Edwards A, et al. Randomised, double-blind, placebo-controlled trial to determine whether steroids reduce the incidence and severity of nephropathy in Henoch-Schonlein purpura (HSP). Arch Dis Child 2013;98(10):756–63.
62. Chartapisak W, Opastiraku S, Willis NS, et al. Prevention and treatment of renal disease in Henoch-Schonlein purpura: a systematic review. Arch Dis Child 2009;94(2):132–7.
63. Huber AM, King J, McLaine P, et al. A randomized, placebo-controlled trial of prednisone in early Henoch Schonlein purpura [ISRCTN85109383]. BMC Med 2004;2:7.
64. Weiss PF, Klink AJ, Localio R, et al. Corticosteroids may improve clinical outcomes during hospitalization for Henoch-Schonlein purpura. Pediatrics 2010; 126(4):674–81.
65. Savino F, Lupica MM, Tarasco V, et al. Acute hemorrhagic edema of infancy: a troubling cutaneous presentation with a self-limiting course. Pediatr Dermatol 2013;30(6):3149–52.
66. Fiore E, Rizzi M, Ragazzi M, et al. Acute hemorrhagic edema of young children (cockade purpura and edema): a case series and systematic review. J Am Acad Dermatol 2008;59(4):684–95.
67. Saraclar Y, Tinaztepe K, Adalioglu G, et al. Acute hemorrhagic edema of infancy (AHEI)–a variant of Henoch-Schonlein purpura or a distinct clinical entity? J Allergy Clin Immunol 1990;86(4 Pt 1):473–83.
68. Paradisi M, Annessi G, Corrado A. Infantile acute hemorrhagic edema of the skin. Cutis 2001;68(2):127–9.
69. Watanabe T, Sato Y. Renal involvement and hypocomplementemia in a patient with acute hemorrhagic edema of infancy. Pediatr Nephrol 2007;22(11):1979–81.
70. AlSufyani MA. Acute hemorrhagic edema of infancy: unusual scarring and review of the English language literature. Int J Dermatol 2009;48(6):617–22.
71. Goraya JS, Kaur S. Acute infantile hemorrhagic edema and Henoch-Schonlein purpura: is IgA the missing link? J Am Acad Dermatol 2002;47(5):801 [author reply: 2].
72. Al Mosawi ZS, Al Hermi BE. Hypocomplementemic urticarial vasculitis syndrome in an 8-year-old boy: a case report and review of literature. Oman Med J 2013;28(4):275–7.
73. Macedo PA, Garcia CB, Schmitz MK, et al. Juvenile systemic lupus erythematosus and dermatomyositis associated with urticarial vasculitis syndrome: a unique presentation. Rheumatol Int 2012;32(11):3643–6.
74. Wisnieski JJ. Urticarial vasculitis. Curr Opin Rheumatol 2000;12(1):24–31.
75. Grotz W, Baba HA, Becker JU, et al. Hypocomplementemic urticarial vasculitis syndrome: an interdisciplinary challenge. Dtsch Arztebl Int 2009;106(46): 756–63.
76. Jara LJ, Navarro C, Medina G, et al. Hypocomplementemic urticarial vasculitis syndrome. Curr Rheumatol Rep 2009;11(6):410–5.

77. Dua J, Nandagudi A, Sutcliffe N. *Mycoplasma pneumoniae* infection associated with urticarial vasculitis mimicking adult-onset Still's disease. Rheumatol Int 2012;32(12):4053–6.
78. Soylu A, Kavukcu S, Uzuner N, et al. Systemic lupus erythematosus presenting with normocomplementemic urticarial vasculitis in a 4-year-old girl. Pediatr Int 2001;43(4):420–2.
79. Abdallah M, Darghouth S, Hamzaoui S, et al. McDuffie hypocomplementemic urticarial vasculitis associated with Sjogren's syndrome. Rev Med Interne 2010;31(7):e8–10 [in French].
80. Kuniyuki S, Katoh H. Urticarial vasculitis with papular lesions in a patient with type C hepatitis and cryoglobulinemia. J Dermatol 1996;23(4):279–83.
81. Wisnieski JJ, Naff GB. Serum IgG antibodies to C1q in hypocomplementemic urticarial vasculitis syndrome. Arthritis Rheum 1989;32(9):1119–27.
82. Wisnieski JJ, Jones SM. Comparison of autoantibodies to the collagen-like region of C1q in hypocomplementemic urticarial vasculitis syndrome and systemic lupus erythematosus. J Immunol 1992;148(5):1396–403.
83. Mehregan DR, Gibson LE. Pathophysiology of urticarial vasculitis. Arch Dermatol 1998;134(1):88–9.
84. Venzor J, Lee WL, Huston DP. Urticarial vasculitis. Clin Rev Allergy Immunol 2002;23(2):201–16.
85. Worm M, Sterry W, Kolde G. Mycophenolate mofetil is effective for maintenance therapy of hypocomplementaemic urticarial vasculitis. Br J Dermatol 2000; 143(6):1324.
86. Saigal K, Valencia IC, Cohen J, et al. Hypocomplementemic urticarial vasculitis with angioedema, a rare presentation of systemic lupus erythematosus: rapid response to rituximab. J Am Acad Dermatol 2003;49(Suppl 5):S283–5.
87. Yamazaki-Nakashimada MA, Duran-McKinster C, Ramirez-Vargas N, et al. Intravenous immunoglobulin therapy for hypocomplementemic urticarial vasculitis associated with systemic lupus erythematosus in a child. Pediatr Dermatol 2009;26(4):445–7.
88. Cadnapaphornchai MA, Saulsbury FT, Norwood VF. Hypocomplementemic urticarial vasculitis: report of a pediatric case. Pediatr Nephrol 2000;14(4):328–31.
89. Renard M, Wouters C, Proesmans W. Rapidly progressive glomerulonephritis in a boy with hypocomplementaemic urticarial vasculitis. Eur J Pediatr 1998; 157(3):243–5.
90. Martini A, Ravelli A, Albani S, et al. Hypocomplementemic urticarial vasculitis syndrome with severe systemic manifestations. J Pediatr 1994;124(5 Pt 1):742–4.
91. Fathalla BM, Miller L, Brady S, et al. Cutaneous polyarteritis nodosa in children. J Am Acad Dermatol 2005;53(4):724–8.
92. Mocan H, Mocan MC, Peru H, et al. Cutaneous polyarteritis nodosa in a child and a review of the literature. Acta Paediatr 1998;87(3):351–3.
93. Kumar L, Thapa BR, Sarkar B, et al. Benign cutaneous polyarteritis nodosa in children below 10 years of age–a clinical experience. Ann Rheum Dis 1995; 54(2):134–6.
94. Boren RJ, Everett MA. Cutaneous vasculitis in mother and infant. Arch Dermatol 1965;92(5):568–70.
95. Diaz-Perez JL, De Lagran ZM, Diaz-Ramon JL, et al. Cutaneous polyarteritis nodosa. Semin Cutan Med Surg 2007;26(2):77–86.
96. Williams VL, Guirola R, Flemming K, et al. Distal extremity necrosis as a manifestation of cutaneous polyarteritis nodosa: case report and review of the acute management of a pediatric patient. Pediatr Dermatol 2012;29(4):473–8.

97. Pina T, Blanco R, Gonzalez-Gay MA. Cutaneous vasculitis: a rheumatologist perspective. Curr Allergy Asthma Rep 2013;13(5):545–54.

98. Moreland LW, Ball GV. Cutaneous polyarteritis nodosa. Am J Med 1990;88(4): 426–30.

99. Goslen JB, Graham W, Lazarus GS. Cutaneous polyarteritis nodosa. Report of a case associated with Crohn's disease. Arch Dermatol 1983;119(4):326–9.

100. Pereira BA, Silva NA, Ximenes AC, et al. Cutaneous polyarteritis nodosa in a child with positive antiphospholipid and P-ANCA. Scand J Rheumatol 1995; 24(6):386–8.

101. Valor L, Monteagudo I, de la Torre I, et al. Young male patient diagnosed with cutaneous polyarteritis nodosa successfully treated with etanercept. Mod Rheumatol 2013. [Epub ahead of print].

102. Zoshima T, Matsumura M, Suzuki Y, et al. A case of refractory cutaneous polyarteritis nodosa in a patient with hepatitis B carrier status successfully treated with tumor necrosis factor alpha blockade. Mod Rheumatol 2013;23(5): 1029–33.

103. Schartz NE, Alaoui S, Vignon-Pennamen MD, et al. Successful treatment in two cases of steroid-dependent cutaneous polyarteritis nodosa with low-dose methotrexate. Dermatology 2001;203(4):336–8.

104. Lobo I, Ferreira M, Silva E, et al. Cutaneous polyarteritis nodosa treated with intravenous immunoglobulins. J Eur Acad Dermatol Venereol 2008;22(7):880–2.

105. Kluger N, Guillot B, Bessis D. Ulcerative cutaneous polyarteritis nodosa treated with mycophenolate mofetil and pentoxifylline. J Dermatolog Treat 2011;22(3): 175–7.

106. Till SH, Amos RS. Long-term follow-up of juvenile-onset cutaneous polyarteritis nodosa associated with streptococcal infection. Br J Rheumatol 1997;36(8): 909–11.

107. Calderon MJ, Landa N, Aguirre A, et al. Successful treatment of cutaneous PAN with pentoxifylline. Br J Dermatol 1993;128(6):706–8.

Pediatric Vitiligo

Nanette B. Silverberg, MD

KEYWORDS

- Vitiligo • Depigmentation • Autoimmunity • Vitamin D • Corticosteroids • Tacrolimus

KEY POINTS

- Vitiligo is an autoimmune pigment loss.
- Children with nonsegmental vitiligo have a tendency toward other autoimmune diseases including thyroid disease, not seen with segmental disease. The presence of low 25-hydroxyvitamin D can herald the presence or tendency to secondary autoimmunity in children with vitiligo.
- Psychological sequelae including impaired quality of life are often noted in children, especially adolescents with vitiligo of large surface areas, genitalia, and noticeable locations.
- Therapy for vitiligo in children and adolescents is based on a cyclic model of topical therapies with ultraviolet light adjunctively.

INTRODUCTION

Vitiligo is a cutaneous illness caused by melanocyte destruction or damage, resulting in reduced or absent pigmentation of the skin, hair, and/or mucous membranes. Vitiligo affects 0.5% to 2% of the world's population.[1–4] Vitiligo is caused by a genetic propensity paired with environmental triggering that initiates the self-recognition of melanocytes. Autoimmune destruction of melanocytes is the leading theory supported by patient and family history of autoimmunity, absence or reduction of melanocytes on biopsy, presence of lymphocytes at the periphery of active vitiligo lesions, and the detection of antimelanocyte antibodies in the sera of patients with vitiligo. Other theories of the pathogenesis of vitiligo and include neuronal triggers, Koebner phenomenon,[5] and oxidative damage. Each of these is likely contributory to disease development.[6,7]

The Koebner phenomenon is a traumatic induction of lesions. In the setting of vitiligo, the Koebner phenomenon triggers melanocytorrhagy, a rounding of melanocytes and loss of adhesion to surrounding cells in the epidermis. This process results in functional loss of pigment production. Free radicals and tetrahydrobiopterin pathway–generated oxidative species seem to further induce loss of melanocyte activity and enhance damage to melanocytes. The combination of events results in apoptosis of the melanocyte and cell loss.[8–10]

Department of Dermatology, St. Luke's-Roosevelt Hospital Center, Icahn School of Medicine at Mount Sinai, 1090 Amsterdam Avenue, Suite 11D, New York, NY 10025, USA
E-mail address: nsilverb@chpnet.org

Pediatr Clin N Am 61 (2014) 347–366
http://dx.doi.org/10.1016/j.pcl.2013.11.008
0031-3955/14/$ – see front matter © 2014 Elsevier Inc. All rights reserved.

EPIDEMIOLOGY

One half to two percent of the population has vitiligo worldwide.[1–4] Historically in the American literature, about half of cases of vitiligo begin in childhood, with a slight female predominance.[11] A recently published Chinese population-based survey of more than 17,000 people confirms that this trend is still true, and seems to transcend cultures and countries. The investigators reported that 0.56% of subjects had vitiligo. A slight female predominance was noted in childhood, but lost in adulthood.[12,13]

There are sometimes deviations from this trend in prevalence, as population-based genetic differences and/or environmental factors may affect disease presentation. Prevalence of 0.18% of vitiligo was reported in a population-based study of 2194 Egyptian children living in the Sinai desert, suggesting that lifestyle and socioeconomic status can affect the prevalence.[14]

PATHOPHYSIOLOGY

It has been recently demonstrated that atopy seems to have a linkage to early-onset (ie, childhood) vitiligo in both European and American cohorts. The specific mechanism of interaction is unknown, but this has been demonstrated previously in another pediatric cutaneous autoimmune entity, alopecia areata.[15,16] The only association now noted with atopy is the presence of raised borders, with the notation of inflammatory vitiligo as a subtype.[17] At present, no therapeutic differences in response to treatment have been reported in the literature based on atopy in vitiligo, other than the possible greater severity of disease over time.[16]

Vitiligo is a polygenic or multifactorial disease, 23% of identical twins with vitiligo having an identical twin with vitiligo.[18,19] Genetically vitiligo has been linked to more than a dozen genes in genome-wide association studies in the United States, Europe, and China.[20,21] The genes thus far identified as participatory in vitiligo support a role for different aberrations of immunity in the process of moving from autoimmune antibodies to loss of pigment.

The genetic aberrances that contribute to the development of vitiligo include genetic alteration or polymorphism in pigmentation genes that allow these genes to trigger the recognition of self more easily. Genes involved include tyrosinase, an enzyme that promotes melanin production (TYR), OCA2, the pigment gene that is abnormal in oculocutaneous albinism type 2, the melanin transcription downregulator HERC2, and MC1R, the α–melanocyte-stimulating hormone receptor.[20,22]

These antigens may compete at altered major histocompatibility complex loci that allow for further promotion of self antigens. HLA-A*02:01 has been linked to enhanced development of vitiligo.[21]

Recent studies support the age-old theory that vitiligo is an antibody-dependent cellular immune destruction of pigment cells. First, there are data on production of antibodies to melanocytes by patients with vitiligo[23] and by melanoma patients who develop vitiligo while undergoing therapy.[24] Second, recent biopsy studies have demonstrated that early vitiliginous lesions have dendritic cells consistent with antigen-presenting cells, whereas older lesions contain mature T cells. This finding demonstrates that antigen presentation occurs early on in vitiligo, whereas the inflammatory process may be more cell mediated at a later time.[25] Furthermore, mature T cells have been identified at the border of vitiliginous lesions.[26]

A variety of altered immune processes must occur to generate vitiligo, including autoreactive T-cell augmentation[27] and B-cell activation resulting in autoantibody production, thereby creating a target for aberrant T cells.[28] B- and T-cell genes linked to vitiligo include CTLA4, BACH2, CD44, IKZF4, and LNK.[20] Abnormalities in the innate immune system, such as the NLRP-1 (formerly NALP-1) gene and CASP-7 (an apoptosis gene), have also been described. The exact mechanism by which these play a role in vitiligo is not fully elucidated, but is putatively thought to be related to enhanced inflammatory activity.[29] In a study of 620 Chinese children with vitiligo, abnormalities of humoral and cellular immunity have been noted in children with active vitiligo, the former with segmental active disease and the latter with generalized vitiligo. Lower percentages of CD3+ and CD4+ T cells and a lower CD4+/CD8+ ratio are noted with active generalized disease, and complement C3 and C4 were depressed with segmental disease.[30]

Antioxidant vitamin processing seems to be an issue in some individuals with vitiligo. Postulation of exaggerated oxidative stress in patients with vitiligo has resulted in a plethora of antioxidant vitamin regimens.[31–34]

The final common pathway of melanocyte destruction in vitiligo seems to be associated with melanocytorrhagy, a poor cellular attachment of melanocytes in the epidermis resulting in extreme susceptibility to the Koebner phenomenon, that is, traumatic damage.[35] This phenomenon promotes apoptosis/cellular death of the melanocyte.[36]

Vitamin D deficiency and/or metabolic alterations have been linked to many autoimmune diatheses, such as systemic lupus erythematosis, multiple sclerosis, and diabetes mellitus.[37–39] The role of vitamin D in immunity has not been fully defined, but people with the Apa I-A variant genotype carriers have higher levels of vitamin D and reduced risk of vitiligo.[40] This fact is not surprising, as it has been shown that patients with low vitamin D levels (25-hydroxyvitamin D <15 ng/dL) are more likely to develop polyautoimmunity in the setting of vitiligo.[41] This finding is noted in adults and children older than 3 years. Thus it is clearly important to maintain good levels of vitamin D (as measured by 25-hydroxyvitamin D) in vitiligo patients.[41]

Other triggers of vitiligo include contact allergens such as paraphenylenediamine, an ingredient in hair dyes that seems to trigger both oxidative stress and contact allergy in some individuals. Teenagers with vitiligo or a strong family history of vitiligo may do well to avoid hair dyes.[42] Chemical-induced vitiligo presents most commonly on the head and neck and hands. Recently a group of investigators identified a pathway called the unfolded response, which seems to trigger interleukin (IL)-6 and IL-8, previously implicated as vitiligo-associated immunogenic agents.[43,44]

Tan/brown and hazel/green categories of eye color have been associated with development of vitiligo,[20] demonstrating that pigment type may contribute to disease or perhaps promote allergenicity of melanocytes.

PROGNOSIS

The prognosis of vitiligo depends on the type. Segmental vitiligo tends to spread over a few months to years throughout the entire skin segment involved. Nonsegmental vitiligo has a slow and steady spread gradually with age if not otherwise treated. There are occasional patients with rapidly progressive, generalized color loss termed vitiligo universalis, a very aggressive subtype of nonsegmental disease.

Comorbid autoimmune diseases may develop over time. Such diseases are often associated with larger body surface area, but it is unclear whether these diseases trigger each other or whether they reflect greater genetic tendency to vitiligo.[45]

CLINICAL FEATURES
History

Vitiligo (**Fig. 1**) usually presents in the spring with the appearance of lesions that are hypopigmented or depigmented, or that appear on tanning of the skin in

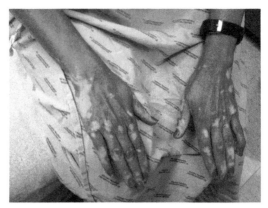

Fig. 1. Nonsegmental vitiligo of the hands. Note the prominence of lesions in an African American patient. Lesions are localized on the fingertips and over joints, extending up the hand toward the wrist.

fair-skinned individuals. Lesions may be segmental along the lines of Blaschko (**Fig. 2**), which are embryonic developmental lines that run like bands around the abdomen and down the extremities, or nonsegmental (ie, generalized) involving the periorificial skin, skin folds (eg, intertriginous), and pressure points of the hips and extremities. Mixed segmental and nonsegmental cases do occur, but are rare and represent a phenomenon of loss of heterozygosity, whereby an individual has the global genetic tendency toward a disease but also locally has a more severe genetic burden in a segment.[46] Segmental cases are most common in childhood, representing one-fifth to one-third of all cases, with 87% of cases presenting by age 20 years, and spread limited to the segment involved.[11,47] When pigmentation is not fully lost, areas of complete, partial, and full repigmentation may create a trichrome pattern known as trichrome vitiligo. The natural history of generalized disease is slow extension of lesions over time if left untreated. Rarely, generalized extension may occur rapidly, resulting in vitiligo universalis, which represents less than 1% of adult and pediatric cases.[48,49]

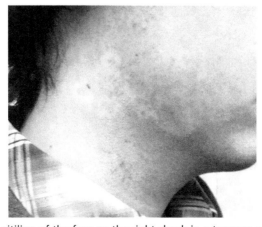

Fig. 2. Segmental vitiligo of the face on the right cheek in a teenage male. Note that the area follows the lines of Blaschko.

Physical Examination

Physical examination is typified by the presence of sharply demarcated areas of hypopigmentation or depigmentation in typical locations. Woods lamp examination will highlight areas of pigment loss and should be done in all cases, especially in light-skinned individuals, to highlight the extent of disease.[50] At least half of children will have oral involvement, which can result in extension onto the face. Dermoscopy, which uses a polarized magnifying lens to identify pigmentation patterns on the skin, or a digital microscope can be used to identify whether hairs are pigmented or not, to aid in deciding whether a good pigment reservoir exists for repigmentation.[51]

COMORBIDITIES

Comorbidities of vitiligo include: (1) secondary autoimmune conditions, (2) deficiencies of vitamins (see pathophysiology section and later discussion), (3) psychological interplay, and (4) symptomatology. These issues are not necessarily mutually exclusive, and the issues are reviewed in this section.

Generalized or nonsegmental vitiligo is associated with a personal and familial tendency to autoimmune illnesses, the most common being thyroid disease (5.4%), rheumatoid arthritis (1.1%), psoriasis (1.1%), and alopecia areata (0.8%) (numbers in parentheses indicate the incidence in children as reported by their parents without sensitive testing). Thyroid disease is more common in girls, and hypothyroidism is 6 times more common than hyperthyroidism.[52,53] Prolonged vitiligo, female sex, and extensive surface area may increase the risk of autoimmune thyroid disease in children with vitiligo.[45] Of children with autoimmune thyroid disease, 2% with Hashimoto thyroiditis and 4.6% with Graves disease will have comorbid vitiligo, with Graves disease being seen with vitiligo in younger patients.[54]

Adults with vitiligo have thyroid disease (12%) and pernicious anemia (1.3%), with 3.7% of patients having elevations of thyroid-stimulating hormone without notable thyroid disease.[55] Outside the United States studies have also linked vitiligo to celiac disease, pemphigus vulgaris, and Addison disease.[56] Family members may also report vitiligo, type 2 diabetes, and Addison disease.[19,20] Polyautoimmunity can rarely be seen in the setting of Schmidt syndrome or one of the other polyglandular autoimmune polyendocrine (polyglandular) syndromes.[57] Other syndromes associated with vitiligo include the rare Vogt-Koyanagi-Harada syndrome, which is a combination of autoimmune attack on multiple pigmented tissues including the eye, ear, meninges, and skin.[58]

Segmental disease involves a limited genetic area, usually on the trunk or hips, and may not be associated with polyautoimmunity unless nonsegmental vitiligo develops. Some children may have segmental vitiligo in the setting of other autoimmune illnesses such as alopecia areata; in this case, the fact that they have alopecia areata confers a risk of autoimmunity. In nonsegmental vitiligo, worldwide data support a strong association with autoimmune thyroid disease on sensitive testing (10.7%–26%).[52,53,59–62]

Vitamin D deficiency is common in the general population, despite addition of vitamin D to milk in the United States. When patients (age ≥3 years) with vitiligo have vitamin D deficiency with levels at or below 15 ng/mL, secondary autoimmune diseases arise more frequently including thyroid problems, type 2 diabetes, and lupus anticoagulant. It is therefore important to screen, treat, and give long-term supplementation according to Institute of Medicine (IOM) and American Academy of Pediatrics (AAP) recommendations to maintain vitamin D levels and, it is hoped, general health in vitiligo patients.[41] Furthermore, vitamin D deficiency should be suspected in the setting of generalized dull coloration and confetti-like hypopigmentation.[63,64]

Psychological impairment affects 51.1% of children with severe emotional impairments, with 10.7% of children aged 4 to 16 years with less than 25% vitiliginous body surface area (BSA) having moderate to severe deficits on the Children's Dermatology Life Quality Index (CDLQI). Psychological comorbidities (eg, poor functioning, poor self-image) become more common with age, with lower rates in younger vitiligo sufferers (<10 years of age) and almost universal presence in teenagers with vitiligo, with 13% of teenagers experiencing severe psychological impairments. Girls aged 8 to 18 years report impairment of quality of life with genital disease, whereas adults report sexual dysfunction in association with larger surface areas and genital involvement.[65] Occurrence of vitiligo during the age of sexual debut may create lifelong psychological issues,[66] suggesting that either early medical therapy, which works better (especially in the first 2–5 years of disease),[67] is required, or early psychological intervention is required.

Although many parents may wish to defer therapy because their child is not bothered by lesions, a recent study demonstrated that whereas 45.6% (0–6 years) and 50% (7–14 years) of children are not bothered by their lesions, only 4.1% of teenagers (15–18 years) feel similarly.[68,69] Therefore, it is reasonable to initiate therapy in an effort to reduce self-consciousness at a later date. As facial and leg lesions seem to be most associated with self-consciousness, these sites should be addressed early.

Pruritus is noted in some cases of vitiligo (30.1%) and can be a sign of psychological distress, including self-consciousness and susceptibility to bullying, in children with vitiligo. Children with pruritus or burning sensation should be observed more carefully, and referred for psychological counseling where appropriate.[68] Teasing and bullying is more common in the setting of facial disease and greater than 25% BSA for children aged 4 to 16 years, and these children and their parents should be offered psychological support.[65,66,70]

Cosmetic therapies are of great importance in helping children avoid unwanted attention. These treatments include self-tanners, cosmetic cover-up, and bleaching in psychologically stable teenagers with extensive disease. The process of bleaching is dramatic psychologically, and mandates prescreening with a psychologist or psychiatrist and a mature age for participation in decision making.[65,71,72]

A simple comorbidity of vitiligo is loss of pigmentation in the nevi, termed the halo nevus. The halo nevus is a melanocytic nevus that develops an immune process, which causes a lightening of the surrounding skin and eventual immune removal by the body. Unless the central nevus is irregular, these are considered benign in nature.[73] Presence of a halo nevus and leukotrichia suggest that a generalized rather than a segmental variant of vitiligo is present.[74,75]

The risk of skin cancer has been feared in the past in patients with vitiligo, owing to the lack of protective melanin; however, in adults the risk seems to be one-third that of spousal controls.[76]

DIFFERENTIAL DIAGNOSIS

Congenital Hypopigmentation (appearing before the age of 2 years in most cases)[77]
- Nevus depigmentosus
- Tuberous sclerosis/hypomelanotic macules
- Waardenburg syndrome
- Piebaldism

Acquired Hypopigmentation
  Inflammatory disorders
  - Pityriasis lichenoides chronica

- Mycosis fungoides

Autoimmune illnesses

- Scleroderma (salt and pepper pigmentation)
- Discoid lupus (scarring associated with dyspigmentation)
- Lichen sclerosus et atrophicus

Infectious reduction in pigmentation

- Progressive macular hypomelanosis
- Tinea versicolor

Postinflammatory pigment alteration

Dermatitis

- Atopic dermatitis
- Pityriasis alba
- Seborrheic dermatitis

Environmental

- Allergic contact dermatitis–induced pigment loss
- Chemical leukoderma (can be induced by hair-dye ingredients, imiquimod, and topical contact sensitizer agents used medically)

DIAGNOSTIC RECOMMENDATIONS
Laboratory Studies

Children with segmental vitiligo do not require screening unless there is suspicion of the occurrence of a generalized autoimmune process. The current data support screening children with nonsegmental vitiligo for thyroid disease and levels of 25-hydroxyvitamin D. Deficiency of the latter may signal the need for broader screening including diabetes, pernicious anemia, and lupus. Screening for celiac disease should be performed when children have extensive abdominal complaints including bloating and cramping, although this can be generally associated with vitiligo and acts as a marker for the risk of being bullied. Children with joint complaints should be screened for rheumatoid arthritis. All children who will be receiving phototherapy, whether natural or medical grade, should be screened with an antinuclear antibody test to avoid precipitation of severe phototoxic reactions that can exacerbate the vitiligo.

Radiology

Radiology is not applicable in the diagnostic workup of vitiligo.

Histology

Cases of mycosis fungoides and pityriasis lichenoides mimicking vitiligo do occur. Differentiation in suspicious cases requires biopsy for histologic examination, which would demonstrate absence of pigment cells in vitiligo with or without inflammatory lymphocytes. Special stains for pigment can be used to highlight the presence or absence of melanocytes in a biopsy specimen.

THERAPEUTIC RECOMMENDATIONS
Pharmacologic Treatment

Treatment of vitiligo remains uncommon among physicians according to the literature, especially because many physicians will not offer any therapy to patients. Studies from 1999 in the Netherlands and 2004 in Belgium reported that only 16% and 36% of dermatologists offered therapies to vitiligo patients.[78,79] This lack of treatment may reflect the light skin tone of the patient population in the countries surveyed; however, since

2004 an improvement in the therapeutics of vitiligo has occurred with the conversion of most patients from psoralen and ultraviolet A (UVA) phototherapy to narrow-band ultraviolet B (UVB) phototherapy, the introduction of topical tacrolimus, the combination of corticosteroids and calcipotriene as a treatment option, and the introduction of the excimer laser to the armamentarium of dermatologists. A recent survey of dermatologists in Saudi Arabia indicated that 76% do not consider vitiligo purely cosmetic and that 69% offer therapy to their patients with vitiligo, suggesting either that physician attitudes and understanding of care have improved, or that physicians treating patients of color are more likely to treat vitiligo.[80]

Unfortunately, long-term outcomes with these therapies are unknown. Similarly, the attitude of dermatologists and primary care physicians in the United States regarding vitiligo has never been reviewed.[81]

The care of vitiligo in childhood is 5-fold. (1) Evaluation at onset to rule out presence of melanoma. At first presentation, a full-body skin examination is merited for all children (especially preteens and adolescents) with vitiligo that is nonsegmental in nature. (2) Identification and therapy for comorbid autoimmune conditions and vitamin deficiencies (reviewed earlier). (3) Therapy for vitiligo using topical and/or oral medications and/or phototherapy (see later discussion). (4) Psychological care of the child and their parents where appropriate. (5) Lifestyle alteration. Brief psychological screening of children and their parents to determine their level of concern should help identify children and parents requiring psychological referral.

Current medical treatments and their side effects (**Table 1**) work through a variety of mechanisms that together can enhance a patient's overall chances of repigmentation. Mechanisms of disease therapy by medications and procedures include rescue of damaged pigment cells, reduction in the inflammatory process, reduction in oxidative damage of pigment cells, induction of repigmentation from the hair follicles or edges of lesions, and grafting of dermal melanocytes using a variety of surgical procedures. Although vitiligo is autoimmune in nature it is a generalized inflammatory process, and as requires such conceptualization to understand the silent destruction of pigment that occurs in this illness. It is unfortunate that many health care providers and medical insurance carriers consider this illness cosmetic and do not offer patients therapy when desired.[82]

Topical therapies

There are no therapies for vitiligo approved by the Food and Drug Administration (FDA). Every topical therapy and/or psoriasis used or reviewed in this article is off-label and is approved for use in other conditions, eg, atopic dermatitis. As a result, despite the need for therapy and the good efficacy of currently available agents, coverage of therapies can be difficult within the United States insurance system. Topical therapies of vitiligo include topical corticosteroids, topical calcineurin inhibitors, topical vitamin D analogues, and topical antioxidant complexes, alone, combined, or paired with a phototherapy and/or surgical technique. Most therapies have been studied as case series, in the absence of randomization or comparison with other agents. Therefore, few data exist on relative efficacies in childhood. One study from Italy identified high-potency corticosteroids as being most efficacious; however, these agents would not be suitable for facial, genital, and/or intertriginous skin because of the risk of atrophy. Furthermore, the timing of the agent's introduction is consequential: early-onset lesions (<2 years) will respond better to calcineurin inhibitors. As a broad overview, the Vitiligo European Task Force (VETF) recommends a class 2 topical corticosteroid (eg, mometasone) for use on the body, and tacrolimus for face and intertriginous areas as well as early-onset lesions. The rest of this article

Table 1
Types of therapy, mechanisms of action, and complications

Therapy	Mechanism of Action	Therapeutic Usage Patterns	Complication
Cosmetics	Cover up	For obvious skin lesions not covered by clothes	Allergy to cosmetics
Topical calcineurin inhibitors (eg, pimecrolimus, tacrolimus)	Anti-inflammatory	Sensitive skin areas: face, eyelids, intertriginous, groin	Irritation, redness, burning, pruritus Black-box warning suggests the product cannot be used before age 2 y and that the products may be associated with risk of skin cancer
Topical corticosteroids	Anti-inflammatory	Continuous or intermittent usage for cutaneous vitiligo alone or in combination with calcipotriene Class II agents preferred for longer-term usage in children (eg, mometasone furoate)	Skin thinning, irritation, contact allergy, risk of absorption, and HPA axis suppression with long-term usage over large body surface areas, no results
Photochemotherapy with psoralens and UVA	Anti-inflammatory, promotes melanocyte movement/migration	For localized resistant plaques unresponsive to other therapeutics; Oral PUVA not advised in children younger than 10 y owing to difficulties of compliance with ocular protection	Risk of phototoxic reaction, erythema, pain, tenderness, premature aging, blistering, Koebnerization of vitiligo, and potential risk of skin cancer based on data from psoriasis patients, no results, ocular toxicity
Narrow-band UVB/excimer (excimer laser risk is focal, Narrow-band UVB risks generalized)	Anti-inflammatory, stabilizing, promotes melanocyte migration, increase vitamin D levels	For generalized disease, unstable vitiligo and/or for lack of response to topical agents; excimer usually for limited surface area resistant to generalized narrow-band UVB or requiring higher dosages focally	Risk of phototoxic reaction, erythema, pain, tenderness, premature aging, blistering, and potential risk of skin cancer, no results, ocular toxicity
Grafting	Places melanocyte source in areas of depigmentation	For stable loss of pigment in a limited surface area (eg, long-standing segmental vitiligo)	Pain, scars, bleeding, secondary infection, cobblestoned skin (ie, irregular texture), no results

Abbreviations: HPA, hypothalamic-pituitary-adrenal; PUVA, psoralen combined with UVA treatment; UVA, ultraviolet A; UVB, ultraviolet B.

is devoted to the nuances of vitiligo therapy; however, the VETF recommendations are generally wise ones for the pediatrician. Variation from this paradigm generally should be handled by a dermatologist or pediatric dermatologist.[83]

Tacrolimus Tacrolimus is a calcineurin inhibitor that was originally used orally or intravenously for the prevention of allograft rejection. The product works by blocking phosphorylation of nuclear factor of activated T cells, producing a broad immunosuppressive and anti-inflammatory effect noted systemically with oral or intravenous usage, and cutaneously when applied to the skin. Tacrolimus has been approved for a dozen years in the United States as a topical therapy for moderate to severe atopic dermatitis, with the 0.03% concentration being used for children (age 2–15 years) and the 0.1% concentration for adults (age $\geq$16 years). Tacrolimus is not atrophogenic and can therefore be used on the face, intertriginous regions, and genitalia.[67,83–86]

Tacrolimus topical therapy for pediatric vitiligo was first described in 2003.[67,83,84,87] Results are best on the head and neck, in some patients of color (Fitzpatrick types 3–4 skin types), and in early lesions in patients younger than 5 years.[84,85] Results are often very good when focal or limited disease is noted. Furthermore, the agent is very effective in facial and facial segmental vitiligo, with 89% and 94% response, respectively.[83] Lesser results are noted on the body, especially with acral lesions, with only 63% of children showing a response to the product.[84] Dosage chosen in initial case reports was 0.1%, but the case series from Silverberg and colleagues in 2004 highlighted no statistical benefit to increasing the strength to 0.1% in children aged 2 to 15 years.[67] Furthermore, the case series highlighted a need for a minimum 3-month trial and twice-daily therapy to achieve maximal repigmentation.[67] A recent clinical trial comparing tacrolimus 0.1% and fluticasone 0.05% showed only 15% versus 5% excellent repigmentation,[86] suggesting the product may not be universally effective; however, a trial comparing 2 months of topical tacrolimus and 2 months of clobetasol propionate 0.05% showed approximately 40% repigmentation in both groups, with 58% of children achieving greater than 50% repigmentation on the head and neck and better results with clobetasol propionate 0.05% on the body (39% vs 23% achieved >50% repigmentation).[88,89] Furthermore, a recent clinical study showed children were 9 times more likely than adults to achieve excellent repigmentation with topical tacrolimus 0.01% ointment for vitiligo. These investigators[90] corroborated the Silverberg data of 2004,[67] demonstrating 76.2% response of segmental disease and 56.25% in acrofacial vitiligo. In addition, an excimer laser, a 308-nm laser light source, will enhance the results of tacrolimus and vice versa[91]; however, the combination is controversial because of the black-box warning placed by the FDA on tacrolimus in 2005, which states that usage in children younger than 2 years is not advised, usage should be limited as a second-line agent, and there may be an association with malignancy or lymphoma. Although no statistical association has been made with the topical product and malignancies, there is a reported case of an enlarging melanocytic malignancy resulting from tacrolimus application,[92] and tacrolimus orally or intravenously is associated with Epstein-Barr virus–associated lymphomas. For this reason, the author does not advise usage over pigmented lesions and would exert caution in immunocompromised children. Tacrolimus is a thick topical agent formulated in white petrolatum, so facial acne can occur during therapy for vitiligo of the face. Continued usage and addition of a topical acne therapy are advised in these cases.[93]

Tacrolimus seems to promote melanoblast differentiation. Repigmentation is often more diffuse than follicular, unless phototherapy is added, suggesting that the product may rescue partially damaged melanocytes from entering cell death[94]; this may be why the agent is most effective in newer lesions.

Topical pimecrolimus Pimecrolimus is the sister calcineurin inhibitor to tacrolimus, but is approved in the United States for mild to moderate atopic dermatitis rather than moderate to severe disease for which tacrolimus is approved. The product bears a black-box warning identical to that of tacrolimus. Usage is usually described for facial vitiligo and vitiligo in sensitive skin areas such as the axillae/groin. It is especially helpful for patients who cannot tolerate the ointment formulation of tacrolimus but, like the efficacy in atopic dermatitis cases, tacrolimus may be somewhat more effective for vitiligo as a disease state. A randomized trial in Turkey of pimecrolimus versus mometasone cream (class 4) for facial vitiligo in children showed 42% versus 65% repigmentation at 3 months on the face, with almost no pimecrolimus response for body and extremity lesions.[95] Efficacy of pimecrolimus has been reported to be improved when paired with microdermabrasion. Unfortunately, this regimen also enhances absorption of the agent with a theoretical risk of malignancy.[96] Excimer laser treatment twice weekly over sites of pimecrolimus application statistically improves the repigmentation, but remains controversial because of the black-box warning and the theoretical increased risk of skin cancers.[97]

Corticosteroids and calcipotriene (topical vitamin D analogue) Topical corticosteroids remain an excellent option for repigmenting children with vitiligo, being more effective for children with lesions on the head and neck as well as below the neck.[89] For this reason, the VETF has recommended mometasone as a first-line agent for children on the body.[64,83] Other reports have promoted usage of the highest potency corticosteroids[98,99] for brief time periods, with 90% response in children. Ongoing corticosteroid usage topically can result in thinning, glaucoma, and potential inhibition of pigmentation; therefore, judicious application for limited time periods and avoidance of the eyelids is advised. Acne can also occur with either topical or oral corticosteroids, as a result of the occlusive effects of thick products and effects on the cycling hair follicle. Therapy can be paired with a topical acne medication in these cases. Tretinoin daily therapy has been reported to increase the speed of repigmentation on face and body lesions when paired with topical clobetasol used concurrently in one case series of 50 Korean patients, 12 of whom were younger than 20 years, with the youngest being 7 years old in the study.[100]

Oral corticosteroids can also be used for vitiligo. Mini-pulses are particularly helpful for disease stabilization in rapidly expanding lesions (surface area doubling in a 2–3-month time period or loss of a unit of pigment such as the face or hands in that time frame). Betamethasone/dexamethasone 5 mg (dexamethasone 5 mg monthly in a single dose or 2.5 mg on 2 consecutive days per month by mouth), with an increase to 7.5 mg when ineffective, can be used monthly until stabilization occurs (2–4 months). A small percentage of patients may have excellent repigmentation with this therapy.[101–103]

Phototherapy and surgical therapies

Phototherapy can be very helpful in patients with vitiligo who have unstable disease, extensive involvement, or poor response to topical agents. Psoralens (topical or oral) and UVA (PUVA) originally was the standard of care in vitiligo. These agents were more difficult to use and resulted in more numerous side effects such as redness and blistering. Furthermore, a comparative trial of topical puvasol and clobetasol demonstrated 17.4% versus 68.2% of patients repigmenting more than 50% of their vitiliginous lesions.[104] Systemic PUVA was described to produce 67% repigmentation in 64 sessions in subjects aged 14 to 32 years with vitiligo, representing a more effective therapy than topical psoralens, likely because of the stabilizing effect of systemic therapy.[105,106] PUVA is of limited benefit in younger children, especially school-aged children, who find it difficult to comply with the protective eye wear needed for 24 hours after therapy. The risk of skin cancer related to PUVA is well defined in psoriasis but thus far has not been demonstrated for vitiligo patients. However, counseling of theoretical risk is important for parental counseling in phototherapy cases.

Narrow-band UVB has replaced PUVA as the standard of care in pediatric vitiligo that is unresponsive to topical agents and in expanding or advancing disease, and in children who have a large surface area. Eighty percent of children with advancing disease will stabilize with twice-weekly or thrice-weekly therapy over a 1-year period. Excellent repigmentation (>75%) will be seen in 53% of patients at the 1-year mark, enhanced by patient/parent compliance, with proportionate improvements in quality of life (as measured by the CDLQI).[107] A study of narrow-band UVB for vitiligo in a mixed adult and pediatric population (the youngest patient was 6 years old) of vitiligo demonstrated that therapy was more effective in illness of recent onset.[108] Rapid onset of response (in the first month), facial lesions, and skin types 3 to 4 are associated with better outcomes.[109] If response is not noted by 6 months, therapy should be discontinued.[110] Studies demonstrate that the addition of topical tacrolimus 0.1% twice daily for patients aged 12 years or older enhances the clearance of vitiligo lesions with narrow-band UVB, with a more rapid onset of repigmentation.[111] However, the tacrolimus black-box warning makes this combination more controversial. Another option is the coadministration of topical corticosteroids early on in therapy with narrow-band UVB.[112] Topical calcipotriol has not been found to enhance the response to narrow-band UVB sources, including excimer laser.[113,114] A newer agent not yet approved for vitiligo, the melanocyte-stimulating hormone analogue afamelanotide, administered as quarterly subcutaneous implants, is undergoing phase 2 and phase 3 clinical trials in the United States for vitiligo, combined with narrow-band UVB. In the initial case reports released from this trial, onset of repigmentation in adults, when paired with narrow-band UVB, was as early as 2 weeks and was excellent for patients with skin types 3 or darker. This therapy has not been tested in children, but holds great promise.[115] Broad-band UVA is an emerging therapy that may give better results than narrow-band UVB, but there are no good data from children and the treatment is not currently available in the United States.[116]

For disease that has been stable and depigmented for extended time periods, skin grafting can be performed, although this is not a commonplace therapy in pediatric dermatology. Grafts can be placed in areas that may have no pigmentation and no pigment reservoir, such as the fingertips, especially in segmental vitiligo that has not repigmented over an extended period (>10 years). Grafting is more often done in adulthood owing to the cost, the need for patient maturity and cooperation, and the need for demonstrated long-term stability. Grafting can produce reasonable repigmentation, although irregular texture, mottled coloration, and scarring can be seen in some patients.[117–120] The literature reports that children respond more quickly than adults, especially those with segmental disease.[67,83] Therapies are limited by lack of child cooperation for the procedures in younger children. Excellent results have been reported with some graft techniques, but melanocyte suspension grafts are not readily available in the United States and require the addition of agents that promote melanocyte growth, thereby theoretically increasing the risk of melanoma. Repigmentation advances more rapidly and evenly when grafting is paired with UV therapy, including narrow-band UVB, excimer laser, or PUVA.[121,122] The long-term outcomes (ie, cancer risk, recurrence risk) of these therapies for adults who were treated as children is unknown.[120,123]

Rarely, in teenagers BSA can advance to greater than 30% with lack of response to treatment. In these cases, when children are psychologically able to cope, depigmentation therapy can be performed after careful psychological screening and with close monitoring by a dermatologist.[66] Camouflage makeup can be used to help children achieve maximal self-confidence and reduce self-consciousness in social settings.[124] Although there is no current biological therapy for vitiligo, there is a heat-shock protein 70 analogue in development in animal models that looks extremely promising.[125]

Coordination of Care

Therapy has to be coordinated with parents, and includes strategic partnership toward improvement of a child's general health (eg, vitamin D levels, thyroid screening) and psychological well-being with appropriate referral to pediatric dermatology, pediatric endocrinology, pediatric psychology or psychiatry, and pediatric rheumatology.

Therapy for vitiligo is generally performed in a cyclic manner, with application of topical agents for 3 to 4 months on the face/6 to 8 months on the body, and alteration for lack of or incomplete response. Addition of excimer laser for focal disease can be used for patients with lack of or poor response to topical agents and narrow-band UVB for unstable generalized disease. Observance of a child's social and school schedule may play a role in decision making regarding therapy, and parents and children should be collaborated with accordingly.[126]

Self-Management Strategies

Self-management of vitiligo is not advised in most cases, owing to the nature of pharmacologic therapies. However, patients with disease can do some things themselves for their benefit. First, patients should be on vitamin D supplementation as per AAP and IOM recommendations.

Superoxide dismutase subvariants have been associated with vitiligo, supporting the idea that patients with vitiligo may accumulate high levels of free radicals with resulting peroxidative damage.[127] The role of other vitamins in childhood is not clear, but as there is a body of literature in favor of a variety of B-complex and antioxidant vitamins, a multivitamin is advised in most children undergoing therapy.

Avoidance of certain foods may benefit vitiligo, including hydroquinone-rich foods and phenol-rich foods such as blueberries and pears, and mushrooms that are thought to contain melanin,[128] potentially exacerbating the immune response. Furthermore, it is well advised to avoid hair dye, which often contains chemicals that can exacerbate vitiligo or induce chemical leukoderma of the scalp and forehead/neck.

SUMMARY

Vitiligo of childhood is a systemic illness that requires global attention to health. Therapy should be offered to all parents and patients based on the extent and location of disease. With good continued care, disease control and repigmentation (albeit often partial) can be achieved.

REFERENCES

1. Mehta NR, Shah KC, Theodore C, et al. Epidemiological study of vitiligo in Surat area, South Gujarat. Indian J Med Res 1973;61:145–54.
2. Howitz J, Brodthagen H, Schwartz M, et al. Prevalence of vitiligo. Epidemiological survey on the Isle of Bornholm, Denmark. Arch Dermatol 1977;113:47–52.

3. Boisseau-Garsaud AM, Garsaud P, Cales-Quist D, et al. Epidemiology of vitiligo in the French West Indies (Isle of Martinique). Int J Dermatol 2000;39:18–20.

4. Krüger C, Schallreuter KU. A review of the worldwide prevalence of vitiligo in children/adolescents and adults. Int J Dermatol 2012;51:1206–12.

5. Diallo A, Boniface K, Jouary T, et al. Development and validation of the K-VSCOR for scoring Koebner's phenomenon in vitiligo/non-segmental vitiligo. Pigment Cell Melanoma Res 2013;26:402–7.

6. Silverberg NB. Update on childhood vitiligo. Curr Opin Pediatr 2010;22:445–52.

7. Silverberg NB, Travis L. Childhood vitiligo. Cutis 2006;77:370–5.

8. Kovacs SO. Vitiligo. J Am Acad Dermatol 1998;38:647–66.

9. Lee AY, Youm YH, Kim NH, et al. Keratinocytes in the depigmented epidermis of vitiligo are more vulnerable to trauma (suction) than keratinocytes in the normally pigmented epidermis, resulting in their apoptosis. Br J Dermatol 2004;151: 995–1003.

10. Wang X, Erf GF. Apoptosis in feathers of Smyth line chickens with autoimmune vitiligo. J Autoimmun 2004;22:21–30.

11. Halder RM, Grimes PE, Cowan CA, et al. Childhood vitiligo. J Am Acad Dermatol 1987;16:948–54.

12. Wang X, Du J, Wang T, et al. Prevalence and clinical profile of vitiligo in China: a community-based study in six cities. Acta Derm Venereol 2013;93:62–5.

13. Lerner AB. Vitiligo. J Invest Dermatol 1959;32:285–310.

14. Yamamah GA, Emam HM, Abdelhamid MF, et al. Epidemiologic study of dermatologic disorders among children in South Sinai, Egypt. Int J Dermatol 2012;51: 1180–5.

15. Silverberg JI, Silverberg NB. Association between vitiligo and atopic disorders: a pilot study. JAMA Dermatol 2013;149:963–86.

16. Ezzedine K, Diallo A, Léauté-Labrèze C, et al. Pre- vs. post-pubertal onset of vitiligo: multivariate analysis indicates atopic diathesis association in pre-pubertal onset vitiligo. Br J Dermatol 2012;167:490–5.

17. Sugita K, Izu K, Tokura Y. Vitiligo with inflammatory raised borders, associated with atopic dermatitis. Clin Exp Dermatol 2006;31:80–2.

18. Sun X, Xu A, Wei X, et al. Genetic epidemiology of vitiligo: a study of 815 probands and their families from south China. Int J Dermatol 2006;45:1176–81.

19. Alkhateeb A, Fain PR, Thody A, et al. Mapping of an autoimmunity susceptibility locus (AIS1) to chromosome 1p31.3-p32.2. Hum Mol Genet 2002;11:661–7.

20. Jin Y, Birlea SA, Fain PR, et al. Genome-wide association analyses identify 13 new susceptibility loci for generalized vitiligo. Nat Genet 2012;44:676–80.

21. Quan C, Ren YQ, Xiang LH, et al. Genome-wide association study for vitiligo identifies susceptibility loci at 6q27 and the MHC. Nat Genet 2010;42:614–8.

22. Jin Y, Ferrara T, Gowan K, et al. Next-generation DNA re-sequencing identifies common variants of TYR and HLA-A that modulate the risk of generalized vitiligo via antigen presentation. J Invest Dermatol 2012;132:1730–3.

23. Hann SK, Shin HK, Park SH, et al. Detection of antibodies to melanocytes in vitiligo by Western immunoblotting. Yonsei Med J 1996;37:365–70.

24. Träger U, Sierro S, Djordjevic G, et al. The immune response to melanoma is limited by thymic selection of self-antigens. PLoS One 2012;7:e35005.

25. Sanchez-Sosa S, Aguirre-Lombardo M, Jimenez-Brito G, et al. Immunophenotypic characterization of lymphoid cell infiltrates in vitiligo. Clin Exp Immunol 2013;173:179–83.

26. Horn TD, Abanmi A. Analysis of the lymphocytic infiltrate in a case of vitiligo. Am J Dermatopathol 1997;19:400–2.

27. Ben Ahmed M, Zaraa I, Rekik R, et al. Functional defects of peripheral regulatory T lymphocytes in patients with progressive vitiligo. Pigment Cell Melanoma Res 2012;25:99–109.
28. Lin X, Tian H, Xianmin M. Possible roles of B lymphocyte activating factor of the tumour necrosis factor family in vitiligo autoimmunity. Med Hypotheses 2011;76: 339–42.
29. Levandowski CB, Mailloux CM, Ferrara TM, et al. NLRP1 haplotypes associated with vitiligo and autoimmunity increase interleukin-1β processing via the NLRP1 inflammasome. Proc Natl Acad Sci U S A 2013;110:2952–6.
30. Lin X, Tang LY, Fu WW, et al. Childhood vitiligo in China: clinical profiles and immunological findings in 620 cases. Am J Clin Dermatol 2011;12: 277–81.
31. Jalel A, Yassine M, Hamdaoui MH. Oxidative stress in experimental vitiligo C57BL/6 mice. Indian J Dermatol 2009;54:221–4.
32. Liu L, Li C, Gao J, et al. Genetic polymorphisms of glutathione S-transferase and risk of vitiligo in the Chinese population. J Invest Dermatol 2009;129:2646–52.
33. D'Osualdo A, Reed JC. NLRP1, a regulator of innate immunity associated with vitiligo. Pigment Cell Melanoma Res 2012;25:5–8.
34. Ruiz-Argüelles A, Brito GJ, Reyes-Izquierdo P, et al. Apoptosis of melanocytes in vitiligo results from antibody penetration. J Autoimmun 2007;29:281–6.
35. Kumar R, Parsad D. Melanocytorrhagy and apoptosis in vitiligo: connecting jigsaw pieces. Indian J Dermatol Venereol Leprol 2012;78:19–23.
36. Wu J, Zhou M, Wan Y, et al. CD8+ T cells from vitiligo perilesional margins induce autologous melanocyte apoptosis. Mol Med Rep 2013;7:237–41.
37. Sahin SB, Cetinkalp S, Erdogan M, et al. Fas, Fas Ligand, and vitamin D Receptor FokI gene polymorphisms in patients with type 1 diabetes mellitus in the Aegean region of Turkey. Genet Test Mol Biomarkers 2012;16:1179–83.
38. Cox MB, Ban M, Bowden NA, et al. Potential association of vitamin D receptor polymorphism Taq1 with multiple sclerosis. Mult Scler 2012;18:16–22.
39. Luo XY, Yang MH, Wu FX, et al. Vitamin D receptor gene BsmI polymorphism B allele, but not BB genotype, is associated with systemic lupus erythematosus in a Han Chinese population. Lupus 2012;21:53–9.
40. Li K, Shi Q, Yang L, et al. The association of vitamin D receptor gene polymorphisms and serum 25-hydroxyvitamin D levels with generalized vitiligo. Br J Dermatol 2012;167:815–21.
41. Silverberg JI, Silverberg AI, Malka E, et al. A pilot study assessing the role of 25 hydroxyvitamin D levels in patients with vitiligo vulgaris. J Am Acad Dermatol 2010;62:937–41.
42. Ghosh S. Chemical leukoderma: what's new on etiopathological and clinical aspects? Indian J Dermatol 2010;55:255–8.
43. Toosi S, Orlow SJ, Manga P. Vitiligo-inducing phenols activate the unfolded protein response in melanocytes resulting in upregulation of IL6 and IL8. J Invest Dermatol 2012;132:2601–9.
44. Singh S, Singh U, Pandey SS. Serum concentration of IL-6, IL-2, TNF-α, and IFNγ in Vitiligo patients. Indian J Dermatol 2012;57:12–4.
45. Gey A, Diallo A, Seneschal J, et al. Autoimmune thyroid disease in vitiligo: multivariate analysis indicates intricate pathomechanisms. Br J Dermatol 2013;168: 756–61.
46. Ezzedine K, Gauthier Y, Léauté-Labrèze C, et al. Segmental vitiligo associated with generalized vitiligo (mixed vitiligo): a retrospective case series of 19 patients. J Am Acad Dermatol 2011;65:965–71.

47. Mazereeuw-Hautier J, Bezio S, Mahe E, et al. Segmental and nonsegmental childhood vitiligo has distinct clinical characteristics: a prospective observational study. J Am Acad Dermatol 2010;62(6):945–9.
48. Hann SK, Kim YS, Yoo JH, et al. Clinical and histopathologic characteristics of trichrome vitiligo. J Am Acad Dermatol 2000;42:589–96.
49. Herane MI. Vitiligo and leukoderma in children. Clin Dermatol 2003;21:283–95.
50. Ducharme EE, Silverberg NB. Selected applications of technology in the pediatric dermatology office. Semin Cutan Med Surg 2008;27(1):94–100.
51. Lee DY, Kim CR, Park JH, et al. The incidence of leukotrichia in segmental vitiligo: implication of poor response to medical treatment. Int J Dermatol 2011;50: 925–7.
52. Pagovich OE, Silverberg JI, Freilich E, et al. Thyroid abnormalities in pediatric patients with vitiligo in New York City. Cutis 2008;81:463–6.
53. Iacovelli P, Sinagra JL, Vidolin AP, et al. Relevance of thyroiditis and of other autoimmune diseases in children with vitiligo. Dermatology 2005;210:26–30.
54. Prindaville B, Rivkees SA. Incidence of vitiligo in children with Graves' disease and Hashimoto's thyroiditis. Int J Pediatr Endocrinol 2011;2011:18.
55. Sawicki J, Siddha S, Rosen C. Vitiligo and associated autoimmune disease: retrospective review of 300 patients. J Cutan Med Surg 2012;16:261–6.
56. Palit A, Inamadar A. Childhood vitiligo. Indian J Dermatol Venereol Leprol 2012; 78:30–41.
57. Cutolo M. Autoimmune polyendocrine syndromes. Autoimmun Rev 2014;13(2): 85–9.
58. Greco A, Fusconi M, Gallo A, et al. Vogt-Koyanagi-Harada syndrome. Autoimmun Rev 2013;12:1033–8.
59. Prćić S, Djuran V, Katanić D, et al. Vitiligo and thyroid dysfunction in children and adolescents. Acta Dermatovenerol Croat 2011;19:248–54.
60. Kakourou T, Kanaka-Gantenbein C, Papadopoulou A, et al. Increased prevalence of chronic autoimmune (Hashimoto's) thyroiditis in children and adolescents with vitiligo. J Am Acad Dermatol 2005;53:220–3.
61. Silverberg JI, Silverberg NB. Clinical features of vitiligo associated with comorbid autoimmune disease: a prospective survey. J Am Acad Dermatol 2013; 69(5):824–6.
62. Silverberg N. Segmental vitiligo may not be associated with risk of autoimmune thyroiditis. Skinmed 2011;9:329–30.
63. Silverberg NB. Atlas of cutaneous biodiversity. New York: Springer; 2012. p. 38.
64. Ezzedine K, Lim HW, Suzuki T, et al. Vitiligo global issue consensus conference panelists. Revised classification/nomenclature of vitiligo and related issues: the vitiligo global issues consensus conference. Pigment Cell Melanoma Res 2012; 25:E1–13.
65. Bilgiç O, Bilgiç A, Akiş HK, et al. Depression, anxiety and health-related quality of life in children and adolescents with vitiligo. Clin Exp Dermatol 2011;36: 360–5.
66. Grau C, Silverberg NB. Vitiligo patients seeking depigmentation therapy: a case report and guidelines for psychological screening. Cutis 2013;91(5): 248–52.
67. Silverberg NB, Lin P, Travis L, et al. Tacrolimus ointment promotes repigmentation of vitiligo in children: a review of 57 cases. J Am Acad Dermatol 2004;51: 760–6.
68. Silverberg JI, Silverberg NB. Quality of life impairment in children and adolescents with vitiligo. Pediatr Dermatolog 2013. [Epub ahead of print].

69. Silverberg JI, Silverberg NB. Association between vitiligo extent and distribution and quality-of-life impairment. JAMA Dermatol 2013;149:159–64.
70. Choi S, Kim DY, Whang SH, et al. Quality of life and psychological adaptation of Korean adolescents with vitiligo. J Eur Acad Dermatol Venereol 2010;24:524–9.
71. Ongenae K, Dierckxsens L, Brochez L, et al. Quality of life and stigmatization profile in a cohort of vitiligo patients and effect of the use of camouflage. Dermatology 2005;210:279–85.
72. Silvan M. The psychological aspects of vitiligo. Cutis 2004;73:163–7.
73. Lai C, Lockhart S, Mallory SB. Typical halo nevi in childhood: is a biopsy necessary? J Pediatr 2001;138:283–4.
74. Ezzedine K, Diallo A, Léauté-Labrèze C, et al. Halo nevi association in nonsegmental vitiligo affects age at onset and depigmentation pattern. Arch Dermatol 2012;148:497–502.
75. Ezzedine K, Diallo A, Léauté-Labrèze C, et al. Halo naevi and leukotrichia are strong predictors of the passage to mixed vitiligo in a subgroup of segmental vitiligo. Br J Dermatol 2012;166:539–44.
76. Teulings HE, Overkamp M, Ceylan E, et al. Decreased risk of melanoma and nonmelanoma skin cancer in patients with vitiligo: a survey among 1307 patients and their partners. Br J Dermatol 2013;168:162–71.
77. Tey HL. A practical classification of childhood hypopigmentation disorders. Acta Derm Venereol 2010;90:6–11.
78. Ongenae K, Van Gell N, De Schepper S, et al. Management of vitiligo patients and attitude of dermatologists towards vitiligo. Eur J Dermatol 2004;14:177–81.
79. Njoo MD, Bossuyt PM, Westerhof W. Management of vitiligo. Results of a questionnaire among dermatologists in The Netherlands. Int J Dermatol 1999;38: 866–72.
80. Ismail SA, Sayed DS, Abdelghani LN. Vitiligo management strategy in Jeddah, Saudi Arabia as reported by dermatologists and experienced by patients. J Dermatolog Treat 2014;25(3):205–11.
81. Whitton ME, Pinart M, Batchelor J, et al. Interventions for vitiligo. Cochrane Database Syst Rev 2010;(1):CD003263.
82. Taieb A. Vitiligo as an inflammatory skin disorder: a therapeutic perspective. Pigment Cell Melanoma Res 2011;25:9–13.
83. Taieb A, Alomar A, Böhm M, et al. Guidelines for the management of vitiligo: the European Dermatology Forum consensus. Br J Dermatol 2013;168(1):5–19.
84. Travis LB, Weinberg JM, Silverberg NB. Successful treatment of vitiligo with 0.1% tacrolimus ointment. Arch Dermatol 2003;139:571–4.
85. Silverberg JI, Silverberg NB. Topical tacrolimus is more effective for treatment of vitiligo in patients of skin of color. J Drugs Dermatol 2011;10:507–10.
86. Kathuria S, Khaitan BK, Ramam M, et al. Segmental vitiligo: a randomized controlled trial to evaluate efficacy and safety of 0.1% tacrolimus ointment vs 0.05% fluticasone propionate cream. Indian J Dermatol Venereol Leprol 2012; 78(1):68–73.
87. Grimes PE, Soriano T, Dytoc MT. Topical tacrolimus for repigmentation of vitiligo. J Am Acad Dermatol 2002;47:789–91.
88. Lepe V, Moncada B, Castanedo-Cazares JP, et al. A double-blind randomized trial of 0.1% tacrolimus vs 0.05% clobetasol for the treatment of childhood vitiligo. Arch Dermatol 2003;139:581–5.
89. Ho N, Pope E, Weinstein M, et al. A double-blind, randomized, placebo-controlled trial of topical tacrolimus 0·1%vs. clobetasol propionate 0·05% in childhood vitiligo. Br J Dermatol 2011;165:626–32.

90. Udompataikul M, Boonsupthip P, Siriwattanagate R. Effectiveness of 0.1% topical tacrolimus in adult and children patients with vitiligo. J Dermatol 2011;38:536–40.
91. Berti S, Buggiani G, Lotti T. Use of tacrolimus ointment in vitiligo alone or in combination therapy. Skin Therapy Lett 2009;14:5–7.
92. Mikhail M, Wolchok J, Goldberg SM, et al. Rapid enlargement of a malignant melanoma in a child with vitiligo vulgaris after application of topical tacrolimus. Arch Dermatol 2008;144:560–1.
93. Bakos L, Bakos RM. Focal acne during topical tacrolimus therapy for vitiligo. Arch Dermatol 2007;143:1223–4.
94. Lan CC, Wu CS, Chen GS, et al. FK506 (tacrolimus) and endothelin combined treatment induces mobility of melanoblasts: new insights into follicular vitiligo repigmentation induced by topical tacrolimus on sun-exposed skin. Br J Dermatol 2011;164:490–6.
95. Köse O, Arca E, Kurumlu Z. Mometasone cream versus pimecrolimus cream for the treatment of childhood localized vitiligo. J Dermatolog Treat 2010;21: 133–9.
96. Farajzadeh S, Daraei Z, Esfandiarpour I, et al. The efficacy of pimecrolimus 1% cream combined with microdermabrasion in the treatment of nonsegmental childhood vitiligo: a randomized placebo-controlled study. Pediatr Dermatol 2009;26:286–91.
97. Hui-Lan Y, Xiao-Yan H, Jian-Yong F, et al. Combination of 308-nm excimer laser with topical pimecrolimus for the treatment of childhood vitiligo. Pediatr Dermatol 2009;26:354–6.
98. Kumari J. Vitiligo treated with topical clobetasol propionate. Arch Dermatol 1984;120:631–5.
99. Cockayne SE, Messenger AG, Gawkrodger DJ. Vitiligo treated with topical corticosteroids: children with head and neck involvement respond well. J Am Acad Dermatol 2002;46:964–5.
100. Kwon HB, Choi Y, Kim HJ, et al. The therapeutic effects of a topical tretinoin and corticosteroid combination for vitiligo: a placebo-controlled, paired-comparison, left-right study. J Drugs Dermatol 2013;12:e63–7.
101. Pasricha JS, Khaitan BK. Oral mini-pulse therapy with betamethasone in vitiligo patients having extensive or fast-spreading disease. Int J Dermatol 1993;32: 753–7.
102. Kanwar AJ, Dhar S, Dawn G. Oral minipulse therapy in vitiligo. Dermatology 1995;190:251–2.
103. Kanwar AJ, Mahajan R, Parsad D. Low-dose oral mini-pulse dexamethasone therapy in progressive unstable vitiligo. J Cutan Med Surg 2013;17:259–68.
104. Khalid M, Mujtaba G, Haroon TS. Comparison of 0.05% clobetasol propionate cream and topical Puvasol in childhood vitiligo. Int J Dermatol 1995;34:203–5.
105. Al Aboosi M, Ajam ZA. Oral photochemotherapy in vitiligo: follow-up, patient compliance. Int J Dermatol 1995;34:206–8.
106. Hann SK, Im S, Bong HW, et al. Treatment of stable vitiligo with autologous epidermal grafting and PUVA. J Am Acad Dermatol 1995;32:943–8.
107. Njoo MD, Bos JD, Westerhof W. Treatment of generalized vitiligo in children with narrow-band (TL-01) UVB radiation therapy. J Am Acad Dermatol 2000;42: 245–53.
108. Hallaji Z, Ghiasi M, Eisazadeh A, et al. Evaluation of the effect of disease duration in generalized vitiligo on its clinical response to narrowband ultraviolet B phototherapy. Photodermatol Photoimmunol Photomed 2012;28:115–9.

109. Nicolaidou E, Antoniou C, Stratigos AJ, et al. Efficacy, predictors of response, and long-term follow-up in patients with vitiligo treated with narrowband UVB phototherapy. J Am Acad Dermatol 2007;56:274–8.

110. Percivalle S, Piccinno R, Caccialanza M, et al. Narrowband ultraviolet B phototherapy in childhood vitiligo: evaluation of results in 28 patients. Pediatr Dermatol 2012;29:160–5.

111. Majid I. Does topical tacrolimus ointment enhance the efficacy of narrowband ultraviolet B therapy in vitiligo? A left-right comparison study. Photodermatol Photoimmunol Photomed 2010;26:230–4.

112. Bayoumi W, Fontas E, Sillard L, et al. Effect of a preceding laser dermabrasion on the outcome of combined therapy with narrowband ultraviolet B and potent topical steroids for treating nonsegmental vitiligo in resistant localizations. Br J Dermatol 2012;166:208–11.

113. Gamil H, Attwa E, Ghonemy S. Narrowband ultraviolet B as monotherapy and in combination with topical calcipotriol in the treatment of generalized vitiligo. Clin Exp Dermatol 2010;35:919–21.

114. Goldinger SM, Dummer R, Schmid P, et al. Combination of 308-nm xenon chloride excimer laser and topical calcipotriol in vitiligo. J Eur Acad Dermatol Venereol 2007;21:504–8.

115. Grimes PE, Hamzavi I, Lebwohl M, et al. The efficacy of afamelanotide and narrowband UV-B phototherapy for repigmentation of vitiligo. JAMA Dermatol 2013;149:68–73.

116. El-Mofty M, Mostafa W, Youssef R, et al. BB-UVA vs. NB-UVB in the treatment of vitiligo: a randomized controlled clinical study (single blinded). Photodermatol Photoimmunol Photomed 2013;29:239–46.

117. Kato H, Furuhashi T, Ito E, et al. Efficacy of 1-mm minigrafts in treating vitiligo depends on patient age, disease site and vitiligo subtype. J Dermatol 2011; 38:1140–5.

118. Matsuzaki K, Kumagai N. Treatment of vitiligo with autologous cultured keratinocytes in 27 cases. Eur J Plast Surg 2013;36:651–6.

119. Kim BS, Kim JM, Kim WJ, et al. Circumcised foreskin may be useful as a donor tissue during an autologous, non-cultured, epidermal cell transplantation for the treatment of widespread vitiligo. J Dermatol 2012;39:558–9.

120. Yao L, Li SS, Zhong SX, et al. Successful treatment of vitiligo on the axilla in a 5-year-old child by cultured-melanocyte transplantation. J Eur Acad Dermatol Venereol 2012;26:658–60.

121. Linthorst Homan MW, Spuls PI, Nieuweboer-Krobotova L, et al. A randomized comparison of excimer laser versus narrow-band ultraviolet B phototherapy after punch grafting in stable vitiligo patients. J Eur Acad Dermatol Venereol 2012; 26:690–5.

122. Patel N, O'Haver J, Hansen RC. Vitiligo therapy in children: a case for considering excimer laser treatment. Clin Pediatr (Phila) 2010;49:823–9.

123. Sahni K, Parsad D, Kanwar AJ. Noncultured epidermal suspension transplantation for the treatment of stable vitiligo in children and adolescents. Clin Exp Dermatol 2011;36:607–12.

124. Tedeschi A, Dall'Oglio F, Micali G, et al. Corrective camouflage in pediatric dermatology. Cutis 2007;79:110–2.

125. Taïeb A, Seneschal J. Targeting iHSP 70 in vitiligo: a critical step for cure? Exp Dermatol 2013;22:570–1.

126. Veith W, Deleo V, Silverberg N. Medical phototherapy in childhood skin diseases. Minerva Pediatr 2011;63:327–33.

127. Laddha NC, Dwivedi M, Gani AR, et al. Involvement of superoxide dismutase isoenzymes and their genetic variants in progression of and higher susceptibility to vitiligo. Free Radic Biol Med 2013;65C:1110–25.

128. Dorđić M, Matić IZ, Filipović-Lješković I, et al. Immunity to melanin and to tyrosinase in melanoma patients, and in people with vitiligo. BMC Complement Altern Med 2012;12:109.

Diagnosis and Management of Diaper Dermatitis

Helen T. Shin, MD

KEYWORDS

- Diaper dermatitis • Infant skin care • Barrier creams • Irritant contact dermatitis

KEY POINTS

- Diaper dermatitis is an irritant contact dermatitis that is typically self-limited.
- An impaired barrier function of the skin develops because of the presence of moisture, friction, and irritants from the contents of urine and feces.
- Attempts to minimize irritants with the use of modern disposable diapers and barrier emollients decrease the incidence of diaper dermatitis.

INTRODUCTION

Overview

Diaper dermatitis is the most common skin disorder in infants and is often a concern for parents and caretakers. It is an irritant contact dermatitis secondary to impairment of the normal skin barrier due to the presence of moisture, friction, urine, and feces. The condition typically resolves with conservative management. It is important to distinguish diaper dermatitis from other dermatoses that may develop in the diaper area.

Pathophysiology

The interaction of a variety of factors contributes to the development of diaper dermatitis (**Fig. 1**).[1] The moist environment and presence of friction in the diaper area lead to disruption of the stratum corneum, the outer layer of the skin that provides a barrier from external irritants.[2–4]

The presence of urine allows the skin to become overly hydrated, increasing its permeability to potential irritants. Urine also increases the pH of the diaper environment by breaking down urea when fecal urease is present.[5] Bile salts as well as

Funding Sources: None.
Conflict of Interest: Onset Dermatologics, Advisory Board.
Pediatric Dermatology, The Joseph M. Sanzari Children's Hospital, Hackensack University Medical Center, 155 Polifly Road, Suite 101, Hackensack, NJ 07601, USA
E-mail address: hshin@hackensackumc.org

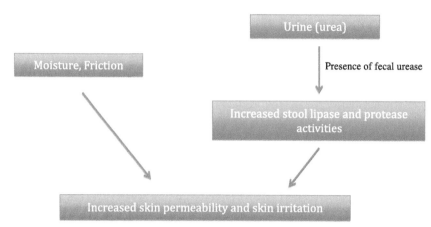

Fig. 1. Pathogenesis of irritant diaper dermatitis.

proteases and lipases from feces also contribute to the erythema and epidermal barrier disruption of the skin.[6,7] A correlation between the number of bowel movements per day and the frequency of diaper dermatitis has been reported.[8,9]

Microbes do not seem to play a direct role in the development of diaper dermatitis. Bacterial counts were evaluated on the skin of infants with and without diaper dermatitis and no difference was found.[10,11] *Candida* sp have also been isolated from the skin and feces of infants with and without diaper dermatitis.[12]

Epidemiology

Diaper dermatitis is a common condition affecting 50% of patients in the at-risk age range of the pediatric population.[9,13] It has been observed most frequently in infants 9 to 12 months in one series and toddlers in the 12- to 24-months age group in another series.[8,13] There is no difference in its prevalence between genders or among races.[13]

With the advent of superabsorbent gel disposable diapers, the overall incidence of diaper dermatitis has decreased.[14] Breast-fed infants seem to be less likely to develop moderate to severe diaper dermatitis in comparison to formula-fed infants.[8,15] Pediatricians and family physicians provide more than 90% of physician services for patients with diaper dermatitis.[13]

Prognosis

The course of diaper dermatitis is typically episodic. Each episode is self-limiting with a mean duration per episode of 2 to 3 days.[16] A small minority of those affected will go on to develop moderate to severe disease. The condition is effectively cured once the child is fully toilet trained and discontinues the use of diapers.

CLINICAL FEATURES
History

A thorough history including the infant's bathing, cleansing, and diapering routine should be obtained. Encourage the patient's family to bring in all of the products that have been used in case specific ingredients need to be checked. Factors to consider when evaluating for diaper dermatitis are listed in **Box 1**.

Box 1
Factors to consider when evaluating for diaper dermatitis

Duration of eruption

Symptoms

  Pain, itch

Cleansing routine

  Frequency

  Cleanser or soap product

  Wash cloth vs baby wipes

    Texture, fragrance

Diapers

  Disposable vs cloth

  Presence of elastics, dyes

  Presence of zinc oxide and petrolatum

  Frequency of changing

    Daytime, overnight

Frequency of urination

Defecation

  Frequency, consistency

Products applied to the diaper area

  Barrier emollient creams and pastes

  Powders

  Home remedies

Amount of time exposed to air

Diet

  Breast milk vs formula

  Introduction of new foods

Medications

  Oral antibiotic

  Senna-containing laxative

Concurrent or recent viral gastroenteritis

Physical Examination

Common areas involved in diaper dermatitis include the convex surfaces in contact with the diaper, such as the buttocks, lower abdomen, medial thighs, labia majora, and scrotum. Due to the passage of feces, the perianal area is also at risk for irritant diaper dermatitis. In classic diaper dermatitis, the skin folds are spared because they are protected from exposure to the contents of the diaper.

Clinical Findings of Diaper Dermatitis

Clinical findings of diaper dermatitis are listed in **Box 2 (Figs. 2–6)**.

Box 2
Clinical findings of diaper dermatitis

Early disease

    Scattered pinpoint erythematous papules

    Asymptomatic

Mild disease

    Mild erythema over limited surface areas

    Minimal maceration and chafing

    Asymptomatic

Moderate disease (see **Fig. 2**)

    More extensive erythema with maceration or superficial erosions

    Pain discomfort

Severe disease

    Punched-out lesions or erosions with elevated borders (Jacquet's)

    Pseudoverrucous eroded papules and nodules (see **Fig. 3**)

    Pain

Consider infection

    Maceration present >72 hours

    Satellite superficial erythematous papules and pustules (*Candida*) (see **Fig. 4**)

    Superficial vesicles or bullae, erosions (bacterial) (see **Fig. 5**)

    Follicular based erythematous papules and pustules (bacterial) (see **Fig. 6**)

    Punched out grouped erosions (HSV)

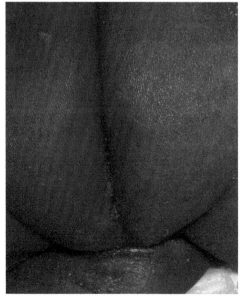

Fig. 2. Irritant contact dermatitis—erythematous patches and superficial erosions on the convex surfaces of the buttocks and perianal area.

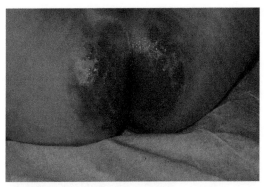

Fig. 3. Pseudoverrucous papules and nodules—painful pseudoverrucous eroded papules and nodules on the convex surfaces of the buttocks and in the perianal area of a patient with persistent loose watery stools.

Comorbidities

Comorbidities for diaper dermatitis include a viral gastroenteritis or a change in diet that leads to a change in stooling frequency and consistency. Fecal incontinence or encopresis secondary to significant constipation or an underlying gastrointestinal disorder may also be present in this population.

DIFFERENTIAL DIAGNOSIS

There is a broad differential for eruptions that may develop in the diaper area (**Table 1**).

Inflammatory Conditions

Several inflammatory conditions present in the diaper area. Intertrigo presents as erythematous patches in the body folds where skin folds are in close opposition. Heat, moisture, sweat retention, and friction contribute to the irritation and maceration in the affected areas. The symptoms typically resolve once the affected areas are exposed to air. A short course of a low-potency topical cortisone may help to alleviate the erythema.

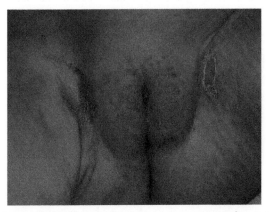

Fig. 4. Candidal diaper dermatitis—erythematous pinpoint papules some with overlying fine scale or collarettes of scale.

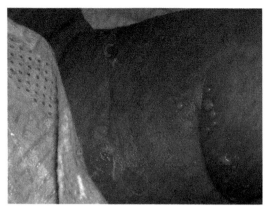

Fig. 5. Bullous impetigo—superficial blisters and pustules on the medial thigh of a neonate. Cultures were positive for methicillin-sensitive *Staphylococcus aureus*.

Seborrheic dermatitis manifests around 3 to 4 weeks of life as asymptomatic erythema and scaling of the scalp that spreads to the face, behind the ears, and to the body folds (**Fig. 7**). It responds well to a short course of a low-potency topical cortisone. Seborrheic dermatitis typically resolves by 3 to 4 months of age. If it persists and is recalcitrant to treatment in the setting of recurrent infections, vomiting, diarrhea, failure to thrive, hepatosplenomegaly, arthritis, adenopathy, and hematologic abnormalities, an immunodeficiency or Langerhans cell histiocytosis should be considered.

Atopic dermatitis commonly presents in the first year of life. Because of the presence of moisture, the diaper area is typically not affected in atopic dermatitis. However, these patients are more susceptible to an irritant contact dermatitis. In infants, the face and extensor surfaces of the extremities develop erythematous scaly plaques that are extremely itchy. In the presence of these findings, an eczematous eruption in the diaper area is also atopic dermatitis. After infancy, the body folds such as the neck and the antecubital and popliteal fossae are involved. Low potency topical corticosteroids such as hydrocortisone acetate cream or ointment along with a proper bathing and moisturizing routine help to control this condition.

Infants have immature immunologic systems that make allergic contact dermatitis rare. There are reports of allergic contact dermatitis of the diaper area to rubber

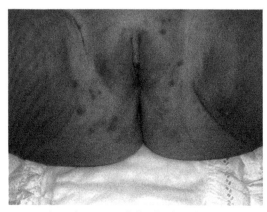

Fig. 6. Folliculitis—scattered erythematous follicular-based pinpoint papules and pustules.

Table 1
Differential diagnosis for diaper dermatitis

Inflammatory conditions	Infectious conditions	Nutritional deficiencies
Intertrigo	Candidiasis	Zinc deficiency
Seborrheic dermatitis	Bacterial infections	Other
Irritant contact dermatitis	Impetigo (bullous)	Langerhans cell
Atopic dermatitis	Folliculitis	histiocytosis
Allergic contact dermatitis	Perianal dermatitis	Child abuse
Psoriasis	Abscess	Burns
Granuloma gluteale infantum	Staphylococcal scalded skin syndrome	
	Viral infections	
	Herpes simplex virus	
	Varicella zoster virus	
	Scabies	

components and dyes found in diapers.[17,18] An allergic contact dermatitis should be considered when a persistent eczematous eruption is present in localized areas where the skin may be in contact with the elastic or dye from the diaper, such as the anterior hips or medial thighs.

Infants and children may develop an allergic contact dermatitis to fragrances and preservatives found in baby wipes and in emollients and barrier creams used in the diaper area.[19] In a more diffuse eczematous eruption of the diaper area, an allergic contact dermatitis to a product being applied to the diaper area should be considered. These eruptions can be remarkably itchy when the infant is continuously exposed to the offending agent.

Psoriasis in infants presents as symmetric, sharply demarcated, erythematous plaques overlying the convex surfaces and within the inguinal folds (**Fig. 8**). The classic silvery scale of psoriasis is absent because of the moist diaper environment. The scalp may also be involved and there is often a family history of psoriasis. This condition is treated with a low-potency topical cortisone and resolves in the diaper area once the child is no longer wearing diapers. Psoriasis of the scalp, face, trunk, and extremities may persist throughout life.

Granuloma gluteale infantum is an inflammatory reaction to potent topical fluorinated steroids and presents as asymptomatic, firm, violaceous papules and nodules.

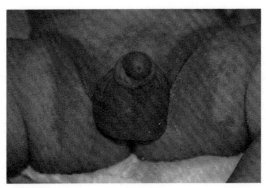

Fig. 7. Seborrheic dermatitis—erythematous patches in the inguinal folds. Similar erythematous patches were present in all of the body folds.

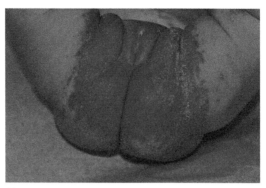

Fig. 8. Psoriasis—diffuse erythematous plaques in the diaper area. Erythematous scaly papules and plaques were also present on the scalp, face, trunk, and extremities.

Prominent areas such as the groin, thighs, abdomen, and genitalia are involved. Once the topical steroid is discontinued, the condition resolves over weeks to months.[20]

Infectious Conditions

Fungal and bacterial infections are commonly seen in the diaper area. Candidiasis is the result of moisture and maceration in the diaper area. It presents as fiery-red, sharply marginated patches with fine peripheral scale involving the inguinal folds, buttocks, genitalia, thighs, and abdomen (see **Fig. 4**). Oral thrush has also been identified in patients with diaper dermatitis.[9] The level of C albicans in the feces of infants with diaper dermatitis has been shown to correlate with the severity of the diaper dermatitis.[21]

Diagnosis can be confirmed with a potassium hydroxide (KOH) preparation that shows pseudohyphae or with a positive fungal culture. Most episodes of candidal diaper dermatitis can be successfully treated with a topical antifungal agent. Nystatin, the first antiyeast agent available, is widely used and has an excellent safety profile. However, topical antifungal agents that were subsequently developed such as azoles (clotrimazole, econazole, ketoconazole, miconazole, oxiconazole) and ciclopirox are more efficacious. In severe cases an oral antifungal medication may be warranted. In low birth-weight neonates or immunocompromised infants, cutaneous Candidal infections may invade the dermis leading to potentially life-threatening systemic Candidal infections.[22]

Bacterial infections can present in a variety of forms. Superficial vesicles, bullae, or erosions that eventually develop a honey-colored crust represent impetigo or its bullous form (see **Fig. 5**). Follicular-based erythematous papules and pustules are suggestive of folliculitis (see **Fig. 6**). Deeper pustules or abscesses may also develop in the diaper area. Perianal erythematous erosions are found in perianal dermatitis secondary to Staphylococcus or Streptococcus. Infants can also develop a diffuse erythema that eventually leads to diffuse scaling particularly in the periorificial areas as well as in the body folds. This condition, Staphylococcal-scalded skin syndrome, occurs from a toxin produced by the bacteria.

When a bacterial infection is suspected, a sample should be taken for Gram stain and bacterial culture to test for the organism present as well as antibiotic sensitivities. Staphylococcus aureus and group A β-hemolytic Streptococcus are typically involved in these infections. S aureus has been found more commonly to be the infecting agent for perianal bacterial dermatitis.[23]

For limited disease, a topical antibiotic should be used. For more diffuse involvement or progression despite topical treatment, a course of an oral antibiotic should be given. The first line of treatment of abscesses is incision and drainage.

Viral infections such as herpes simplex or varicella zoster virus may also present in the diaper area. Herpes simplex virus infections present as grouped vesicles or punched out erosions that eventually crust over. Varicella presents as a vesicle in the center of an erythematous papule and these lesions are not necessarily grouped. When suspected, a viral culture, Tzanck smear, and if available, direct fluorescent antibody or herpes simplex virus polymerase chain reaction (HSV PCR), should be done to confirm the diagnosis. Although these infections are self-limited, oral acyclovir may shorten its course. For extensive disease, admitting the patient for intravenous acyclovir and monitoring should be considered.

When a herpes infection presents in the first few weeks of life, additional blood culture and spinal tap need to be done to determine systemic involvement and the length of treatment with intravenous acyclovir treatment necessary. Neonates infected with the herpes virus are at risk for keratoconjunctivitis, disseminated infection, meningoencephalitis, or pneumonia.

Scabies infection occurs when there is an infestation of the scabies mite, *Sarcoptes scabiei*. It is highly contagious and presents as extremely pruritic diffuse erythematous papules that may become nodular and crusted. The finger webs, areola, periumbilical area, genitalia, and body folds are the most common areas involved. In an infant, the head can also be affected.

Diagnosis is made by microscopically observing the mite, ova, or fecal matter in a scraping of a suspicious lesion. First-line treatment of scabies is permethrin 5% cream applied head to toe on nonambulating infants older than 2 months and from the neck down on ambulating children and adults. The medication should be left on overnight and washed off in the morning. The treatment should be repeated 1 week later. For infants less than 2 months old, 5% to 6% precipitated sulfur compounded in petrolatum should be applied 3 consecutive nights. Each application should be rinsed off after 8 to 12 hours. All close contacts require treatment and all linens and clothing should be laundered once undergoing treatment.

Nutritional Deficiencies

Nutritional deficiencies such as a zinc deficiency may present with an eruption in the diaper area. Acrodermatitis enteropathica may occur when there is an insufficient amount of zinc in the patient's diet, as the result of an inherent lack of zinc-binding ligands in the intestine or impaired excretion into breast milk. It presents as sharply demarcated, scaly, erythematous, annular plaques in periorificial areas, on the distal extremities, and in the diaper area (**Fig. 9**). Vesicles or bullae can also appear in these affected areas. These infants tend to be very irritable, have diarrhea, and also develop alopecia. Serum zinc level can be tested and the patient can be supplemented orally.

Other

Langerhans cell histiocytosis is an idiopathic reactive disorder of dendritic cells that affects the skin and can also have systemic involvement such as diarrhea, anemia, hepatosplenomegaly, lymphadenopathy, and bony involvement. In the skin, it presents as erythematous papules, vesiculopustules, petechiae, and erosions often in the diaper area. Patients with Langerhans cell histiocytosis can also develop thick scaling on the scalp and in the postauricular areas. Diagnosis is made by skin biopsy. Systemic workup and treatment plan should be done in conjunction with a pediatric

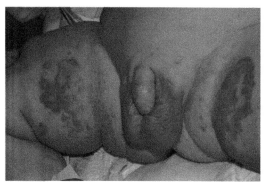

Fig. 9. Acrodermatitis enteropathica—erythematous annular scaly plaques and erythematous scaly papules on the medial thighs and in the diaper area.

oncologist. Potential treatments include systemic corticosteroids, vinblastine, etoposide, methotrexate, cyclosporine, and radiation.[24]

Child abuse or burns can present in the diaper area. Physical abuse can present as unexplained purpura. Burns may present as blisters and erosions diffusely on the buttocks and legs from immersion in scalding hot water or as discrete circular lesions from a cigarette burn or candle dripping. Discrete geometric-shaped burns may occur from an iron. These changes should be documented and one should work with the local child protective services to ensure the safety of the child.

DIAGNOSTIC RECOMMENDATIONS
Laboratory Studies

The diagnosis of irritant diaper dermatitis is based on clinical findings. If there are erosions, erythematous papules, or pustules present, a workup for an infection should be considered. Depending on the index of suspicion, a Gram-stain and bacterial culture, KOH preparation, and fungal culture or a Tzanck smear, direct fluorescent antibody or HSV PCR and viral culture may be warranted. A skin biopsy should be considered when an eruption is resistant to treatment, is atypical, or if Langerhans cell histiocytosis is suspected.

Histology

Diaper dermatitis is a clinical diagnosis and there is limited information on its histology. The histologic findings of different types of diaper dermatitis have been summarized by Montes.[25] Papillary edema and an inflammatory infiltrate of varying degrees were reported. In the setting of classic diaper dermatitis, a biopsy is not warranted for a diagnosis. It is only when proper management fails to improve the condition that a skin biopsy may be warranted.

THERAPEUTIC RECOMMENDATIONS

Management of irritant diaper dermatitis involves gentle cleansing, choice of diapers, and minimizing exposure to potential irritants, such as moisture, friction, urine, and feces. Once inflammation is present, measures should be taken to calm the inflammation and if present treat any secondary infections. There are a lack of controlled trial data to support any particular treatment regimen.[26,27] Parent education and support are essential when treating this typically self-limited condition (**Table 2**).

Table 2 Therapeutic recommendations for diaper dermatitis		
Pharmacologic Treatment	**Nonpharmacologic Treatment**	**Self-Management Strategies**
Topical corticosteroids	Barrier preparations	Cleansing routine
Lowest potency (class 7)	Zinc oxide	Diapers
Hydrocortisone acetate	Petrolatum	Wipes
0.5, 1, 2.5%	Powders	Compresses
Low potency (class 6)	Cornstarch	
Aclometasone	Caution: risk of aspiration	
Desonide		
Fluocinolone		

Pharmacologic Treatment

Topical corticosteroids and antifungal agents are frequently prescribed for the treatment of diaper dermatitis.[13] However, there is only one prescription medication approved by the Food and Drug Administration (FDA) for the treatment of diaper dermatitis and it is only indicated when it is complicated by *Candidiasis*.

Topical corticosteroid therapy

A low-potency topical corticosteroid can help the inflammation present in diaper dermatitis persisting despite conservative measures. In this case, a low potency, nonhalogenated corticosteroid such as hydrocortisone acetate 0.5, 1, or 2.5% cream or ointment should be applied twice a day sparingly to the affected areas before any barrier preparation. Topical corticosteroids should not be used for longer than 2 weeks unless under the supervision of a dermatologist.

Due to the presence of moisture and occlusive properties of the diaper, the absorption and potency of medications are enhanced. There are multiple reports of infants who developed Cushing syndrome with the overuse of clobetasol, a class I topical cortisone.[28,29] Infants also have a relatively higher body surface area-to-volume ratio, making them more prone to absorption of topical medications. Combination products that contain clotrimazole and betamethasone dipropionate or nystatin and triamcinolone acetonide should be avoided and the former is specifically labeled by the FDA not to be used in patients younger than 17 years or in pediatric patients with diaper dermatitis.[30]

Topical inhibitors of calcineurin were developed for the treatment of mild to moderate (pimecrolimus) or moderate to severe (tacrolimus) atopic dermatitis as a second-line treatment. In 2006, a black box warning was issued by the FDA warning of the potential risks of lymphoma and skin cancer with this class of medications. These medications are not approved for use in children less than 2 years of age, the population most likely to experience diaper dermatitis.

Antifungal therapy

When the presence of yeast is suspected, a topical antifungal agent should be part of the treatment regimen. Nystatin is the most common topical agent prescribed for diaper dermatitis.[13] A product that contains miconazole in a zinc oxide and petrolatum formulation is the only FDA-approved medication for the treatment of diaper dermatitis. It is only indicated when it is complicated by Candidiasis.[31]

Other topical antifungal agents effective against *Candida* include clotrimazole, econazole, ketoconazole, miconazole, oxiconazole, sertaconazole, and ciclopirox.

Potential side effects of these medications include irritation, burning, and itching. Some topical antifungals including terbinafine, naftifine, and tolnaftate are not effective against *Candida*.

In a randomized, controlled study, an antifungal paste containing clotrimazole was found to be superior to one with nystatin with respect to reduction in symptom score and global assessment of diaper dermatitis in infants.[32] There was no evidence of development of resistance to miconazole in Candidal diaper dermatitis in a prospective, open-label trial of chronic intermittent use.[33]

Infants with Candidal diaper dermatitis should be checked for oral thrush. When present, these infants can be treated with 1 mL of nystatin suspension (100,000 units/mL) 4 times a day for 1 week or, in more resistant cases, fluconazole (40 mg/mL) may be given at a dose of 6 mg/kg/d for the first dose and then 3 mg/kg/d for 7 to 14 days. Griseofulvin is not effective against *Candida* species.

Antibacterial therapy
Topical antibiotics, such as mupirocin, bacitracin, polysporin, or retapamulin, should be added when a bacterial infection is suspected. These agents should be applied 3 times a day until the infected area clears. If there is no improvement on this regimen, an oral antibiotic effective against *Staphylococcus* (cephalexin) and *Streptococcus* (penicillin or a macrolide for those who are penicillin allergic) is recommended. When methicillin-resistant *Staphylococcus* is cultured, treatment with trimethoprim/sulfamethoxazole or clindamycin should be considered.

Decreasing bacterial colonization
Some patients are at risk for recurrent infection in the diaper area. *S aureus* is able to colonize in the skin particularly in the nares, perianal areas, and body folds. Adding sodium hypochlorite (bleach) to the bath water ($^1/_8$ to $^1/_2$ cup in a full tub) twice a week along with applying mupirocin to the nares twice a day for 5 days of every month has been shown to decrease colonization.[34,35]

Nonpharmacologic Treatment
Barrier preparations that typically contain zinc oxide and petrolatum are used for the prevention and treatment of diaper dermatitis. Other ingredients in barrier creams include titanium oxide, white soft paraffin, or a water-repellent substance, such as dimethicone or other silicones. These barrier products create a lipid film that penetrates into the stratum corneum to protect the surface of the skin.[36] For dermatitis-prone infants, a barrier preparation should be applied with every diaper change to be effective.

Preservatives, fragrances, and other additives such as vitamins, aloe, and herbals may also be present in products developed for use in the diaper area. Some of these ingredients have the potential to be irritating or may lead to allergic contact sensitization.[37] A Cochrane database analysis of the use of topical vitamin A or its derivatives to treat and prevent diaper dermatitis determined that there was only one randomized controlled trial comparing a topical vitamin A product to vehicle. In this study, there was no difference in the prevention, severity, or treatment of diaper dermatitis when comparing vitamin A group to the vehicle group.[27,38]

Powders are used to reduce friction and absorb moisture. There is evidence that cornstarch provides protection from frictional injury and does not enhance the growth of *C albicans*.[39] Caution must be used with powders because there are reports of aspiration of cornstarch leading to pneumonitis in children.

Self-Management Strategies

Cleansing routine

A gentle cleansing routine should be developed for infants and toddlers prone to irritation in the diaper area. The skin barrier is easily damaged by excessive cleansing and scrubbing with harsh soaps or products that contain alcohol. When using a disposable diaper, minimal cleansing is necessary after urination. After defecation, gentle rinsing with plain warm water and a small amount of a mild soap or a mild liquid cleanser without water may be used. Once cleansed, the area should be gently patted dry as opposed to rubbing and if possible left open to air until completely dry.

When erosions are present, the area may be cleansed with gentle irrigation with water from a plastic squeeze bottle or by squeezing a washcloth soaked in water over the affected area. Mineral oil on a cotton ball is useful to remove dried feces or thick pastes. If the bath water stings, a $1/4$ cup of salt or baking soda may be added to the bath water to minimize the discomfort.

Diapers

Today's disposable diapers with superabsorbent gels, an external porous cloth layer, and a breathable outer layer have been shown to decrease the incidence of diaper dermatitis.[40] These disposable diapers are also less likely to cause an irritant diaper dermatitis relative to cloth diapers.[14,41] More recently, a diaper was developed that delivers a petrolatum-based formulation continuously to the skin and was shown to decrease irritation.[42] In a Cochrane review of randomized controlled trials evaluating disposable diapers, the authors found that there was not enough evidence to support or refute the use and type of disposable napkins (diapers) for the prevention of napkin dermatitis in infants.[26]

Cloth diapers allow the urine and feces to mix and to come in contact with the skin. An optional disposable top sheet acts as a moisture barrier with cloth diapers to minimize contact skin. Interestingly, in China, thin pieces of cloth are cut from other garments and are held in place with an elastic band around a child's waist. The cloth serves as a signal when urination or defecation has occurred and is changed almost immediately once soiled. The prevalence and severity of diaper dermatitis in this population were looked at and found to be rare in the buttocks and genital area but was common in the perianal and intertriginous regions.[43] The incidence of diaper rash was found to be less in infants who wore disposable diapers exclusively versus those who used cloth diapers exclusively or intermittently.[8]

The length of time diapers are worn influences the development of diaper dermatitis. The frequency of diaper dermatitis decreases with an increased number of diaper changes.[8] When possible, the diaper should be changed immediately after urinating or defecating and can be as frequent as every hour in neonates. Tight-fitting diapers should be avoided. If possible, diaper-free time with exposure to air is needed to completely dry the affected areas.

Wipes

Wipes today are soft and clothlike with low abrasion potential.[44] Using baby wipes for cleansing was found to be equally as mild as using water with no overall change in skin condition.[45] Baby wipes contain preservatives, fragrances, or aloe that are potentially topically sensitizing.[37] The use of wipes should be discontinued when the skin is broken open.

Compresses

Compresses may be added to the treatment regimen when there is an acute exudative eruption. A paper towel, gauze, or soft washcloth should be soaked in tap water or saline and applied before medications or barrier preparations.

COMPLICATIONS

Potential complications of diaper dermatitis when the skin barrier is compromised include pain, and Candidal or bacterial (*Staphylococcal* or *Streptococcal*) superinfections. These conditions are addressed above in the differential diagnosis and management section.

SUMMARY

Diaper dermatitis is a common condition with most cases being self-limited. Prevention and treatment should be directed against moisture, friction, and irritation. With parent education and support, most mild to moderate cases of diaper dermatitis can be controlled with a gentle cleansing routine, frequent diaper changes, air exposure, and thick barrier preparations that contain zinc oxide and/or petrolatum. When an infant fails to respond to these measures, one must consider if the family is taking all measures to minimize aggravating factors or an incorrect diagnosis. Fortunately this is a condition that is cured once the child has been toilet trained.

REFERENCES

1. Atherton DJ. A review of the pathophysiology, prevention and treatment of irritant diaper dermatitis. Curr Med Res Opin 2004;20(5):645–9.
2. Berg RW, Milligan MC, Sarbagh FC. Association of skin wetness and pH with diaper dermatitis. Pediatr Dermatol 1994;11:18–20.
3. Zimmerer RE, Lawson KD, Calvert CJ. The effects of wearing diapers on skin. Pediatr Dermatol 1986;3:95–101.
4. Stamatas GN, Zerweck C, Grove G, et al. Documentation of impaired epidermal barrier in mild and moderate diaper dermatitis in vivo using noninvasive methods. Pediatr Dermatol 2011;28(2):99–107.
5. Berg RW, Buckingham KW, Stewart RL. Etiologic factors in diaper dermatitis: the role of urine. Pediatr Dermatol 1986;3:102–6.
6. Andersen PH, Bucher AP, Saeed I, et al. Faecal enzymes: in vivo human skin irritation. Contact Dermatitis 1994;30:152–8.
7. Buckingham KW, Berg RW. Etiologic factors in diaper dermatitis: the role of feces. Pediatr Dermatol 1986;3:107–12.
8. Jordan WE, Lawson KD, Berg RW, et al. Diaper dermatitis: frequency and severity among a general infant population. Pediatr Dermatol 1986;3:198–207.
9. Adalat S, Wall D, Goodyear H. Diaper dermatitis – frequency and contributory factors in hospital attending children. Pediatr Dermatol 2007;24(5):483–8.
10. Brookes DB, Hubbert RM, Sarkany I. Skin flora of infants with napkin rash. Br J Dermatol 1971;85:250–3.
11. Montes LF, Pittillo RF, Hunt D, et al. Microbial flora of infant's skin. Comparison of types of microorganisms between normal skin and diaper dermatitis. Arch Dermatol 1971;103:400–6.
12. Leyden JJ, Kligman AM. The role of microorganisms in diaper dermatitis. Arch Dermatol 1978;114:56–9.
13. Ward DB, Fleischer AB Jr, Feldman SR, et al. Characterization of diaper dermatitis in the Unites States. Arch Pediatr Adolesc Med 2000;154(9):943–6.
14. Akin F, Spraker M, Aly R, et al. Effects of breathable disposable diapers: reduced prevalence of Candida and common diaper dermatitis. Pediatr Dermatol 2001;18:282–90.

15. Pratt AG, Reed WT. Influence of type of feeding on pH of stool, pH of skin and the incidence of perianal dermatitis in the newborn infant. J Pediatr 1955;46:539–43.
16. Benjamin L. Clinical correlates with diaper dermatitis. Pediatrician 1987;14:21–6.
17. Roul S, Ducombs G, Leute-Labreze C, et al. "Lucky Luke" contact dermatitis due to rubber components of diapers. Contact Dermatitis 1998;38:363–4.
18. Alberta L, Sweeney SM, Wiss K. Diaper dye dermatitis. Pediatrics 2005;116:e450–2.
19. Smith WJ, Jacob SE. The role of allergic contact dermatitis in diaper dermatitis. Pediatr Dermatol 2009;26:369–70.
20. Bonifazi E, Garofalo I, Lospalluti M, et al. Granuloma gluteale infantum with atrophic scars: clinical and histological observations in 11 cases. Clin Exp Dermatol 1981;6:23–9.
21. Ferrazzini G, Kaiser RR, Hirsig Cheng SK, et al. Microbiological aspects of diaper dermatitis. Dermatology 2003;206:136–41.
22. Passeron T, Desruelles F, Gari-Toussaint M, et al. Invasive fungal dermatitis in a 770 gram neonate. Pediatr Dermatol 2004;21:260–1.
23. Heath C, Desai N, Silberberg N. Recent microbiological shifts in perianal bacterial dermatitis: staphylococcus aureus predominance. Pediatr Dermatol 2009; 26(6):696–700.
24. Minkov M. Multisystem Langerhans cell histiocytosis in children: current treatment and future directions. Paediatr Drugs 2011;13(2):75–86.
25. Montes LF. The histopathology of diaper dermatitis. Historical review. J Cutan Pathol 1978;5:1–4.
26. Baer EL, Daview MW, Easterbrook KJ. Disposable nappies for preventing napkin dermatitis in infants. Cochrane Database Syst Rev 2006;(3):CD004262. http://dx.doi.org/10.1002/14651858.CD004262.pub2.
27. Davies MW, Dore AJ, Perissinotto KL. Topical vitamin A, or its derivatives, for treating and preventing napkin dermatitis in infants. Cochrane Database Syst Rev 2005;(4):CD004300.
28. Ermis B, Ors R, Tastekin A, et al. Cushing's syndrome secondary to topical corticosteroids abuse. Clin Endocrinol (Oxf) 2003;58:795–6.
29. Semiz S, Balci YI, Ergin S, et al. Two cases of Cushing's syndrome due to overuse of topical steroid in the diaper area. Pediatr Dermatol 2008;25(5):544–7.
30. Fleischer AB, Feldman SR. Prescription of high-potency corticosteroid agents and clotrimazole-betamethasone dipropionate by pediatricians. Clin Ther 1999; 21:1725–31.
31. Spraker MK, Gisoldi EM, Siegfried EC, et al. Topical miconazole nitrate ointment in the treatment of diaper dermatitis complicated by candidiasis. Cutis 2006;77:113–20.
32. Hoeger PH, Stark S, Jost G. Efficacy and safety of two different antifungal pastes in infants with diaper dermatitis: a randomized, controlled study. J Eur Acad Dermatol Vener 2010;24:1094–8.
33. Blanco D, van Rossen K. A prospective two-year assessment of miconazole resistance in candida spp. with repeated treatment with 0.25% miconazole nitrate ointment in neonates and infants with moderate to severe diaper dermatitis complicated by cutaneous candidiasis. Pediatr Dermatol 2013;30(6):717–24.
34. Huang JT, Abrams M, Tlougan B, et al. Treatment of Staphylococcus aureus colonization in atopic dermatitis decreases disease severity. Pediatrics 2009;123(5): e808–14.
35. Fritz SA, Camins BC, Eisenstein KA, et al. Effectiveness of measures to eradicate Staphylococcus aureus carriage in patients with community-associated skin and soft-tissue infections: a randomized trial. Infect Control Hosp Epidemiol 2011; 32(9):872–80.

36. Clark C, Hoare C. Making the most of emollients. Pharm J 2001;266:227–9.
37. Manzini BM, Ferdani G, Simonetti V, et al. Contact sensitization in children. Pediatr Dermatol 1998;15:12–7.
38. Bosch-Banyeras JM, Catala M, Mas P, et al. Diaper dermatitis. Value of vitamin A topically applied. Clin Pediatr 1988;27(9):448–50.
39. Leyden JJ. Cornstarch, Candida albicans, and diaper rash. Pediatr Dermatol 1984;1:322–5.
40. Davis JA, Leyden JJ, Grove GL, et al. Comparison of disposable diapers with fluff absorbent and fluff plus absorbent polymers: effects on skin hydration, skin pH, and diaper dermatitis. Pediatr Dermatol 1989;6:102–8.
41. Campbell RL, Bartlett AV, Sarbugh FC, et al. Effects of diaper types on diaper dermatitis associated with diarrhea and antibiotic use in children in day-care centers. Pediatr Dermatol 1988;5:83–7.
42. Baldwin S, Odio MR, Haines SL, et al. Skin benefits from continuous topical administration of a zinc oxide/petrolatum formulation by a novel disposable diaper. J Eur Acad Dermatol Venereol 2001;15:16–21.
43. Liu N, Wang X, Odio M. Frequency and severity of diaper dermatitis with use of traditional Chinese cloth diapers: observations in 3- to 9-month-old children. Pediatr Dermatol 2011;28(4):380–6.
44. Odio M, Friedlander SF. Diaper dermatitis and advances in diaper technology. Curr Opin Pediatr 2000;12:342–6.
45. Ehretsmann C, Schaefer P, Adam R. Cutaneous tolerance of baby wipes by infants with atopic dermatitis, and comparison of the mildness of baby wipe and water in infant skin. J Eur Acad Dermatol Venereol 2001;15:16–21.

Diagnosis and Management of Infantile Hemangiomas

Katherine B. Püttgen, MD

KEYWORDS

- Infantile hemangioma • Propranolol • β-Blocker • Timolol • PHACE syndrome

KEY POINTS

- Infantile hemangiomas (IH) show great heterogeneity in size, morphology, growth, residua remaining after involution, and in degree of response to therapy.
- Propranolol is now preferred first-line therapy, given that its efficacy, tolerability, and safety are superior to that of oral corticosteroids.
- The period of most rapid proliferation is complete by 8 weeks after birth, suggesting that referral to specialists should occur early, within the first month of life for concerning IH.
- More infants are now treated with propranolol than were previously treated with oral corticosteroids, and the full implications of this shift in practice are not yet clear.

INTRODUCTION

Infantile hemangiomas (IH) are both the most common benign vascular tumors and the most common soft tissue tumors in children,[1] characterized by a unique tripartite growth cycle of proliferation, plateau, and involution. Although most involute without intervention, many require medical or surgical treatment. They are marked by a great heterogeneity in morphology, size, growth, residua remaining after involution, and in degree of response to therapy. The treatment algorithm and approach to the management of IH have undergone a dramatic shift since 2008, with the advent of propranolol as a treatment option. After an initial report published in the *New England Journal of Medicine*,[2] physicians worldwide rapidly changed decades of practice, seemingly within months. Despite the initial recommendation for caution from some circles, physicians from multiple specialties proceeded in treating many thousands of infants, despite lack of randomized controlled trials or large prospective studies. Propranolol has definitively unseated corticosteroids as preferred first-line therapy, for reasons of both efficacy and safety. Consensus guidelines for its use now exist,[3] but there are many lessons to be learned by the medical community from the haphazard manner

Disclosure: Advisory Board Member, Pierre Fabre.

Division of Pediatric Dermatology, Department of Dermatology, Johns Hopkins University School of Medicine, 200 North Wolfe Street, Unit 2107, Baltimore, MD 21287, USA

E-mail address: kateputtgen@jhmi.edu

Pediatr Clin N Am 61 (2014) 383–402

http://dx.doi.org/10.1016/j.pcl.2013.11.010

pediatric.theclinics.com

in which the primacy of propranolol was established. More recently, the topical β-blocker timolol, which is available as an ophthalmic preparation, has been proposed as an alternative to oral propranolol for smaller IH.[4–6] The last decade has provided evidence-based data about natural history, epidemiology, and syndromes associated with IH. Information continues to emerge about the as yet not fully understood pathogenesis of IH and mechanism of action for therapeutics. The most pressing issue for the clinician treating children with IH is to understand current data to develop an individualized risk stratification for each patient and determine the likelihood of complications and need for treatment.

DIAGNOSIS

Proper diagnosis of IH hinges on a solid understanding of the classification structure for vascular anomalies, and the most comprehensive and widely accepted classification schema is put forth by the International Society for the Study of Vascular Anomalies (ISSVA). The classification rests primarily on distinguishing vascular tumors, of which IH are the most common, from vascular malformations (**Fig. 1**, **Table 1**). In all but a few cases, the diagnosis of IH can be determined by good history taking and physical examination.

EPIDEMIOLOGY

The incidence of IH has remained unclear, because they are not often present at the time of hospital discharge after birth (when most registries for birth defects are completed.) Current evidence from a prospective study that followed nearly 600 pregnant women and their infants until the infants were 9 months of age suggests an overall incidence of IH of 4.5%, and up to 9.8% in premature infants.[7] Although the cause of IH is not yet fully known, there are several important risk factors for development of IH that have been elucidated and corroborated among multiple studies.[8,9] The most important risk factor is that of low birth weight, which, although often associated with prematurity, is a risk factor exclusive of gestational age at birth. For every 500-g decrease in birth weight, Drolet and colleagues[10] showed that the risk of developing an IH increases by 40%, which is in line with previous data showing that hemangiomas occur in nearly 1 in 4 infants weighing less than 1000 g at birth.[11] IH are significantly more common in female infants, with most studies showing a female predominance of 1.8 to 2.4:1.[8,12] White (non-Hispanic) race is another well-established risk factor; additional reported risk factors include multiple gestation pregnancy, advanced maternal age, placenta previa, preeclampsia,[8] chorionic villus

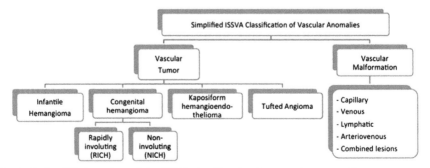

Fig. 1. A simplified version of the ISSVA classification for vascular anomalies.

Table 1 Differential diagnosis of IH			
Vascular Tumors and Malformations			
KHE	Congenital to infancy or later	Firm, reddish brown to violaceous, plaque or nodule	May be associated with Kasabach Merritt phenomenon: increased D-dimer, low fibrinogen, low or very low platelets
TA	As for KHE	Similar to KHE ± associated hair	Similar to KHE, although considered less severe on spectrum
RICH	Congenital; full size at birth	Often symmetric blue nodule with coarse telangiectasia; rim of pallor	High flow
Noninvoluting congenital hemangiomas	Congenital; full size at birth or minimal postnatal growth	Similar to RICH	High flow
Pyogenic granuloma	Infancy or childhood (more commonly)	Friable vascular papule with brisk intermittent bleeding	Rarely may be multiple and congenital
Multifocal lymphangioendo-theliomatosis	Congenital	Varied appearance of papules, plaques, or nodules	Thrombocytopenia (waxing and waning), potentially severe gastrointestinal bleeding
Blue rubber bleb nevus syndrome	Congenital, infancy or later	Small compressible blue to purple papulonodules	May be confused for multifocal IH. Associated with gastrointestinal bleeding ± larger venous malformation, often in thigh or pelvis
Capillary malformation (PWS)	Congenital	Confluent pink to dusky pink; reticulated possible	Reticulated may appear similar to minimal growth IH
Venous malformation	Congenital but may not be noted until later	Blue-purple compressible; growth gradual and progressive	Low flow; may be confused with deep IH
Glomuvenous malformation	Congenital in segmental plaque presentation; multifocal lesions present later	Segmental thin plaque pink to violaceous; papules/nodules firm ± tender	Autosomal dominant; limited to skin and soft tissue

(continued on next page)

Table 1
(continued)

Vascular Tumors and Malformations			
Lymphatic malformation	Macrocystic head and neck present at birth; microcystic often noted later	Deep skin-colored nodule ± vascular appearing pink to purple blebs	Low flow; may be confused with deep IH
Verrucous hemangioma	Congenital	Plaque, papule, or nodule with keratotic change over time	Are subtype of lymphatic malformation
Cutis marmorata telangiectatica congenita	Congenital	Reticulated, marbled pink to dusky purple ± ulceration ± limb undergrowth	May be confused with minimal growth IH or reticulated PWS
Nonvascular Lesions			
Myofibroma	Congenital to infancy	Small to large plaques and nodules	May be ulcerated, mimicking ulcerated IH
Spitz nevus	Infancy rarely; childhood commonly	Pink to red-brown papule	Typically solitary, although may have agminated presentation
Juvenile xanthogranuloma	Congenital to infancy	Pink to red-brown papules or nodules	Become yellow with time; central ulceration possible in larger lesions
Dermoid cyst	Congenital	Skin-colored to slightly bluish, firm, typically mobile nodule face and scalp at sites of suture closure/ embryonic fusion	May be confused with deep IH
Encephalocele	Congenital	Bluish nodule, may transilluminate in midline frontal or occipital scalp	Consider with midline deep blue nodule
Rhadomyosarcoma	Congenital to first year for most	Firm tumoral nodule with overlying telangiectasias; embryonal rhabdomyosarcoma is multifocal and congenital	May be confused with deep or mixed IH
Infantile fibrosarcoma	Congenital to first 2 y	Red to blue, firm and fixed to underlying tissue	May be confused with mixed IH, but more often KHE/ TA or RICH/NICH

(continued on next page)

Table 1 (continued)			
Nonvascular Lesions			
Langerhans cell histiocytosis	Congenital, infancy or later	Seborrheic distribution in scalp and diaper area especially; red to brown papules, nodules, petechial papules	Congenital presentation more favorable prognosis than presentation in infancy or later. Presentation with larger nodule, often on scalp, possible
Neuroblastoma	Congenital to early infancy	Blue to violaceous nodule	Increased urine homovanillic ± vanillylmandelic acid
Congenital leukemia cutis	Congenital to neonatal	Pink, blue, or violaceous firm plaques and nodules	May be confused with multifocal IH

Abbreviations: KHE, kaposiform hemangioendothelioma; NICH, noninvoluting congenital hemangiomas; PWS, port wine stain; RICH, rapidly involuting congenital hemangiomas; TA, tufted angioma.

Adapted from Frieden IJ, Rogers M, Garzon MC. Conditions masquerading as infantile haemangioma: part 1. Australas J Dermatol 2009;50(2):77–97, with permission; and Frieden IJ, Rogers M, Garzon MC. Conditions masquerading as infantile haemangioma: part 2. Australas J Dermatol 2009;50(3):153–68, with permission.

sampling,[13] and antenatal vaginal bleeding.[14] Although IH have traditionally been discussed as a sporadic disorder, there is mounting evidence of IH occurring in kindreds, suggesting there is a role for genetic predisposition in the pathogenesis of IH.[15]

NATURAL HISTORY

The growth cycle of IH is unique among vascular tumors and malformations, showing proliferation and preprogrammed involution. IH start with a nascent phase as either an area of pallor, a telangiectatic patch, or something mistaken for an ecchymosis or birth trauma.[16] They may present anywhere on the body surface but are present most commonly on the head and neck, a finding which is also true of vascular malformations.[17] Typically, most begin to proliferate to a noticeable degree at between 2 and 4 weeks of life, although IH that are located primarily in the subcutis, known as deep IH, presenting as bluish or skin-colored nodules (**Fig. 2**), may not be noted until even a few months of age.

IH morphology can be described by the following 2 complementary concepts (**Fig. 3**). First, the concept of depth of involvement in the dermis, fat, and soft tissue is informative not only in establishing the diagnosis but can help to predict concern for future deformity and residua. In addition to deep lesions, IH can present as superficial, with bright pink, fuchsia, or red on the surface of a papule, plaque, or nodule (**Fig. 4**). Most IH present as mixed morphology, with both superficial and deep components, with a pink surface overlying a soft tissue swelling with a pink to bluish hue (**Fig. 5**). Second, the outline and distribution of IH on the body surface, in addition

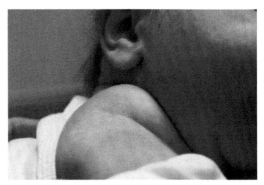

Fig. 2. A deep focal IH on the right shoulder of this 3-month-old infant was first noted at 2 months of age.

to the anatomic depth, provide valuable prognostic information about the possible need for treatment and potential associated complications. In this schema, IH are regarded as localized when they seem to arise from an isolated focal point as with a solitary nodule; these are the most common presentation (see **Fig. 5**). IH are deemed segmental when they occupy a subunit of a body part such as the forearm (**Fig. 6**) or a broad region on the face (**Fig. 7**). Segmental IH are more often, but not always, plaques as opposed to nodules.

Significant work has elucidated the segments of the face through reproducible mapping of photographs of affected children.[18] The segments are labeled 1 (frontotemporal), 2 (maxillary), 3 (mandibular), and 4 (frontonasal). Segments 2, 3, and 4 correlate with established embryologic placodes[19]; however, segment 1 is similar but not

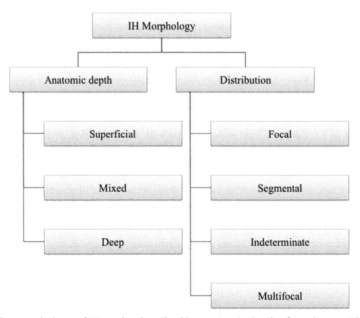

Fig. 3. The morphology of IH can be described by anatomic depth of involvement (*left*) and by the pattern of distribution on the body surface (*right*).

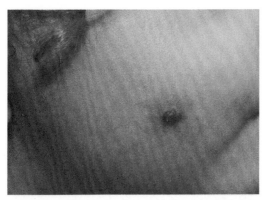

Fig. 4. A superficial IH on the right cheek of a 2-year-old girl, which has not yet shown signs of involution.

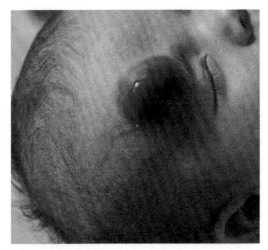

Fig. 5. A rapidly growing mixed focal IH on the right forehead of a 6-week-old girl, which was firm and minimally compressible.

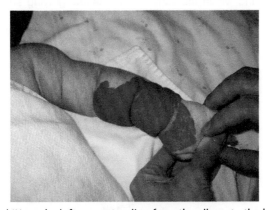

Fig. 6. A segmental IH on the left arm extending from the elbow to the hand has a plaque-like appearance.

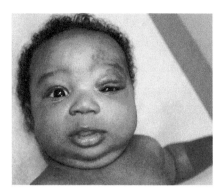

Fig. 7. A primarily deep segmental IH on the left eye, temple, and scalp comprising discrete and coalescing superficial pink papules. The infant did not fulfill criteria for PHACE despite full workup.

identical to distribution of the first branch of the trigeminal nerve (V1.) The reason for this lack of conformity with known facial planes on the upper face is not fully understood. The concept of facial segments for IH is important, because it relates to associated syndromes, complications, and necessity of therapeutic intervention. The category of indeterminate IH encompasses those lesions that appear more geographic in morphology than localized lesions but that do not clearly occupy a known mapped segment (**Fig. 8**). Multifocal IH (**Fig. 9**) are defined differently by different investigators, but are generally held to be small, relatively monomorphic lesions, at least 5 to 10 in number, distributed over the skin surface.

During the first 2 months of life, nearly all hemangiomas double in size, and newer evidence suggests that the most rapid period of growth occurs between 5.5 and 7.5 weeks of age, with most rapid proliferation complete in the first 8 weeks of life.[16] Most reach 80% of maximum size at between 3 and 5 months of age, although segmental and deep IH have a more prolonged growth phase.[20] Maximum size is generally fulfilled at 9 months and almost always by 12 months of age, although rare reports exist of growth extending beyond age 2 years.[21] Plateau in growth then occurs and is followed by involution, which occurs over several years, with the most rapid phase of involution occurring between ages 1 and 4 years. The growth cycle is dynamic, and within the same lesion, central graying and regression may begin to occur as the periphery is still proliferating. This improved understanding of the growth cycle informs the clinician's ability to offer anticipatory guidance to

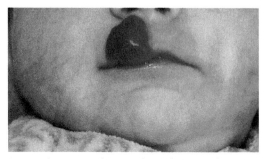

Fig. 8. An indeterminate subsegmental IH on the right upper lip.

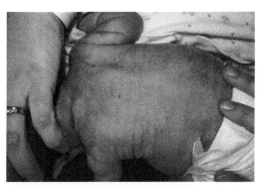

Fig. 9. This infant with multifocal IH had similar multifocal IH throughout the liver paren-chyma; both the cutaneous and visceral IH responded well to propranolol.

families about expected future growth and to plan for the likelihood of need for, and duration of, intervention and workup based on age at presentation, size, and morphology of IH.

Although radiologic imaging is not necessary in most cases of IH, IH are high-flow lesions that show the features presented in **Table 2**, which can help to confirm diag-nosis in challenging cases and with presurgical planning, most often during involution.[17]

COMPLICATIONS

Most IH follow a benign course without the need for intervention aside from anticipa-tory guidance, but evidence shows that approximately 12% are complex and war-rant referral for specialist evaluation; of those seen at tertiary care centers, nearly a quarter developed complications, ranging from ulceration to obstruction of the eye, airway, or auditory canal to cardiac compromise, in a study based on a cohort of more than 1000 infants.[9] The same study documented that segmental IH are 11 times more likely to have complications and have an 8-fold increased likelihood of receiving treatment. Size and location on the face are the other most important pre-dictors of complications and need for treatment. The risk of permanent disfigurement is the most common reason that therapy is initiated, for the purpose of preventing the development of further distortion or destruction of anatomy. A severity scale has been developed that may help with determining need for treatment[22]; in practice, the decision to institute therapy is typically based on a gestalt of the IH size, location, subtype, extent of growth, and likelihood of future growth along with discussion with

Table 2	
Radiologic appearance of IH	
Radiologic Imaging Characteristics of IH	
Ultrasonography	High flow, low resistance, variable echogenicity, high vessel density, no arteriovenous shunting
Computed tomography	Lobular soft tissue mass, intensely staining
Magnetic resonance imaging	Isointense (T1), hyperintense (T2), homogeneously enhancing soft tissue mass, can see flow voids within and surrounding IH; no phleboliths

the family about their wishes for a more proactive or laissez-faire approach. The concept of slope is important, because it pertains to the height and volume of IH and risk of residual lesion; those with a minimal slope tend to involute with less risk of fibrofatty residuum, whereas those with a steep slope at the junction of normal and affected skin have a higher risk of anetodermic scar tissue.[23] Both can be complicated by skin wrinkling and telangiectasias. **Table 3** shows high-risk locations for IH.

Ulceration is the most frequently occurring complication, occurring in up to 25% of patients at referral centers.[9] The first 4 months of life are the period of highest risk for the development of ulceration, and the occurrence of a gray-white discoloration akin to that typically seen and described as graying in the involuting IH can herald impending ulceration and should be a cause for worry, because it seems to represent necrosis of the overlying epidermis. The cause for ulceration is not fully understood, but areas at highest risk for skin breakdown are those with constant exposure to moisture and potential maceration, such as the lip, diaper area, neck, and axillae (**Fig. 10**).[24–26] In a large prospective study, 50% of IH in the diaper area ulcerated and 30% of lower lip lesions ulcerated, as did 25% of neck lesions.[24] Parents frequently question whether IH are painful for infants; they are not, unless ulceration occurs, in which case, they can cause exquisite pain and can make normal activities of daily living such as feeding and diapering difficult. As with any ulcer, because the ulcer extends to the dermis or deeper, scarring occurs and typically results in a white smooth surface after healing (**Fig. 11**). Severe bleeding is a rare complication, occurring in less than 1% of cases.

MULTIFOCAL IH

Infants can present with multiple, often small, focal IH; clinically, some infants present with monomorphic small superficial His, sometimes numbering in the hundreds, whereas others present with multiple focal IH of various sizes and appearance. This phenomenon has been referred to as benign neonatal hemangiomatosis when it

Table 3
Anatomic locations of IH associated with increased morbidity

High-Risk IH Presentations	
Large, facial segmental	PHACE
Segment 3 (mandibular or beard area)	Airway IH, PHACE, risk of coarctation of the aorta
Segment 1 and 4 (frontotemporal and frontonasal)	Risk of cerebrovascular anomalies, structural brain abnormalities
Nasal tip, ear, large facial	Disfigurement, destruction of anatomic landmarks, scarring
Lip, perioral	Ulceration, disfigurement, feeding difficulties
Periorbital or retrobulbar	Ocular axis occlusion, astigmatism, amblyopia, tear duct obstruction
Lumbosacral	LUMBAR syndrome, tethered cord, genitourinary anomalies
Perineal, axilla, neck, perioral	Ulceration
Multifocal	Visceral involvement (liver, gastrointestinal tract)
Hepatic	Congestive heart failure, consumptive hypothyroidism

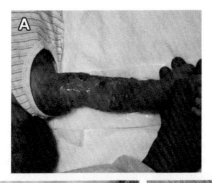

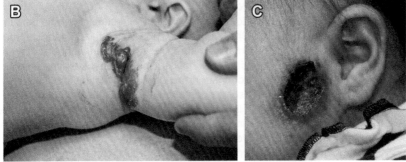

Fig. 10. (*A*) This infant presented with an unusually severe ulceration down to muscle. (*B*) This infant presented with painful ulceration in the left axilla, which required addition of propranolol after failure of wound care alone. (*C*) A deep ulcer on the left cheek of an infant girl.

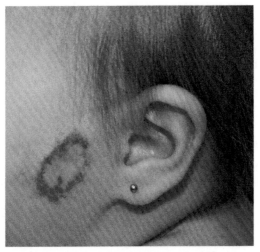

Fig. 11. Excellent outcome after a course of propranolol for the patient in **Fig. 10**C shows a smooth white scar.

occurs without visceral involvement and as diffuse or disseminated neonatal hemangiomatosis (DNH) when it is accompanied by symptomatic IH internally, in the liver, gastrointestinal tract, lung, or central nervous system. Originally, DNH was proposed to be the occurrence of multiple IH in neonates, affecting 3 organ systems and with no concurrent malignancy.[27] Over time, the term DNH has been used to apply to multifocal IH with 1 extracutaneous site, typically liver. More recently, Glick and colleagues[28] suggested that better terminology would refer to this phenomenon as multifocal IH with or without extracutaneous disease. Historically, the reported mortality for DNH has been very high, between 60% and 81%[29]; however, newer evidence suggests that those cases associated with high mortality were not IH, but were other vascular tumors or disorders. Multifocal lymphangioendotheliomatosis with thrombocytopenia is a recently described entity, which likely accounts for many of the fatal cases previously categorized as DNH.[30–32]

Just as morphologic categorization is informative in IH, infantile hepatic hemangiomas (IHH) are characterized by Christison-Lagay and colleagues[33] as focal, multifocal, or diffuse. Focal hepatic hemangiomas occur most often without cutaneous involvement and may be diagnosed on prenatal ultrasonography; their clinical course suggests that they are the hepatic counterparts of rapidly involuting congenital hemangiomas (RICH), because they resolve spontaneously within several months of life and are generally asymptomatic; like congenital hemangiomas, they are glucose transporter 1 negative, differentiating them from IH. Multifocal and diffuse IHH are IH and follow an identical growth cycle of nascency, growth, and involution. Multifocal hepatic hemangiomas can be complicated by high-output heart failure from associated portovenous or arteriovenous shunts, but multifocal lesions are often asymptomatic. There are several reports detailing positive response to therapy with propranolol and corticosteroids, separately or in combination.[34–36]

Diffuse IHH is the more ominous presentation, characterized by subtotal replacement of the liver parenchyma by vascular tumor. Abdominal compartment syndrome, respiratory and cardiac compromise, and multiorgan dysfunction are possible. Diffuse IHH can be associated with profound hypothyroidism from production of type III iodothyronine deiodinase, placing infants at risk for mental retardation and cardiac compromise.[37] A recent retrospective study of 121 hepatic hemangiomas showed that cutaneous IH were present in more than 75% of multifocal IHH, more than half of diffuse IHH, and in 15% of focal hepatic hemangiomas. Kulungowski and colleagues[38] found hypothyroidism in all patients with diffuse lesions, in 21% with multifocal IHH, and in no patients with focal disease. Recent evidence also supports the long-held dogma that infants with 5 or more cutaneous IH deserve screening abdominal ultrasonography to look for hepatic involvement.[39] Although there are reports of gastrointestinal tract involvement complicating multifocal IH, it has been suggested that involvement here is associated with segmental IH instead of multifocal IH.

COMPLICATIONS ASSOCIATED WITH SEGMENTAL IH

PHACE (OMIM 606519), a neurocutaneous syndrome of skin, brain, eye, and ventral body anomalies, is the most well-documented segmental IH syndrome occurring in the setting of segmental facial IH (**Fig. 12**), although a few cases have been reported with nonfacial IH and systemic complications relevant to PHACE.[40–43] Diagnostic criteria were published in 2009 and help to risk stratify patients into definite, possible, or probable PHACE syndrome, based on organ involvement at presentation.[44] PHACE has an impressive nearly 90% female predominance. However, unlike nonsyndromic IH, patients with PHACE are more likely to be of normal gestational age and birth

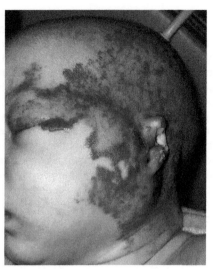

Fig. 12. This infant had both cerebrovascular anomalies and gastrointestinal bleeding as manifestations of her PHACE syndrome.

weight, and the product of singleton pregnancy. In the largest prospective study to date,[42] almost one-third of 108 patients with facial segmental IH met diagnostic criteria for PHACE. All patients with facial segmental IH should undergo evaluation with magnetic resonance imaging (MRI) and magnetic resonance angiography (MRA) (**Box 1**) at or near the time of presentation, given that structural brain and cerebrovascular anomalies are the most common extracutaneous finding in patients with PHACE, occurring in between 72% and 94% of patients in the literature. Those lesions with the highest association with brain involvement occur on the lateral forehead (segment 1) or mandible (segment 3).[42,45] Cerebrovascular anomalies in PHACE have been described, from most to least common, as dysgenesis (56%), anomalous origin or course of vessel (47%), vessel narrowing (39%), nonvisualization from occlusion or aplasia (20%), or embryonic artery persistence (20%) in a study of 70 patients with documented PHACE.[44] As with Sturge-Weber syndrome, cerebrovascular anomalies overwhelmingly occur on the side ipsilateral to the cutaneous IH. The internal cerebral artery was the most commonly affected artery in this cohort. Although rare, progressive stenoses have been reported.[45] Structural brain abnormalities were less common, although as the name suggests, posterior fossa abnormalities (hypoplasia)

Box 1
The protocol for MRI/MRA imaging of vascular anomalies used at Johns Hopkins Hospital

Johns Hopkins Pediatric Vascular Anomaly MRI Protocol

- Axial, coronal, and sagittal T2-weighted imaging with fat saturation

- Precontrast axial T1

- Postcontrast axial T1

- Postcontrast coronal and sagittal T1 with fat-saturation time-resolved angiography with interleaved stochastic trajectories (dynamic MRA/magnetic resonance venography) were the most common. Developmental delay, seizure, headache, and stroke have been reported as persistent neurologic deficits. A review of 22 cases of acute ischemic stroke in the context of PHACE syndrome reported that nonvisualization or severe narrowing of at least 1 major cerebral artery was present in all but 1 reported case.[46]

In the largest study to date of 150 patients with cardiovascular disease in PHACE,[47] 41% showed aortic arch, intracardiac, or anomalies of the brachiocephalic vessels. In this cohort, aberrant takeoff of the subclavian artery was slightly more common (21%) than coarctation (19%.) The investigators emphasized that coarctation may be overlooked because of the combined occurrence of the 2 anomalies, such that both subclavian arteries arise beyond the site of obstruction, which renders the standard physical examination technique of obtaining blood pressures in each extremity nondiagnostic. Ninety-two percent of patients with cardiac involvement had anomalies of the cerebral or cervical vasculature, an association known to increase risk of cerebrovascular accident. When coarctation does occur in PHACE, it is notably different from nonsyndromic coarctation, characterized by narrowing of long segments of the transverse arch and is adjacent to aneurismal dilation. Eye involvement in PHACE occurs in 7% to 17% of cases[41,42]; major criteria for diagnosis include the posterior segment anomalies of morning glory disk anomaly, hypoplasia of the optic nerve, retinal vascular abnormalities, persistent embryonic vasculature, coloboma, and peripapillary staphyloma. Anterior segment anomalies such as cataract and microphthalmia are minor criteria in the consensus guidelines,[43] and 1 case report suggests the addition of congenital glaucoma as a diagnostic criterion.[48] Supraumbilical raphe and sternal clefting are reported in up to 15% of patients. Arteriovenous malformation is another rare association with PHACE.[49]

The lower body correlate of PHACE syndrome has been reported under 3 different acronyms: LUMBAR, PELVIS, and SACRAL.[50–52] Because the investigators who proposed the term LUMBAR have reported on the greatest number of cases, it is discussed here. It is a constellation of lower body IH and skin defects such as lipoma, urogenital anomalies, ulceration, myelopathy (tethered cord was the most common extracutaneous manifestation overall), bony deformities, anorectal malformations (most commonly imperforate anus), arterial anomalies, and renal anomalies.[52] The investigators suggest that in infants presenting younger than 3 months screening ultrasonography of the affected areas of the abdomen, pelvis, and spine is warranted, and beyond 3 months of age, MRI and a time-resolved MRA should be pursued with the area of imaging based on the location of the cutaneous IH and other anomalies.[52]

THERAPY

Although there have been impressive and fundamental changes in our understanding of the heterogeneous presentations and pathogenesis of IH in the last decade, clearly the most dramatic changes have occurred in the realm of therapy, with the complete shift toward β-blockers as the standard of care. An important simultaneous but perhaps less obvious effect of the use of propranolol, which is widely accepted to be a safer and more well-tolerated drug than oral corticosteroids (OCS), is that therapy is now offered to more patients than those treated in decades past.[53] OCS were generally prescribed only to patients with very large or obviously function-threatening IH, and watchful waiting was the preferred therapy for most other infants. The long-term implications of this latter change are not yet fully clear. There is evidence that propranolol is in addition distinguished from OCS in its effectiveness in treating infants who are beyond the proliferative phase of growth, well beyond 2 years of age.[54] Indications for systemic therapy include threat to a vital function (vision, feeding, stooling, cardiac function), risk of disfigurement, ulceration, and bleeding. The concept of disfigurement is one that has shifted significantly in the β-blocker era, in part because of the availability of a treatment viewed as safe and in part because of the theory that medical intervention with propranolol may obviate further therapy, such as pulsed dye laser or surgery.

The proposed mechanism of action of propranolol includes rapid vasoconstriction, which corresponds to the color change from pink to violaceous typically seen in the first 1 to 2 days of therapy. Inhibition of angiogenesis by downregulation of proangiogenic growth factors vascular endothelial growth factor, basic fibroblast growth factor, and matrix metalloproteinases 2 and 9 seems to correspond to growth arrest. Third, hastening of the induction of apoptosis of endothelial cells, known to occur in natural involution, has been proposed to result in the stimulation of IH regression.[55,56] In addition to propranolol, nadolol and atenolol have been suggested as alternative systemic β-blockers for IH.[57–59] Topical timolol[4–6] (generally preferred in the 0.5% gel forming solution formulation) is an alternative for smaller, cosmetically sensitive lesions and can be used as an adjunct to systemic therapy in some cases, either to postpone initiation of systemic therapy or to speed tapering of propranolol with subsequent transition to timolol to prevent posttreatment rebound growth.

The most commonly used dosage of propranolol is 2 mg/kg/d, although some evidence suggests that infants may respond well at 1 to 1.5 mg/kg/d or require as much as 3 mg/kg/d.[3,34,60] Doses are typically divided 2 to 3 times a day to coincide with feedings. The mean duration of propranolol therapy in a meta-analysis of 41 studies of more than 1200 infants was 6.4 months,[61] but the optimal length of treatment has yet to be determined prospectively. There are reports of rebound growth of IH after stopping propranolol,[62] and it seems prudent to continue therapy until beyond the proliferative phase (9–12 months of age) to decrease the chance of this occurring. The same review found a reported rebound rate of 17%, although many early reports discussed patients who were still on therapy at the time of publication, potentially underestimating the frequency of rebound growth. Response rate in this series was 98%, although response was defined loosely as any improvement on therapy.[61] The most common adverse events were changes in sleep and acrocyanosis. Serious adverse events were rare, with 5 reports of symptomatic hypotension, 4 of hypoglycemia, and 1 of symptomatic bradycardia. A study of 50 infants hospitalized for propranolol initiation[63] showed that infants older than 6 months were more likely to have bradycardia than younger infants and that periods of bradycardia with or without hypotension do occur during dose escalation but are asymptomatic.

Consensus guidelines now exist for pretreatment workup, initiation, and monitoring during propranolol therapy. Drolet and colleagues noted that the guidelines are intentionally conservative and as experience and data mount, more evidence-based and likely less stringent guidelines will replace these. Recommendations for inpatient versus outpatient monitoring are presented in **Fig. 13**.

The most frequent non−β-blocker therapeutic intervention is wound care for ulceration.[24,64] Barrier creams with petrolatum or zinc oxide can ease pain and help to prevent contamination, especially in the diaper area, which can cause irritation and impede healing. Hydrocolloid dressings (eg, Duoderm), silver impregnated dressings (eg, AquacelAg), and petrolatum gauze can be helpful to protect and gently debride the ulcer. In the appropriate setting of odor or purulent discharge, topical or oral

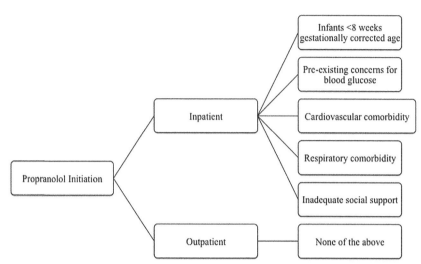

Fig. 13. Recommendations for inpatient versus outpatient initiation of propranolol. (*Data from* Drolet BA, Frommelt PC, Chamlin SL, et al. Initiation and use of propranolol for infantile hemangioma: report of a consensus conference. Pediatrics 2013;131(1):135.)

antibiotics may be necessary. Pulsed dye laser has also been used to treat ulcerated IH, although the mechanism of action is poorly understood.[65] The ability of propranolol to speed ulcer healing has been widely reported.[66–70] **Table 4** presents less frequently used therapeutics.

Table 4
Non−β-blocker treatments for IH

Therapy	Comments
OCS	Should not be forgotten as a valuable treatment option in the propranolol era. Useful as occasional adjunct with propranolol to increase speed on effect onset; aid in healing difficult ulceration; for propranolol nonresponders; for those with absolute contraindications to propranolol use
Intralesional steroids	Rarely used but still favored by some in small, but slightly bulky focal IH; should not be used periorbitally because of risk of blindness
Topical steroids	Used less given the effectiveness of timolol for small, cosmetically sensitive lesions
Pulsed dye laser	Most frequently used to treat residual telangiectasias during involution; for ulcerated IH; can be an early adjunct with propranolol if early resolution on systemic therapy
Excisional surgery	Performed during involution phase primarily, or when maximal β-blocker effect is achieved; rarely necessary during proliferative phase but may be used in exceptional circumstances (severe threat to function or pedunculated lesion)
Interferon	Rarely used given up to 20% risk of spastic diplegia; age at highest risk for spastic diplegia is younger than 12 mo
Vincristine	Rarely used given need for indwelling catheter, slow onset of effect, immunosuppression

SUMMARY

Improved insight into the natural history, associated complications, and response to propranolol has helped to advance IH research and practice. In many cases, the decision to treat is made obvious by associated complications. For most patients whose indication for therapy is risk of disfigurement, it is a fundamentally important concept to decide at which stage within the growth cycle of the IH to intervene with close monitoring, topical, systemic, adjunctive (laser or intralesional) therapy, or surgery. For most, the ideal time for intervention is the point at which the IH shows capacity for significant ongoing growth, but before significant, potentially irreversible distortion of soft tissue.

REFERENCES

1. Kilcline C, Frieden IJ. Infantile hemangiomas: how common are they? A systematic review of the medical literature. Pediatr Dermatol 2008;25(2):168–73.
2. Léauté-Labrèze C, Dumas de la Roque E, Hubiche T, et al. Propranolol for severe hemangiomas of infancy. N Engl J Med 2008;358(24):2649–51.
3. Drolet BA, Frommelt PC, Chamlin SL, et al. Initiation and use of propranolol for infantile hemangioma: report of a consensus conference. Pediatrics 2013; 131(1):128–40.
4. Chakkittakandiyil A, Phillips R, Frieden IJ, et al. Timolol maleate 0.5% or 0.1% gel-forming solution for infantile hemangiomas: a retrospective, multicenter, cohort study. Pediatr Dermatol 2012;29(1):28–31.
5. Chan H, McKay C, Adams S, et al. RCT of timolol maleate gel for superficial infantile hemangiomas in 5- to 24-week-olds. Pediatrics 2013;131(6):e1739–47.
6. Chambers CB, Katowitz WR, Katowitz JA, et al. A controlled study of topical 0.25% timolol maleate gel for the treatment of cutaneous infantile capillary hemangiomas. Ophthal Plast Reconstr Surg 2012;28(2):103–6.
7. Kanada KN, Merin MR, Munden A, et al. A prospective study of cutaneous findings in newborns in the United States: correlation with race, ethnicity, and gestational status using updated classification and nomenclature. J Pediatr 2012; 161(2):240–5.
8. Haggstrom AN, Drolet BA, Baselga E, et al. Prospective study of infantile hemangiomas: demographic, prenatal, and perinatal characteristics. J Pediatr 2007; 150(3):291–4.
9. Haggstrom AN, Drolet BA, Baselga E, et al. Prospective study of infantile hemangiomas: clinical characteristics predicting complications and treatment. Pediatrics 2006;118(3):882–7.
10. Drolet BA, Swanson EA, Frieden IJ. Infantile hemangiomas: an emerging health issue linked to an increased rate of low birth weight infants. J Pediatr 2008; 153(5):712–5, 715.e1.
11. Amir J, Metzker A, Krikler R, et al. Strawberry hemangioma in preterm infants. Pediatr Dermatol 1986;3(4):331–2.
12. Li J, Chen X, Zhao S, et al. Demographic and clinical characteristics and risk factors for infantile hemangioma: a Chinese case-control study. Arch Dermatol 2011;147(9):1049–56.
13. Bauland CG, Smit JM, Bartelink LR, et al. Hemangioma in the newborn: increased incidence after chorionic villus sampling. Prenat Diagn 2010;30(10):913–7.
14. Chen XD, Ma G, Chen H, et al. Maternal and perinatal risk factors for infantile hemangioma: a case-control study. Pediatr Dermatol 2013;30(4):457–61.

15. Grimmer JF, Williams MS, Pimentel R, et al. Familial clustering of hemangiomas. Arch Otolaryngol Head Neck Surg 2011;137(8):757–60.
16. Tollefson MM, Frieden IJ. Early growth of infantile hemangiomas: what parents' photographs tell us. Pediatrics 2012;130(2):e314–20.
17. Puttgen KB, Pearl M, Tekes A, et al. Update on pediatric extracranial vascular anomalies of the head and neck. Childs Nerv Syst 2010;26(10):1417–33.
18. Haggstrom AN, Lammer EJ, Schneider RA, et al. Patterns of infantile hemangiomas: new clues to hemangioma pathogenesis and embryonic facial development. Pediatrics 2006;117(3):698–703.
19. Waner M, North PE, Scherer KA, et al. The nonrandom distribution of facial hemangiomas. Arch Dermatol 2003;139(7):869–75.
20. Chang LC, Haggstrom AN, Drolet BA, et al. Growth characteristics of infantile hemangiomas: implications for management. Pediatrics 2008;122(2):360–7.
21. Brandling-Bennett HA, Metry DW, Baselga E, et al. Infantile hemangiomas with unusually prolonged growth phase: a case series. Arch Dermatol 2008;144(12):1632–7.
22. Haggstrom AN, Beaumont JL, Lai JS, et al. Measuring the severity of infantile hemangiomas: instrument development and reliability. Arch Dermatol 2012;148(2):197–202.
23. Holland KE, Drolet BA. Approach to the patient with an infantile hemangioma. Dermatol Clin 2013;31(2):289–301.
24. Chamlin SL, Haggstrom AN, Drolet BA, et al. Multicenter prospective study of ulcerated hemangiomas. J Pediatr 2007;151(6):684–9, 689.e1.
25. Maguiness SM, Hoffman WY, McCalmont TH, et al. Early white discoloration of infantile hemangioma: a sign of impending ulceration. Arch Dermatol 2010;146(11):1235–9.
26. Hermans DJ, Boezeman JB, Van de Kerkhof PC, et al. Differences between ulcerated and non-ulcerated hemangiomas, a retrospective study of 465 cases. Eur J Dermatol 2009;19(2):152–6.
27. Holden KR, Alexander F. Diffuse neonatal hemangiomatosis. Pediatrics 1970;46(3):411–21.
28. Glick ZR, Frieden IJ, Garzon MC, et al. Diffuse neonatal hemangiomatosis: an evidence-based review of case reports in the literature. J Am Acad Dermatol 2012;67(5):898–903.
29. Golitz LE, Rudikoff J, O'Meara OP. Diffuse neonatal hemangiomatosis. Pediatr Dermatol 1986;3(2):145–52.
30. North PE, Kahn T, Cordisco MR, et al. Multifocal lymphangioendotheliomatosis with thrombocytopenia: a newly recognized clinicopathological entity. Arch Dermatol 2004;140(5):599–606.
31. Yeung J, Somers G, Viero S, et al. Multifocal lymphangioendotheliomatosis with thrombocytopenia. J Am Acad Dermatol 2006;54(Suppl 5):S214–7.
32. Esparza EM, Deutsch G, Stanescu L, et al. Multifocal lymphangioendotheliomatosis with thrombocytopenia: phenotypic variant and course with propranolol, corticosteroids, and aminocaproic acid. J Am Acad Dermatol 2012;67(1):e62–4.
33. Christison-Lagay ER, Burrows PE, Alomari A, et al. Hepatic hemangiomas: subtype classification and development of a clinical practice algorithm and registry. J Pediatr Surg 2007;42(1):62–7 [discussion: 67–8].
34. Tan ST, Itinteang T, Leadbitter P. Low-dose propranolol for multiple hepatic and cutaneous hemangiomas with deranged liver function. Pediatrics 2011;127(3):e772–6.

35. Mazereeuw-Hautier J, Hoeger PH, Benlahrech S, et al. Efficacy of propranolol in hepatic infantile hemangiomas with diffuse neonatal hemangiomatosis. J Pediatr 2010;157(2):340–2.

36. Mhanna A, Franklin WH, Mancini AJ. Hepatic infantile hemangiomas treated with oral propranolol–a case series. Pediatr Dermatol 2011;28(1):39–45.

37. Huang SA, Tu HM, Harney JW, et al. Severe hypothyroidism caused by type 3 iodothyronine deiodinase in infantile hemangiomas. N Engl J Med 2000; 343(3):185–9.

38. Kulungowski AM, Alomari AI, Chawla A, et al. Lessons from a liver hemangioma registry: subtype classification. J Pediatr Surg 2012;47(1):165–70.

39. Frieden IJ, Reese V, Cohen D. PHACE syndrome. The association of posterior fossa brain malformations, hemangiomas, arterial anomalies, coarctation of the aorta and cardiac defects, and eye abnormalities. Arch Dermatol 1996; 132(3):307–11.

40. Nabatian AS, Milgraum SS, Hess CP, et al. PHACE without face? Infantile hemangiomas of the upper body region with minimal or absent facial hemangiomas and associated structural malformations. Pediatr Dermatol 2011;28(3):235–41.

41. Haggstrom AN, Garzon MC, Baselga E, et al. Risk for PHACE syndrome in infants with large facial hemangiomas. Pediatrics 2010;126(2):e418–26.

42. Metry DW, Haggstrom AN, Drolet BA, et al. A prospective study of PHACE syndrome in infantile hemangiomas: demographic features, clinical findings, and complications. Am J Med Genet A 2006;140(9):975–86.

43. Metry D, Heyer G, Hess C, et al. Consensus statement on diagnostic criteria for PHACE syndrome. Pediatrics 2009;124(5):1447–56.

44. Hess CP, Fullerton HJ, Metry DW, et al. Cervical and intracranial arterial anomalies in 70 patients with PHACE syndrome. AJNR Am J Neuroradiol 2010;31(10): 1980–6.

45. Heyer GL, Dowling MM, Licht DJ, et al. The cerebral vasculopathy of PHACES syndrome. Stroke 2008;39(2):308–16.

46. Siegel DH, Tefft KA, Kelly T, et al. Stroke in children with posterior fossa brain malformations, hemangiomas, arterial anomalies, coarctation of the aorta and cardiac defects, and eye abnormalities (PHACE) syndrome: a systematic review of the literature. Stroke 2012;43(6):1672–4.

47. Bayer ML, Frommelt PC, Blei F, et al. Congenital cardiac, aortic arch, and vascular bed anomalies in PHACE syndrome (from the International PHACE Syndrome Registry). Am J Cardiol 2013;112(12):1948–52.

48. Coats DK, Paysse EA, Levy ML. PHACE: a neurocutaneous syndrome with important ophthalmologic implications: case report and literature review. Ophthalmology 1999;106(9):1739–41.

49. Brandon K, Burrows P, Hess C, et al. Arteriovenous malformation: a rare manifestation of PHACE syndrome. Pediatr Dermatol 2011;28(2):180–4.

50. Stockman A, Boralevi F, Taïeb A, et al. SACRAL syndrome: spinal dysraphism, anogenital, cutaneous, renal and urologic anomalies, associated with an angioma of lumbosacral localization. Dermatology 2007;214(1):40–5.

51. Girard C, Bigorre M, Guillot B, et al. PELVIS syndrome. Arch Dermatol 2006; 142(7):884–8.

52. Iacobas I, Burrows PE, Frieden IJ, et al. LUMBAR: association between cutaneous infantile hemangiomas of the lower body and regional congenital anomalies. J Pediatr 2010;157(5):795–801.e7.

53. Gomulka J, Siegel DH, Drolet BA. Dramatic shift in the infantile hemangioma treatment paradigm at a single institution. Pediatr Dermatol 2013;30(6):751–2.

54. Zvulunov A, McCuaig C, Frieden IJ, et al. Oral propranolol therapy for infantile hemangiomas beyond the proliferation phase: a multicenter retrospective study. Pediatr Dermatol 2011;28(2):94–8.
55. Storch CH, Hoeger PH. Propranolol for infantile haemangiomas: insights into the molecular mechanisms of action. Br J Dermatol 2010;163(2):269–74.
56. Wong A, Hardy KL, Kitajewski AM, et al. Propranolol accelerates adipogenesis in hemangioma stem cells and causes apoptosis of hemangioma endothelial cells. Plast Reconstr Surg 2012;130(5):1012–21.
57. Pope E, Chakkittakandiyil A, Lara-Corrales I, et al. Expanding the therapeutic repertoire of infantile haemangiomas: cohort-blinded study of oral nadolol compared with propranolol. Br J Dermatol 2013;168(1):222–4.
58. De Graaf M, Raphael MF, Breugem CC, et al. Treatment of infantile haemangiomas with atenolol: comparison with a historical propranolol group. J Plast Reconstr Aesthet Surg 2013;66(12):1732–40.
59. Raphaël MF, de Graaf M, Breugem CC, et al. Atenolol: a promising alternative to propranolol for the treatment of hemangiomas. J Am Acad Dermatol 2011;65(2):420–1.
60. Ma X, Zhao T, Xiao Y, et al. Preliminary experience on treatment of infantile hemangioma with low-dose propranolol in China. Eur J Pediatr 2013;172(5):653–9.
61. Marqueling AL, Oza V, Frieden IJ, et al. Propranolol and infantile hemangiomas four years later: a systematic review. Pediatr Dermatol 2013;30(2):182–91.
62. Shehata N, Powell J, Dubois J, et al. Late rebound of infantile hemangioma after cessation of oral propranolol. Pediatr Dermatol 2013;30(5):587–91.
63. Puttgen KB, Summerer B, Schneider J, et al. Cardiovascular and blood glucose parameters in infants during propranolol initiation for treatment of symptomatic infantile hemangiomas. Ann Otol Rhinol Laryngol 2013;122(9):550–4.
64. Kim HJ, Colombo M, Frieden IJ. Ulcerated hemangiomas: clinical characteristics and response to therapy. J Am Acad Dermatol 2001;44(6):962–72.
65. David LR, Malek MM, Argenta LC. Efficacy of pulse dye laser therapy for the treatment of ulcerated haemangiomas: a review of 78 patients. Br J Plast Surg 2003;56(4):317–27.
66. Hermans DJ, van Beynum IM, Schultze Kool LJ, et al. Propranolol, a very promising treatment for ulceration in infantile hemangiomas: a study of 20 cases with matched historical controls. J Am Acad Dermatol 2011;64(5):833–8.
67. Hong E, Fischer G. Propranolol for recalcitrant ulcerated hemangioma of infancy. Pediatr Dermatol 2012;29(1):64–7.
68. Kim LH, Hogeling M, Wargon O, et al. Propranolol: useful therapeutic agent for the treatment of ulcerated infantile hemangiomas. J Pediatr Surg 2011;46(4):759–63.
69. Naouri M, Schill T, Maruani A, et al. Successful treatment of ulcerated haemangioma with propranolol. J Eur Acad Dermatol Venereol 2010;24(9):1109–12.
70. Saint-Jean M, Léauté-Labrèze C, Mazereeuw-Hautier J, et al. Propranolol for treatment of ulcerated infantile hemangiomas. J Am Acad Dermatol 2011;64(5):827–32.

Cutaneous Drug Reactions in the Pediatric Population

Lucero Noguera-Morel, MD, Ángela Hernández-Martín, PhD,
Antonio Torrelo, MD, PhD*

KEYWORDS

- Drug allergy • Hypersensitivity • Exanthems • Urticaria • DRESS syndrome
- Stevens-Johnson syndrome • Toxic epidermal necrolysis

KEY POINTS

- Adverse drug reactions (ADRs) frequently manifest on the skin. Cutaneous ADRs (CADRs) in children are a diagnostic challenge because CADRs can mimic many other childhood eruptions.
- Urticaria is an immediate hypersensitivity reaction, usually immunoglobulin E–mediated, predominantly manifesting as wheals.
- Maculopapular morbilliform exanthems are the most frequent form of hypersensitivity reactions in children.

OVERVIEW

Any unintended harmful reaction to a medicine or drug is known as an adverse drug reaction (ADR) according to the definition by the World Health Organization.[1,2] ADRs are classified as type A (augmented) or type B (bizarre) according to whether it is a predictable side effect related to the pharmacologic action of a drug or if it is an idiosyncratic reaction, respectively (**Fig. 1**).[3–5] There are several examples of each type of reaction, many of which manifest on the skin. Therefore, the dermatologist plays an important role in the team management of these patients. This article discusses the clinical manifestations of cutaneous ADRs (CADRs) and their pathophysiology.

In children, ADRs represent a diagnostic challenge. On the one hand, children are more susceptible than adults to drug-dosage errors because of their smaller body size[1]; on the other hand, ADRs can mimic other skin diseases of children, especially viral exanthems, frequently appearing as a maculopapular or morbilliform rash sometimes indistinguishable from a CADR.[6]

Department of Dermatology, University Hospital of the Infant Jesus, Avda. Menéndez Pelayo 65, Madrid 28009, Spain
* Corresponding author.
E-mail address: atorrelo@aedv.es

Pediatr Clin N Am 61 (2014) 403–426
http://dx.doi.org/10.1016/j.pcl.2013.12.001   **pediatric.theclinics.com**
0031-3955/14/$ – see front matter © 2014 Elsevier Inc. All rights reserved.

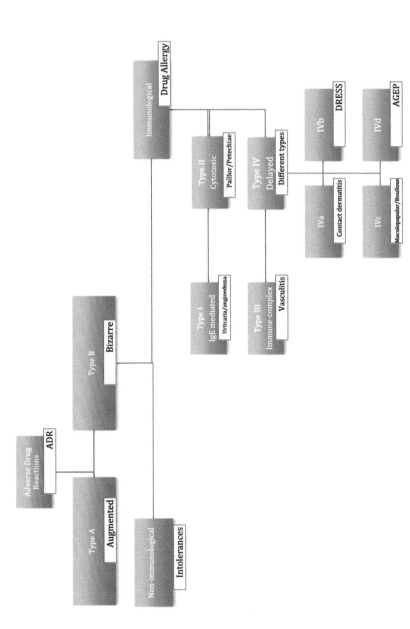

Fig. 1. Summary of adverse drug reactions according to the new concepts. DRESS, drug reactions with eosinophilia and systemic symptoms; AGEP, acute generalized exanthematic pustulosis.

PATHOPHYSIOLOGY

In ADRs of type A, a predictable side effect is related to the pharmacologic action of the drug, hence this type of reaction is considered nonimmunologic. It can be produced by overdose, cumulative or delayed toxicity, drug interactions, abnormalities in patient metabolism, or exacerbation of a preexisting disease (**Table 1**).

Alternatively, drugs can bind covalently to proteins and then induce an immune response. These reactions are different in nature and severity depending on the patient's specific metabolic pathways. An example of such variations and how they are influenced genetically is the increased incidence of induced systemic lupus

Table 1
Adverse drug reactions produced by nonimmunologic mechanisms

Nonimmunologic Factor	Mechanism	Drug Example	Manifestation on Skin
Overdose	Exaggeration of drug's pharmacologic actions		
Side effect	Undesirable or toxic effects that cannot be separated from the desired pharmacologic actions	Chemotherapeutic agents	Chemotherapeutic agents producing alopecia, mucositis
Cumulative toxicity	Prolonged exposure to a medication may lead to cumulative toxicity	Minocycline, amiodarone	Discoloration of skin
Delayed toxicity (nonimmunologic)	Dose-dependent effect that occurs months to years after the discontinuation of a medication	Arsenic	Squamous cell carcinomas and palmoplantar keratoses
Drug interactions	Interactions between 2 or more drugs administered simultaneously	Tetracycline and calcium, methotrexate and sulfonamides, cyclosporine and azoles, and methotrexate and probenecid	
Alteration in metabolism	Drugs may induce cutaneous changes by their effects on the nutritional or metabolic status of the patient	Bexarotene, isoniazid	Bexarotene may induce severe hypertriglyceridemia and eruptive xanthomas, whereas isoniazid may be associated with pellagra-like changes
Exacerbation of disease	Exacerbation of preexisting dermatologic disease	Androgen, lithium, interferon	Acne vulgaris (androgens), psoriasis (lithium and interferon)

syndrome by sulfonamide/procainamide in slow acetylators in comparison with rapid acetylators. In addition, certain human leukocyte antigen (HLA) alleles increase the risk of ADRs (see later discussion). Immunologically mediated reactions are considered drug hypersensitivity reactions, and are included as 4 types in the basic immune classification by Coombs and Gell[7] (see **Fig. 1**):

1. Type I: Cross-linked reactions with high-affinity immunoglobulin (Ig)E receptor, whereby mast cells and basophils release mediators responsible for anaphylaxis; for example, urticarial reactions.
2. Type II: IgG-mediated cytotoxic mechanisms against an antigenic component of the cell surface; for example, hemolytic anemia, thrombocytopenia.
3. Type III: Circulating immune complexes lead to endothelial damage and complement activation, and usually manifest as vasculitis, which can be seen on the skin.
4. Type IV: All delayed hypersensitivity reactions are included in this category, subclassified as[8]:
   a. IVa: Mediators such as interferon (IFN)-γ and tumor necrosis factor α (from T-helper 1 cells) produce macrophage activation and immune response; for example, contact dermatitis, tuberculin reactions.
   b. IVb: Certain cytokines (interleukin [IL]-5, IL-4, IL-13) interact with eosinophils, which become the main cells involved; clinical manifestations include maculopapular exanthems with eosinophilia (drug reactions with eosinophilia and systemic symptoms [DRESS syndrome]).
   c. IVc: Perforins, granzyme-B, and Fas ligand are incriminated, activating cytotoxic T cells, natural killer (NK)/T cells, and NK cells clinically manifesting as contact dermatitis, maculopapular rash, and Stevens-Johnson syndrome (SJS)/toxic epidermal necrosis (TEN) exhanthems.[9] In bullous exanthems there is a higher percentage of perforin-positive CD8$^+$ killer T cells in the epidermis and dermis.[10]
   d. IVd: CxCL8 and granulocyte macrophage colony-stimulating factor induce neutrophil activation, and can manifest on the skin as acute generalized exanthematic pustulosis (AGEP).

According to several studies, the most frequent cause of ADRs is antibiotics, including β-lactams and macrolides, followed by nonsteroidal anti-inflammatory drugs (NSAIDs) and barbiturates/antiepileptic drugs.[11] A genetic predisposition has been demonstrated to exist in many of these reactions; for example, abacavir hypersensitivity is linked to HLA-B*5701. The pharmacogenetics of these reactions is currently being investigated, with promising results in the screening of patients before the administration of medications with high risk for severe ADRs (**Box 1**).[12]

EPIDEMIOLOGY

CADRs represent a major pediatric health problem frequently encountered in clinical practice.[3] However, few epidemiologic studies have addressed the incidence of common, non–life-threatening CADRs, including reactions of both delayed and immediate hypersensitivity, such as maculopapular exanthem, fixed drug eruption, or urticaria.[13] CADRs represent 35% to 36% of any ADRs in children, only being surpassed by gastrointestinal symptoms (39%). In 2000, Menniti-Ippolito and colleagues[14] performed an active monitoring system of ADRs in children through a network of family pediatricians; more than 24,000 patients were recruited, and the reported incidence of ADRs was 15.1 per 1000 children.[6,14]

| Box 1 |
| Drugs frequently related to cutaneous adverse drug reactions |

Antibiotics

  Penicillins

  Cephalosporins

  Carbapenems

  Fluoroquinolones

  Macrolides

  Sulfonamides

  β-Lactam inhibitors

  Glycopeptides

Nonsteroidal anti-inflammatories

  Metamizole sodium

  Diclofenac

  Acetylsalicylic acid

  Ibuprofen

Anticonvulsants

  Carbamazepine

  Lamotrigine

  Phenobarbital

Antifungals

  Clotrimazole

  Terbinafine

Data from Heinzerling LM, Tomsitz D, Anliker MD. Is drug allergy less prevalent than previously assumed? A 5-year analysis. Br J Dermatol 2012;166(1):107–14.

It is of great importance that parents often report drug hypersensitivity events in their children that are not confirmed by diagnostic tests. In a study by Rebelo Gomes and colleagues,[15] 94% of patients diagnosed with hypersensitivity reactions were actually able to tolerate the initially suspected drug. The authors believe that it is important to confirm and document any self-reported drug reaction. Identification of the harmful drug can limit potentially life-threatening reexposure and will also prevent avoidance of innocent drugs that can be life-saving.

PROGNOSIS

The spectrum of drugs causing CADRs differs substantially when the various clinical conditions are considered.[13] Most ADRs with cutaneous involvement are mild, and resolve on withdrawal of the causative drug. The most common forms of CADRs are maculopapular exanthems and urticarial reactions, both of which have excellent outcomes. Less frequent, but more severe reactions may have a risk of mortality, estimated at 10% for DRESS syndrome, 1% to 5% for SJS, 25% to 35% for TEN,[16] and less than 5% for acute generalized exanthematic pustulosis.[17]

CLINICAL FEATURES
Urticaria

Urticaria is a common disorder in children and adults, usually caused by IgE-mediated or direct degranulation of mast cells in response to antigens, drugs, chemical compounds, or proteases.[18] In children the main cause of urticaria is infection, although when antibiotics or other drugs have been administered, it is difficult to determine whether drugs play a role because of the time line. Drug-induced urticaria can appear within the first 2 weeks after starting a drug. β-Lactam antimicrobials, sulfonamides, and NSAIDs are the most common reported causes.[19] NSAIDs can produce urticarial reactions resulting from both immunologic and nonimmunologic intolerance, the latter attributable to enhanced synthesis of leukotrienes.[20] Characteristically, nonimmunologic urticarial reactions are usually retarded, starting 24 hours after drug intake, unlike type I immunologic reactions that are usually immediate.

Acute urticaria is manifested by wheals or hives (**Fig. 2**) that appear as pruritic erythematous or pale-pink edematous patches, which coalesce into plaques of varying size. Individual lesions last less than 24 to 36 hours but reappear in subsequent attacks with asymmetric distribution. The condition is self-limiting and can last up to 6 weeks, resolving without residual signs. There are some particularities of urticaria in children; pruritus is an inconstant symptom and angioedema is relatively frequent. Annular or polycyclic giant lesions are not uncommon in infants.[21] The wheals can evolve into purpuric macules because of capillary fragility (**Fig. 3**). Usually children with urticaria have a good general status.[22] Angioedema describes large subcutaneous swellings of the eyelids, hands and feet, genitalia, or even mucous membranes; it can co-occur with urticaria or appear isolated.[23]

These types of reactions are mild and, in general, non–life-threatening, but cause discomfort and parent anxiety.[24] Anaphylaxis, also a type I hypersensitivity reaction, is a life-threatening condition that may follow a course with urticarial lesions plus systemic symptoms including weakness, dyspnea, hypotension, abdominal pain, diarrhea, vomiting, and circulatory collapse.[23] It often occurs after ingestion of food, but

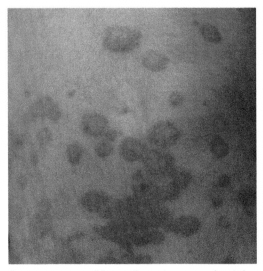

Fig. 2. Typical wheals appear as pruritic, erythematous or pale pink, edematous patches, which coalesce into plaques of varying size.

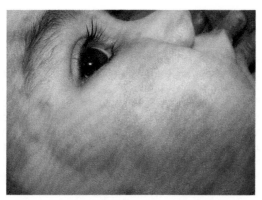

Fig. 3. Wheals or hives can look like annular or polycyclic lesions in infants.

can also be drug related. Although incidence varies according to different reports, approximately 9% of the cases of drug-induced anaphylaxis occur in children younger than 18 years.[25] There have been reports of anaphylaxis following immunizations, although this remains a rare adverse event. No cases were related to vaccines given as part of the routine infant and preschool immunization program, despite more than 5.5 million vaccines being delivered per year.[26]

Treatment consists of withdrawal of the causative drug and antihistamines to control pruritus. A short course of oral steroids can be used to control symptoms in refractory cases. Anaphylaxis treatment goes beyond the aims of this article, and consists of rapid administration of epinephrine and life-support therapy.

Serum Sickness–Like Reactions

Serum sickness–like reaction (SSLR) is considered a drug reaction characterized by the triad of rash, arthralgia, and fever, without evidence of cutaneous or systemic vasculitis. It may occur within the first 3 weeks after a drug is started. Its pathophysiology is not well known and is not thought to be a type III hypersensitivity reaction.[27] Historically cefaclor was frequently associated with SSLR, with an estimated frequency of 1% to 2% of all children who received cefaclor. Despite a decline in the use of cefaclor, SSLR continues to occur in the pediatric population in association with a variety of antibiotic agents such as penicillins, tetracyclines, cefprozil, sulfonamides, macrolides, griseofulvin, and itraconazol.[23,28]

SSLR produces a rash that can be urticarial, or may take the form of polycyclic hives with central clearing that may appear ecchymotic or morbilliform. In contrast to true urticaria, lesions are fixed and do not fade within 24 to 36 hours.[29] Accompanying symptoms are frequent, including malaise, fever, lymphadenopathy, splenomegaly, proteinuria, and arthralgia.[23] Differential diagnosis with these symptoms must be made with DRESS syndrome, which usually manifests also with facial edema and eosinophilia. The biopsy of SSLR shows edema on the dermis, with superficial perivascular urticarial lymphocytic infiltrate and no evidence of vasculitis.[27]

The rash usually resolves between 1 and 6 weeks after the causative drug is withdrawn, and the treatment is symptomatic, with antihistamines to control pruritus and NSAIDs to relieve pain and fever.

Maculopapular Exanthems

Maculopapular exanthems are the most common type of drug-induced eruption, usually beginning 7 to 14 days after initiation of medication in nonsensitized patients. If a patient has been previously sensitized, the first signs of this CADR on the skin can appear as soon as 6 to 12 hours after drug intake.[6,30] Drugs frequently associated with this condition include penicillins, sulfonamides, cephalosporins, and antiepileptic medications. This type of reaction is more frequent in the presence of viral infections, especially acute Epstein-Barr virus (EBV) infections, although its incidence in well-designed studies may be no higher than 33%,[31] much lower than the previously reported 90% to 100%.[23] Clinically the eruption starts on the trunk and progresses to the face and extremities, producing diffuse erythroderma in some cases. The maculopapular exanthem is usually morbilliform (**Fig. 4**). Signs of alarm such, as mucous membrane involvement or the Nikolsky sign, do not occur. Palms and soles may be mildly affected, and other symptoms may include low-grade fever and pruritus. The evolution to resolution usually takes about 2 weeks, with the exanthem turning brownish-red and resolving with desquamation.

The pathophysiology is thought to be a T-cell–mediated hypersensitivity reaction, type IVc according to the modified Coombs and Gell classification (see earlier discussion).[3]

Differential diagnoses include viral infections, mostly indistinguishable from CADRs and very frequent in children (EBV, human herpesvirus 6, adenovirus), bacterial infections (*Streptococcus pyogenes*), systemic juvenile arthritis (Still disease), Kawasaki syndrome, graft-versus-host disease in hematopoietic stem cell transplant recipients, and erythema multiforme.[32]

Most of these skin reactions are not severe or life-threatening,[30] and thus need only symptomatic treatment. If the rash is mild and the drug cannot be discontinued, it can be kept under strict monitoring. It is important to remark here that maculopapular exanthems do not progress to severe CADR, but sometimes these severe reactions may resemble at onset an innocent exanthem or a morbilliform maculopapular eruption. Assessing the likelihood of a severe CADR can be very challenging at the beginning, and the caring physician should be alert for alarm signs, such as mucous membrane lesions, bullae, Nikolsky sign, facial edema, or fever.

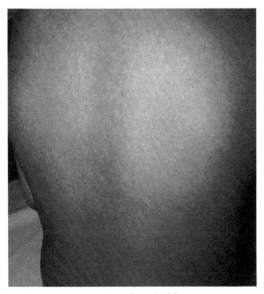

Fig. 4. Macules and erythematous papules of morbilliform appearance.

DRUG REACTION WITH EOSINOPHILIA AND SYSTEMIC SYMPTOMS

DRESS syndrome is a potentially life-threatening severe ADR, with a potential 10% mortality rate.[33] Its exact mechanism of production remains unknown. A type IVb hypersensitivity reaction[8] has been proposed, but reactivation of viral infections, particularly herpesvirus 6, has also been shown to play a role.[34] It is also well determined that individuals with specific HLA haplotypes are predisposed to develop DRESS syndrome when exposed to certain medications.[35]

The European Registry of Severe Cutaneous Adverse Reaction study group (RegiSCAR), a multinational registry of severe CADR, found that antiepileptic drugs, especially carbamazepine but also lamotrigine, phenobarbital, phenytoin, valproic acid, and zonisamide, were involved in 35% of the cases, allopurinol in 18%, antimicrobial sulfonamides and dapsone in 12%, and other antibiotics in 11%. The median time interval after drug intake was 22 days for all drugs with very probable causality, with differences existing between drugs.[36]

DRESS usually starts with unspecific prodromal symptoms such as asthenia, pruritus, and fever. Unexplained fever of 38° to 40°C can precede by several weeks the cutaneous rash, which usually appears as a widespread, unspecific maculopapular morbilliform exanthem. The rash is present in 95% of patients,[36] starting on the face and upper trunk, then expanding quickly downward and developing a violaceous hue. Intense facial edema is seen in 25% of patients (**Fig. 5**).[33]

Systemic involvement includes lymph node enlargement, hematologic abnormalities with eosinophilia or atypical lymphocytes, and multiple internal organ dysfunction.[37] The liver is the most frequently affected organ, but renal failure, pulmonary impaired function, pneumonitis, heart failure secondary to myocarditis, neurologic symptoms manifesting as meningitis or encephalitis, gastroenteritis, and thyroid or pancreatic dysfunction can also occur.[33,38]

Skin histopathology shows a perivascular lymphocytic infiltrate in the papillary dermis, with eosinophils, atypical lymphocytes, and spongiosis.

Diagnosis is based on proposed diagnostic criteria by RegiSCAR or the Japanese Research Committee on Severe Cutaneous Adverse Reaction (J-SCAR) (**Boxes 2 and 3**).[39]

Vesiculobullous Eruptions (SJS and TEN)

TEN and SJS are severe adverse mucocutaneous drug reactions producing epidermal and mucosal detachment. These reactions are considered a continuum of the same disease. There are approximately 1 or 2 cases of SJS/TEN per 1,000,000 individuals annually, and it is considered a medical emergency as it is potentially fatal.

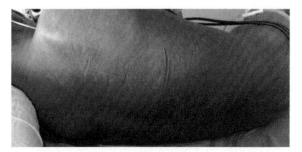

Fig. 5. Generalized, violaceous maculopapular exanthem in a patient with DRESS syndrome.

Box 2
Diagnostic criteria for DRESS established by the J-SCAR group

1. Maculopapular rash developing >3 weeks after starting with a limited number of drugs

2. Prolonged clinical symptoms 2 weeks after discontinuation of the causative drug

3. Fever (>38°C)

4. Liver abnormalities[a] (alanine aminotransferase >100 U/L)

5. Leukocyte abnormalities (at least 1 present)

    a. Leukocytosis (>11 × 10^9/L)

    b. Atypical lymphocytosis (>5%)

    c. Eosinophilia (>1.5 × 10^9/L)

6. Lymphadenopathy

7. Human herpesvirus–6 reactivation

For correct "typical" diagnosis, all 7 criteria must be met; for atypical hypersensitivity syndrome the presence of criteria 1 to 5 is necessary.
  [a] This can be replaced by other organ involvement such as renal involvement.

The main causes of SJS/TEN are drugs, but some infections such as *Mycoplasma pneumoniae* and herpes simplex virus are well documented.[9] In children, the most common causative drugs are antibiotics (sulfonamides, penicillins, cephalosporins, and macrolides), followed by antiepileptics (phenobarbital, valproic acid, lamotrigine, carbamazepine), benzodiazepines, NSAIDs (salicylates, acetaminophen, and others), and more rarely corticosteroids, antihistamines H1, mucolytic agents, vitamins, or even vaccines.[40]

There is a strong genetic association between HLA and a specific drug-induced SJS/TEN.[41] There have been some studies suggesting that HLA testing before starting therapy would be effective to identify individuals at risk of hypersensitivity (**Fig. 6, Table 2**).[42]

Box 3
Diagnostic criteria for DRESS proposed by the RegiSCAR

1. Acute rash

2. Reaction suspected drug related

3. Hospitalization

4. Fever (>38°C)

5. Laboratory abnormalities (at least 1 present)

    a. Lymphocytes above or below normal

    b. Low platelets

    c. Eosinophilia

6. Involvement or >1 internal organ

7. Enlarged lymph nodes >2 sites

The first 3 criteria are necessary for diagnosis, and the presence of 3 out of the other 4.

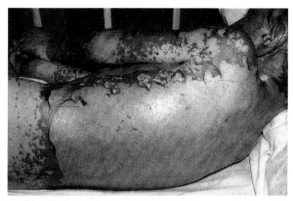

Fig. 6. Epidermal detachment presenting as blisters and areas of denuded skin. The extension of skin detachment determines the diagnosis of Stevens-Johnson syndrome or toxic epidermal necrosis.

Clinical manifestations at the beginning can be unspecific. Patients can manifest fever, discomfort, stinging in the eyes, and difficulty swallowing. A few days later, erythema and purpuric annular macules may appear on the trunk and face, followed by mucocutaneous tenderness with hemorrhagic erosions and epidermal detachment presenting as blisters and areas of denuded skin. The extension of skin detachment determines the diagnosis; if skin detachment affects less than 10% of the body surface area (BSA), a diagnosis of SJS is made; if more than 30% BSA, TEN is diagnosed; and if between 10% and 30% BSA is involved, SJS/TEN overlap is considered.

Diagnosis is mainly clinical. The epidermal detachment can be revealed by exerting a tangential mechanical pressure on the erythematous zones (Nikolsky sign), although it should be noted that this sign is positive in other bullous disorders.[16] The histologic analysis of a skin biopsy shows full-thickness epidermal necrosis and detachment caused by extensive keratinocyte apoptosis.

Management of patients with SJS/TEN requires rapid diagnosis and evaluation of the prognosis using the scoring system (SCORTEN) based on independent clinical

Table 2
Genetic associations between human leukocyte antigens (HLA) and a specific drug-induced Stevens-Johnson syndrome/toxic epidermal necrosis

Population	HLA	Drug/Medication
Asian	HLA-B*1511 HLA-B*1518	Carbamazepine
European	HLA-B*73 HLA-B*12 HLA-A*2	Oxicam
	HLA-B*12 HLA-A*29 HLA DR7	Sulfamethoxazole
Asian and European	HLA-B*5801	Allopurinol
	HLA-B*1502	Carbamazepine/lamotrigine/ oxcarbazepine/phenytoin
	HLA-B*3101	Carbamazepine

and laboratory variables within 24 hours of admission and at day 3; these variables include age, malignancy, BSA detached, tachycardia, and serum glucose, bicarbonate, and urea.[43] Treatment implies the identification and interruption of the suspected causative drug. Patients with suspicion of SJS/TEN should be referred to a burns unit or pediatric intensive care unit with expertise in caring for such patients within 7 days of diagnosis. It is important to bear in mind that the different countries and centers may have different protocols for management, with which physicians should be familiar. This knowledge has been shown to dramatically decrease the mortality rate. Prophylactic antibiotics are not routinely advised.[44] Wound care is important, but no specific approach has been shown to significantly modify survival rates or reepithelialization of the skin. Surgical debridement with nonadherent silver-impregnated gauze[45] and biosynthetic skin substitutes such as Biobrane have been used with success.[46] An eminently feasible way of managing the skin in these patients is antishear wound care, which consists of puncturing bullae with a sterile needle and leaving the skin on top to act as a biological dressing; this provides an effective alternative approach to wound care with equivalent success.[47] Intravenous Ig (IVIg), cyclosporin, corticosteroids, and even biological therapies have been used, with varying rates of success. More than 50% of patients surviving TEN suffer from long-term sequelae of the disease,[16] mostly ocular complications including dry eyes, trichiasis, symblepharon, distichiasis, visual loss, and corneal ulceration. It should be noted that the diagnosis of TEN does not imply a more severe ocular involvement than SJS, and an appropriate intervention during acute ocular disease is key to preventing late complications (see **Fig. 6**).[48]

Acute Generalized Exanthematous Pustulosis

AGEP is a serious cutaneous reaction, considered to be a type IVd hypersensitivity reaction.[4] Its incidence is about 1 to 5 cases per million inhabitants per year. It has been rarely described in children and is usually related to infections, both viral (parvovirus B19, Coxsackie, cytomegalovirus) and bacterial (*Chlamydia pneumoniae, M pneumoniae*), or even vaccinations.[6] When drugs are involved, penicillins, cefixime, clindamycin, vancomycin, and macrolides are the most common agents.[49]

AGEP presents as an acute onset of asymptomatic or mildly pruritic erythema with hundreds of superimposed sterile, nonfollicular pustules, smaller than 5 mm in diameter. Fever and asthenia are often associated. In very rare cases, children may present with overlapping features of other ADRs such as DRESS (with facial edema) or SJS/TEN (some epidermal detachment) (**Fig. 7**).[6]

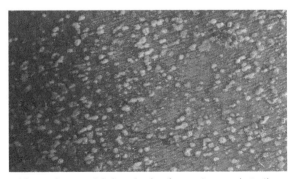

Fig. 7. Mildly pruritic erythema with hundreds of superimposed sterile, nonfollicular pustules, smaller than 5 mm, in a patient with AGEP.

Typical histologic findings include subcorneal pustules with neutrophils, along with marked dermal edema, and perivascular infiltrates with occasional neutrophils. Eosinophils in the superficial dermis and focal necrosis of keratinocytes can also be seen.[50]

Differential diagnosis must be made with pustular psoriasis, DRESS syndrome with pustules, and subcorneal pustular dermatosis (Sneddon-Wilkinson disease).

Withdrawal of the offending factor is the main therapy, with expected spontaneous resolution in 1 to 2 weeks, with a pattern of punctate scaling. Scarring is absent or limited. Antihistamines can be used for pruritus, and a short course of oral corticosteroids may be helpful.[51]

Miscellaneous

Fixed drug eruption

Fixed drug eruption is a drug reaction presenting clinically as a localized, circumscribed, round to oval erythematous or violaceous patch, sometimes with vesicles and blisters.[52] Its main characteristic is that it recurs in the same site each time a particular drug is administered.[53] It may be very difficult to determine the causative drug because most parents often think that trivial over-the-counter medications are harmless,[1] and do not relate the medication with the episode. The pathogenesis is not clear, but cytotoxic memory CD8 cells in the epidermis may play a major role by releasing proinflammatory cytokines on stimulation by drug intake.[54] The most common drugs implicated in fixed drug eruption are antibiotics, especially trimethoprim-sulfamethoxazole, NSAIDs, and paracetamol.[55,56]

The clinical presentation is a single patch or multiple ones with erythema and edema accompanied by pruritus or pain on the lesion. The patch usually turns dusky or violaceous, and resolves after the discontinuation of the medication involved, leaving residual hyperpigmentation. Some lesions may contain vesicles or large bullae. The diagnostic hallmark is the recurrence at previously affected sites.[53] Lesions first occur within 2 weeks of original ingestion of the medication, but subsequent intakes lead to much more rapid reappearance (**Fig. 8**).[57]

Acneiform eruptions

These eruptions are types of pustular reactions in acne-prone areas. The key medications producing this type of reaction are the corticosteroids, with a risk directly proportional to the dose and duration of therapy. It can also be elicited after intake of androgens, lithium, iodides, phenytoin, and isoniazid.[57] New drugs used for the treatment of solid tumors, such as the inhibitors of epidermal growth factor receptor (EGFR/HER1) cetuximab, erlotinib, and panitumumab, are therapeutic agents with a high incidence of acneiform eruptions.[58]

Typical lesions are follicular papules and sterile pustules in acne-prone sites with no mucosal changes. In contrast to acne vulgaris, the acneiform reactions can also appear in atypical areas for acne, such as the arms and legs. The lesions are characteristically monomorphous and heal without scarring.[51]

Benzoyl peroxide preparations with topical or oral antibiotics, as well as topical tretinoin cream can be helpful, but in such cases it will be necessary to withdraw the medication.

Others

Other less frequent or milder drug reactions that may involve the skin of children include drug-induced lupus, lichenoid drug reactions, psoriasiform reactions, vasculitis, bullous pemphigoid, linear IgA bullous dermatosis (LABD), pseudoporphyria, dyschromatosis, nail abnormalities, gingival enlargement, phototoxic and photoallergic reactions, cutaneous lymphoid hyperplasia (pseudolymphoma), warfarin-induced

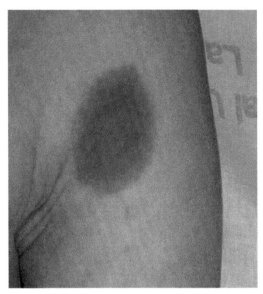

Fig. 8. Fixed drug eruption can be seen as an erythematous round or oval patch that usually turns dusky or violaceous.

necrosis (WIN), and heparin-induced necrosis (HIN), among others.[58,59] WIN or HIN are easily recognized because of necrosis in acral or fat-rich areas such as the abdomen in patients receiving these medications; erythema occurs, followed by purpura and necrosis. WIN is due to protein C deficiency, and patients affected by HIN have heparin antibodies with or without thrombocytopenia.[60,61]

LABD deserves special mention because of the singularity of its clinical presentation. It has been reported that almost two-thirds of LABD cases may be drug induced, but this is rare in children, in whom LABD behaves as an idiopathic autoimmune blistering disease. Commonly implicated medications include antibiotics (frequently vancomycin), NSAIDs, and diuretics.[62] The clinical picture consists in the acute development of vesicles and bullae often on sites of noninflamed skin. Frequently new blisters form at the periphery of the resolving lesions forming rosette-like plaques, widely distributed on the face, trunk, and extremities, especially around the genitals and perioral areas.[63] The prognosis is excellent, with rapid resolution following cessation of the offending drug; there have been some reports of high morbidity because of pruritus.[62]

Children with malignancy are very much exposed to drugs and are at risk of skin reactions. Such reactions can include mild and well-known reactions such as anagen effluvium, mucositis, and skin pigmentation changes,[64] or be truly life-threatening, such as severe and generalized acneiform reactions (**Fig. 9**), DRESS, SJS/TEN, or AGEP.

DIFFERENTIAL DIAGNOSIS

Assigning a cutaneous reaction to a particular drug can be very difficult, because many patients with skin conditions such as viral exanthems or Kawasaki disease may have received oral medications before their rash has appeared.[65] When examining a child with a suspected CADR, personal history (allergies or previous diseases), and history of recent medications and their doses should be recorded. Assessment of

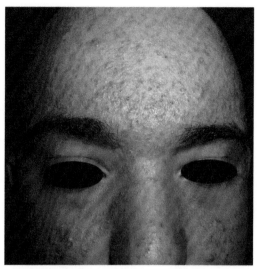

Fig. 9. Generalized acne-like reaction in an adolescent with malignant recurrent glioma receiving adjuvant chemotherapy with bevacizumab and steroids.

the general status is also very important. The chronology of onset and evolution of the skin lesions allows an estimation of the type of hypersensitivity reaction and the causative drug.[30]

The authors suggest an approach based on the type of skin lesions: wheals, macules and papules, pustules, and vesicles and bullae. Wheals indicate an urticarial rash, and thus common urticarial reactions and SSLRs are likely. The presence of fever, arthralgia, and asthenia suggest an SSLR. Mucous involvement with angioedema and anaphylaxis are the most harmful complications in this group.

If the rash is maculopapular, an incipient vesiculobullous disease and mucosal involvement must be ruled out. Mucosal involvement or minimal epidermal detachment might indicate severe CADR such as SJS/TEN. If a true maculopapular reaction is observed, a common morbilliform rash must be differentiated from DRESS syndrome. The presence of fever, lymphadenopathy, and liver or spleen enlargement suggest the latter.

If the Nikolsky sign is positive or there are vesicles or bullae or mucous membrane involvement, a bullous exanthem is considered, and SJS/TEN is strongly suggested. The presence of pustules over a diffuse erythema should lead one to consider AGEP **(Fig. 10)**.

DIAGNOSTIC RECOMMENDATIONS
Laboratory Studies

Because many ADRs are systemic hypersensitivity reactions involving not only the skin, a thorough investigation is mandatory to rule out internal organ involvement **(Fig. 11)**.[30] This evaluation can be done in the emergency room fairly quickly, with a complete blood count panel, basic serum chemistry for renal and liver function, and urinalysis. Radiology tests are not usually necessary unless a severe ADR is suspected. For example, if DRESS syndrome is suspected, a chest radiograph or computed tomography scan is mandatory to search for interstitial pneumonitis or pleural effusion.[66]

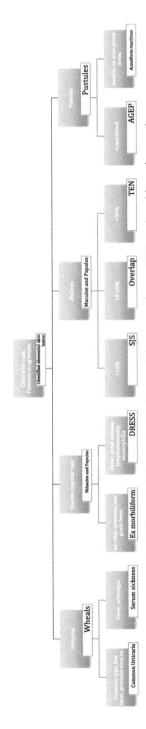

Fig. 10. Initial approach with simplified differential diagnosis. SJS, Stevens-Johnson syndrome; TEN, toxic epidermal necrosis.

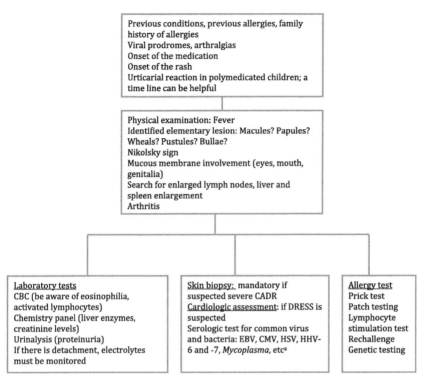

Fig. 11. Approach to the patient with suspected drug reaction. [a] It is important that a positive serologic test does not exclude the diagnosis of a CADR, because some of these reactions may occur in the context of a viral infection or reactivation (eg, DRESS with HHV-6 or maculopapular exanthema with EBV, and antibiotics). CBC, complete blood count; CMV, cytomegalovirus; EBV, Epstein-Barr virus; HHV, human herpesvirus; HSV, herpes simplex virus.

Skin biopsy can be helpful, but is not indicated in all cases. In urticarial reactions and maculopapular exanthems biopsies are often unspecific and unhelpful, and are not routinely recommended. If DRESS syndrome, SJS/TEN, or AGEP is suspected, a skin biopsy must be performed immediately.

Identifying the suspected causative drug is important in avoiding reexposure. After complete recovery and within an interval of 6 weeks to 6 months, diagnostic procedures can be undertaken. Allergy evaluation with skin prick and intracutaneous testing is indicated for immediate reactions. Patch testing for delayed reactions and, in special cases, the lymphocytic transformation test (LTT), usually performed by an immunologist or allergist, can help identify causes of severe reactions. The LTT attempts to quantify T-cell activation in response to a drug. Unfortunately this test cannot be routinely recommended because it is not yet standardized,[67] although it has been shown to be a reliable test when performed at the appropriate time depending on the type of drug reaction. A lymphocyte transformation test should be performed within 1 week after the onset of rashes in patients with maculopapular exanthems and SJS/TEN, and after 5 to 8 weeks in patients with DRESS.[68] Finally, challenging with drug reexposure should be carefully considered and conducted by an allergist. It is important that this is not indicated in cases of DRESS or SJS/TEN because of the greater severity of the recurring reaction.[65]

Although all the data found in recent studies about HLA testing and specific drug reactions need further investigation and clinical correlation before general genetic testing can be recommended, it is thought that this approach will lead to improved prevention of severe ADRs and a more personalized medicine. The Food and Drug Administration recently approved the recommendation of genetic testing before starting abacavir (HLA B*5701) and carbamazepine (HLA B*1502 in patients with Asian ancestry) before starting therapy.[69]

THERAPEUTIC RECOMMENDATIONS
Nonpharmacologic Treatment

The main goal of treatment is to discontinue the suspected drug, although this is not always possible. If a patient is on several medications, it may be difficult to identify exactly which is the causative drug. In such cases one might opt for sequential withdrawal considering the type of reaction, the temporal relation, and the frequency with which the drug has been associated with the patient's cutaneous reaction, always keeping in mind that the patient should be monitored closely.

Pharmacologic Treatment

Treatment varies according to the type of reaction and its severity. Urticarial reactions and mild cases of maculopapular morbilliform exanthems can be managed only symptomatically with antihistamines, but if the rash is very symptomatic, topical corticosteroids can help to reduce skin inflammation and pruritus. When the reaction is moderate to severe, systemic corticosteroids can be helpful, usually 1 mg/kg/d until resolution with careful tapering.[22] For severe CADRs, because they are rare and there are no available randomized controlled trials, the management is based on cohort series and case reports. AGEP can also be manage empirically with corticosteroids.[3]

For DRESS syndrome the treatment of choice depends on the severity and response to the withdrawal of the suspected drug. Oral steroids at 1 mg/kg/d, intravenous methylprednisolone bolus at 30 mg/kg/d, and corticosteroid-sparing agents such as IVIg, plasmapheresis, cyclophosphamide, and cyclosporine have all been used, with variable results.[70–72]

No clear therapeutic guidelines regarding the use of medications for the treatment of SJS/TEN in children exist.[73] Undoubtedly, appropriate skin and mucosal care along with life support are essential. Patients should be transferred to the pediatric intensive care unit. Systemic corticosteroids, plasmapheresis, IVIg, and immunosuppressive agents have been reported to be effective, with no evidence favoring any of them in particular.[74] The use of cyclosporin based on the capability of calcineurin inhibitors to rapidly block the functions of cytotoxic T cells has been advocated.[75]

CADRs in children on chemotherapy for cancer may pose important problems, because suspected drugs may be life-saving and cannot be withdrawn. The goal in these cases is to keep the patient comfortable and treat the CADR while maintaining the medication, unless a severe or even fatal reaction occurs. For example, acneiform drug reactions attributable to EGFR inhibitors can be treated with oral corticosteroids and topical and oral retinoids, or can be prevented with oral doxycycline or minocycline before and during treatment.[58]

SUMMARY

- ADRs frequently manifest on the skin. CADRs in children are a diagnostic challenge because these reactions can mimic many other childhood eruptions.

- Urticaria is an immediate hypersensitivity reaction, usually IgE mediated, predominantly manifesting as wheals.
- Maculopapular morbilliform exanthems are the most frequent form of hypersensitivity reactions in children.
- DRESS syndrome is a systemic and potentially fatal CADR manifesting as fever, rash, lymph node enlargement, eosinophilia, and multiorgan dysfunction.
- SJS and TEN are severe CADRs characterized mainly by mucous and cutaneous necrosis with epidermal detachment.
- Fixed drug eruption is a curious drug reaction presenting clinically as a circumscribed, erythematoviolaceous, round to oval plaque, recurring in the same place after drug reexposure.
- AGEP is a severe CADR characterized by erythroderma and numerous small, sterile, nonfollicular pustules.
- New and old chemotherapeutic agents continue to have a high incidence in CADRs.
- Diagnostic testing after resolution should be aimed at identifying the causative drug so as to prevent morbidity and mortality associated with reexposure.
- A high index of suspicion should be maintained to make a rapid diagnosis and in managing children with severe CADRs.

ACKNOWLEDGMENTS

I am very grateful to Drs P. Herranz and R. deLucas for their contribution of interesting cases (**Figs. 5**, **8** and **9**) for this article.

REFERENCES

1. Koren G. Protecting young children from life-threatening drug toxicity. J Pediatr 2013;163(5):1249–50. Available at: http://www.ncbi.nlm.nih.gov/pubmed/23809045. Accessed August 11, 2013.
2. WHO Media centre. Medicines: safety of medicines—adverse drug reactions. Fact sheet. 2008 (October).
3. Ott H. Hypersensitivity reactions to drugs. In: Irvine AD, Hoeger PH, Yan AC, editors. Harper's textbook of pediatric dermatology. 3rd edition. Blackwell Publishing Ltd; 2011. p. 2816.
4. Posadas SJ, Pichler WJ. Delayed drug hypersensitivity reactions—new concepts. Clin Exp Allergy 2007;37(7):989–99. Available at: http://www.ncbi.nlm.nih.gov/pubmed/17581192. Accessed August 11, 2013.
5. Pichler WJ, Adam J, Daubner B, et al. Drug hypersensitivity reactions: pathomechanism and clinical symptoms. Med Clin North Am 2010;94(4):645–64 xv. Available at: http://www.ncbi.nlm.nih.gov/pubmed/20609855. Accessed August 11, 2013.
6. Heelan K, Shear NH. Cutaneous drug reactions in children: an update. Paediatr Drugs 2013;15(6):493–503. Available at: http://www.ncbi.nlm.nih.gov/pubmed/23842849. Accessed August 11, 2013.
7. Coombs P, Gell P. Classification of allergic reactions responsible for clinical hypersensitivity and disease. In: Gell P, editor. Clinical aspects of immunology. Oxford (United kingdom): Oxford University Press; 1968. p. 575–96.
8. Lerch M, Pichler WJ. The immunological and clinical spectrum of delayed drug-induced exanthems. Curr Opin Allergy Clin Immunol 2004;4(5):411–9. Available at: http://www.ncbi.nlm.nih.gov/pubmed/15349041.
9. Lee HY, Chung WH. Toxic epidermal necrolysis: the year in review. Curr Opin Allergy Clin Immunol 2013;13(4):330–6. Available at: http://www.ncbi.nlm.nih.gov/pubmed/23799330. Accessed August 11, 2013.

10. Yawalkar N. Drug-induced exanthems. Toxicology 2005;209(2):131–4. Available at: http://www.ncbi.nlm.nih.gov/pubmed/15767025. Accessed November 1, 2013.

11. Khaled A, Kharfi M, Ben Hamida M, et al. Cutaneous adverse drug reactions in children. A series of 90 cases. Tunis Med 2012;90(1):45–50. Available at: http://www.ncbi.nlm.nih.gov/pubmed/22311448. Accessed August 25, 2013.

12. Pirmohamed M. Genetics and the potential for predictive tests in adverse drug reactions. Chem Immunol Allergy 2012;97:18–31.

13. Mockenhaupt M. Epidemiology of cutaneous adverse drug reactions. Chem Immunol Allergy 2012;97:1–17. Available at: http://www.ncbi.nlm.nih.gov/pubmed/22613850. Accessed August 24, 2013.

14. Menniti-Ippolito G, Raschetti R, Da Cas R, et al. Active monitoring of adverse drug reactions in children. Italian Paediatric Pharmacosurveillance Multicenter Group. Lancet 2000;355(9215):1613–4. Available at: http://www.ncbi.nlm.nih.gov/pubmed/10821367. Accessed August 24, 2013.

15. Rebelo Gomes E, Fonseca J, Araujo L, et al. Drug allergy claims in children: from self-reporting to confirmed diagnosis. Clin Exp Allergy 2008;38(1):191–8. Available at: http://www.ncbi.nlm.nih.gov/pubmed/18028465. Accessed August 24, 2013.

16. Harr T, French LE. Toxic epidermal necrolysis and Stevens-Johnson syndrome. Orphanet J Rare Dis 2010;5:39. Available at: http://www.pubmedcentral.nih.gov/articlerender.fcgi?artid=3018455&tool=pmcentrez&rendertype=abstract. Accessed August 24, 2013.

17. Mockenhaupt M. Severe drug-induced skin reactions: clinical pattern, diagnostics and therapy. J Dtsch Dermatol Ges 2009;7(2):142–60 [quiz: 161–2]. Available at: http://www.ncbi.nlm.nih.gov/pubmed/19371237. Accessed October 11, 2013.

18. Peroni A, Colato C, Schena D, et al. Urticarial lesions: if not urticaria, what else? The differential diagnosis of urticaria: part I. Cutaneous diseases. J Am Acad Dermatol 2010;62(4):541–55 [quiz: 555–6]. Available at: http://www.ncbi.nlm.nih.gov/pubmed/20227576. Accessed October 7, 2012.

19. Bigby M. Rates of cutaneous reactions to drugs. Arch Dermatol 2001;137(6):765–70. Available at: http://www.ncbi.nlm.nih.gov/pubmed/11444258.

20. Díaz Jara M, Pérez Montero A, Gracia Bara MT, et al. Allergic reactions due to ibuprofen in children. Pediatr Dermatol 2001;18(1):66–7. Available at: http://www.ncbi.nlm.nih.gov/pubmed/11207978.

21. Tamayo-Sanchez L, Ruiz-Maldonado R, Laterza A. Acute annular urticaria in infants and children. Pediatr Dermatol 1997;14(3):231–4. Available at: http://www.ncbi.nlm.nih.gov/pubmed/9192421.

22. Peroni A, Colato C, Zanoni G, et al. Urticarial lesions: if not urticaria, what else? The differential diagnosis of urticaria: part II. Systemic diseases. J Am Acad Dermatol 2010;62(4):557–70 [quiz: 571–2]. Available at: http://www.ncbi.nlm.nih.gov/pubmed/20227577. Accessed October 7, 2012.

23. Paller AS, Mancini AJ. Allergic reactions. In: Paller AS, Mancini AJ, editors. Hurwitz clinical pediatric dermatology. 4th edition. Philadelphia: Elsevier Saunders; 2011. p. 454–82. Available at: www.expertconsult.com. Accessed August 11, 2013.

24. Ibia EO, Schwartz RH, Wiedermann BL. Antibiotic rashes in children. Arch Dermatol 2000;136:849–54.

25. Ribeiro-Vaz I, Marques J, Demoly P, et al. Drug-induced anaphylaxis: a decade review of reporting to the Portuguese Pharmacovigilance Authority. Eur J Clin Pharmacol 2013;69(3):673–81. Available at: http://www.ncbi.nlm.nih.gov/pubmed/22915040. Accessed September 28, 2013.

26. Erlewyn-Lajeunesse M, Hunt LP, Heath PT, et al. Anaphylaxis as an adverse event following immunisation in the UK and Ireland. Arch Dis Child 2012; 97(6):487–90. Available at: http://www.ncbi.nlm.nih.gov/pubmed/22275307. Accessed September 28, 2013.

27. Tolpinrud WL, Bunick CG, King BA. Serum sickness-like reaction: histopathology and case report. J Am Acad Dermatol 2011;65(3):e83–5. Available at: http://www.ncbi.nlm.nih.gov/pubmed/21839305. Accessed September 8, 2013.

28. Patel S, Mancini AJ. Serum sickness-like reaction in children: a retrospective review. J Am Acad Dermatol 2009;60(Suppl 1):AB1–276.

29. Emer JJ, Bernardo SG, Kovalerchik O, et al. Urticaria multiforme. J Clin Aesthet Dermatol 2013;6(3):34–9. Available at: http://www.pubmedcentral.nih.gov/articlerender.fcgi?artid=3613272&tool=pmcentrez&rendertype=abstract.

30. Bircher AJ. Uncomplicated drug-induced disseminated exanthemas. Chem Immunol Allergy 2012;97:79–97. Available at: http://www.ncbi.nlm.nih.gov/pubmed/22613855.

31. Chovel-Sella A, Ben Tov A, Lahav E, et al. Incidence of rash after amoxicillin treatment in children with infectious mononucleosis. Pediatrics 2013;131(5): e1424–7. Available at: http://www.ncbi.nlm.nih.gov/pubmed/23589810. Accessed September 29, 2013.

32. Segal AR, Doherty KM, Leggott J, et al. Cutaneous reactions to drugs in children. Pediatrics 2007;120(4):e1082–96. Available at: http://www.ncbi.nlm.nih.gov/pubmed/17908729. Accessed August 15, 2013.

33. Husain Z, Reddy BY, Schwartz RA. DRESS syndrome: part I. Clinical perspectives. J Am Acad Dermatol 2013;68(5):693.e1–14 [quiz: 706–8]. Available at: http://www.ncbi.nlm.nih.gov/pubmed/23602182. Accessed August 8, 2013.

34. Ferrero NA, Pearson KC, Zedek DC, et al. Case report of drug rash with eosinophilia and systemic symptoms demonstrating human herpesvirus-6 reactivation. Pediatr Dermatol 2013;30(5):608–13. Available at: http://www.ncbi.nlm.nih.gov/pubmed/24016284. Accessed October 19, 2013.

35. Pavlos R, Mallal S, Phillips E. HLA and pharmacogenetics of drug hypersensitivity. Pharmacogenomics 2012;13(11):1285–306. Available at: http://www.ncbi.nlm.nih.gov/pubmed/22920398. Accessed August 24, 2013.

36. Kardaun SH, Sekula P, Valeyrie-Allanore L, et al. Drug reaction with eosinophilia and systemic symptoms (DRESS): an original multisystem adverse drug reaction. Results from the prospective RegiSCAR study. Br J Dermatol 2013; 169(5):1071–80. Available at: http://www.ncbi.nlm.nih.gov/pubmed/23855313. Accessed August 24, 2013.

37. Chiou CC, Yang LC, Hung SI, et al. Clinicopathological features and prognosis of drug rash with eosinophilia and systemic symptoms: a study of 30 cases in Taiwan. J Eur Acad Dermatol Venereol 2008;22(9):1044–9. Available at: http://www.ncbi.nlm.nih.gov/pubmed/18627428. Accessed August 3, 2013.

38. Cacoub P, Musette P, Descamps V, et al. The DRESS syndrome: a literature review. Am J Med 2011;124(7):588–97. Available at: http://www.ncbi.nlm.nih.gov/pubmed/21592453. Accessed August 3, 2013.

39. Tohyama M, Hashimoto K. New aspects of drug-induced hypersensitivity syndrome. J Dermatol 2011;38(3):222–8. Available at: http://www.ncbi.nlm.nih.gov/pubmed/21342223. Accessed August 3, 2013.

40. Levi N, Bastuji-Garin S, Mockenhaupt M, et al. Medications as risk factors of Stevens-Johnson syndrome and toxic epidermal necrolysis in children: a pooled analysis. Pediatrics 2009;123(2):e297–304.

41. Chung WH, Hung SI. Recent advances in the genetics and immunology of Stevens-Johnson syndrome and toxic epidermal necrosis. J Dermatol Sci 2012;66(3):190–6. Available at: http://www.ncbi.nlm.nih.gov/pubmed/22541332. Accessed August 24, 2013.

42. Yip VL, Marson AG, Jorgensen AL, et al. HLA genotype and carbamazepine-induced cutaneous adverse drug reactions: a systematic review. Clin Pharmacol Ther 2012;92(6):757–65. Available at: http://www.ncbi.nlm.nih.gov/pubmed/23132554. Accessed September 17, 2013.

43. Guégan S, Bastuji-Garin S, Poszepczynska-Guigné E, et al. Performance of the SCORTEN during the first five days of hospitalization to predict the prognosis of epidermal necrolysis. J Invest Dermatol 2006;126(2):272–6. Available at: http://www.ncbi.nlm.nih.gov/pubmed/16374461. Accessed October 19, 2013.

44. Palmieri TL, Greenhalgh DG, Saffle JR, et al. A multicenter review of toxic epidermal necrolysis treated in U.S. burn centers at the end of the twentieth century. J Burn Care Rehabil 2002;23(2):87–96. Available at: http://www.ncbi.nlm.nih.gov/pubmed/11882797. Accessed November 5, 2013.

45. Huang SH, Yang PS, Wu SH, et al. Aquacel Ag with Vaseline gauze in the management of toxic epidermal necrolysis (TEN). Burns 2010;36(1):121–6. Available at: http://www.ncbi.nlm.nih.gov/pubmed/19477595. Accessed November 5, 2013.

46. Boorboor P, Vogt PM, Bechara FG, et al. Toxic epidermal necrolysis: use of Biobrane or skin coverage reduces pain, improves mobilisation and decreases infection in elderly patients. Burns 2008;34(4):487–92. Available at: http://www.ncbi.nlm.nih.gov/pubmed/17919820. Accessed November 5, 2013.

47. Dorafshar AH, Dickie SR, Cohn AB, et al. Antishear therapy for toxic epidermal necrolysis: an alternative treatment approach. Plast Reconstr Surg 2008;122(1):154–60. Available at: http://www.ncbi.nlm.nih.gov/pubmed/18594400. Accessed November 5, 2013.

48. Yip LW, Thong BY, Lim J, et al. Ocular manifestations and complications of Stevens-Johnson syndrome and toxic epidermal necrolysis: an Asian series. Allergy 2007;62(5):527–31. Available at: http://www.ncbi.nlm.nih.gov/pubmed/17313402. Accessed October 3, 2013.

49. Ersoy S, Paller AS, Mancini AJ. Acute generalized exanthematous pustulosis in children. Arch Dermatol 2004;140(9):1172–3.

50. Meadows KP, Egan CA, Vanderhooft S. Acute generalized exanthematous pustulosis (AGEP), an uncommon condition in children: case report and review of the literature. Pediatr Dermatol 2000;17(5):399–402. Available at: http://doi.wiley.com/10.1046/j.1525-1470.2000.017005399.x. Accessed August 25, 2013.

51. Lansang P, Weinstein M, Shear N. Drug reactions. In: Schachner LA, Hansen RC, editors. Pediatric dermatology. 4th edition. London: Mosby Elsevier; 2011. p. 1698–711.

52. Fathallah N, Ben Salem C, Slim R, et al. Acetaminophen-induced cellulitis-like fixed drug eruption. Indian J Dermatol 2011;56(2):206–8. Available at: http://www.pubmedcentral.nih.gov/articlerender.fcgi?artid=3108524&tool=pmcentrez&rendertype=abstract. Accessed August 26, 2013.

53. Nussinovitch M, Prais D, Ben-Amitai D, et al. Fixed drug eruption in the genital area in 15 boys. Pediatr Dermatol 2002;19(3):216–9. Available at: http://www.ncbi.nlm.nih.gov/pubmed/12047640.

54. Bilgili SG, Calka O, Karadag AS, et al. Nonsteroidal anti-inflammatory drugs-induced generalized fixed drug eruption: two cases. Hum Exp Toxicol 2012;

31(2):197–200. Available at: http://www.ncbi.nlm.nih.gov/pubmed/21677025. Accessed August 26, 2013.

55. Mahboob A, Haroon TS. Drugs causing fixed eruptions: a study of 450 cases. Int J Dermatol 1998;37(11):833–8. Available at: http://www.ncbi.nlm.nih.gov/pubmed/9865869. Accessed November 5, 2013.

56. Brahimi N, Routier E, Raison-Peyron N, et al. A three-year-analysis of fixed drug eruptions in hospital settings in France. Eur J Dermatol 2010;20(4):461–4. Available at: http://www.ncbi.nlm.nih.gov/pubmed/20507840. Accessed November 5, 2013.

57. Paller AS, Mancini AJ. Hurwitz clinical pediatric dermatology: a textbook of skin disorders of childhood and adolescence. In: Paller AS, Mancini AJ, editors. 4th edition. Philadelphia: Elsevier Inc; 2011. p. 624. Available at: www.expertconsult.com. Accessed August 11, 2013.

58. Revuz J, Valeyrie-Allanore L. Drug reactions in dermatology. In: Jean L, Bolognia M, Julie V, et al, editors. Dermatology. 3rd edition. Philadelphia: Elsevier Inc; 2012. p. Cp21.

59. Wolverton SE. Comprehensive dermatologic drug therapy. 3rd edition. Philadelphia: Elsevier Saunders; 2013.

60. Gatti L, Carnelli V, Rusconi R, et al. Heparin-induced thrombocytopenia and warfarin-induced skin necrosis in a child with severe protein C deficiency: successful treatment with dermatan sulfate and protein C concentrate. J Thromb Haemost 2003;1(2):387–8. Available at: http://www.ncbi.nlm.nih.gov/pubmed/12871519. Accessed November 7, 2013.

61. Warkentin TE. Heparin-induced skin lesions. Br J Haematol 1996;92(2):494–7. Available at: http://www.ncbi.nlm.nih.gov/pubmed/8603024. Accessed November 7, 2013.

62. Ho JC, Ng PL, Tan SH, et al. Childhood linear IgA bullous disease triggered by amoxicillin-clavulanic acid. Pediatr Dermatol 2007;24(5):E40–3. Available at: http://www.ncbi.nlm.nih.gov/pubmed/17958778. Accessed November 7, 2013.

63. Mintz EM, Morel KD. Clinical features, diagnosis, and pathogenesis of chronic bullous disease of childhood. Dermatol Clin 2011;29(3):459–62 ix. Available at: http://www.ncbi.nlm.nih.gov/pubmed/21605812. Accessed November 7, 2013.

64. Cardoza-Torres MA, Liy-Wong C, Welsh O, et al. Skin manifestations associated with chemotherapy in children with hematologic malignancies. Pediatr Dermatol 2012;29(3):264–9. Available at: http://www.ncbi.nlm.nih.gov/pubmed/22044286. Accessed August 12, 2013.

65. Heinzerling LM, Tomsitz D, Anliker MD. Is drug allergy less prevalent than previously assumed? A 5-year analysis. Br J Dermatol 2012;166(1):107–14. Available at: http://www.ncbi.nlm.nih.gov/pubmed/21916887. Accessed August 25, 2013.

66. Guillon JM, Joly P, Autran B, et al. Minocycline-induced cell-mediated hypersensitivity pneumonitis. Ann Intern Med 1992;117(6):476–81. Available at: http://www.ncbi.nlm.nih.gov/pubmed/1503350. Accessed November 5, 2013.

67. Stern RS. Clinical practice. Exanthematous drug eruptions. N Engl J Med 2012; 366(26):2492–501. Available at: http://www.ncbi.nlm.nih.gov/pubmed/22738099. Accessed November 5, 2013.

68. Kano Y, Hirahara K, Mitsuyama Y, et al. Utility of the lymphocyte transformation test in the diagnosis of drug sensitivity: dependence on its timing and the type of drug eruption. Allergy 2007;62(12):1439–44. Available at: http://www.ncbi.nlm.nih.gov/pubmed/17983378. Accessed November 5, 2013.

69. Amur S, Frueh FW, Lesko LJ, et al. Integration and use of biomarkers in drug development, regulation and clinical practice: a US regulatory perspective.

Biomark Med 2008;2(3):305–11. Available at: http://www.ncbi.nlm.nih.gov/pubmed/20477416.

70. Husain Z, Reddy BY, Schwartz RA. DRESS syndrome: part II. Management and therapeutics. J Am Acad Dermatol 2013;68(5):709.e1–9 [quiz: 718–20]. Available at: http://www.ncbi.nlm.nih.gov/pubmed/23602183. Accessed August 8, 2013.

71. Laban E, Hainaut-Wierzbicka E, Pourreau F, et al. Cyclophosphamide therapy for corticoresistant drug reaction with eosinophilia and systemic symptoms (DRESS) syndrome in a patient with severe kidney and eye involvement and Epstein-Barr virus reactivation. Am J Kidney Dis 2010;55(3):e11–4. Available at: http://www.ncbi.nlm.nih.gov/pubmed/20110143. Accessed July 31, 2012.

72. Zuliani E, Zwahlen H, Gilliet F, et al. Vancomycin-induced hypersensitivity reaction with acute renal failure: resolution following cyclosporine treatment. Clin Nephrol 2005;64(2):155–8. Available at: http://www.ncbi.nlm.nih.gov/pubmed/16114793.

73. Reese D, Henning JS, Rockers K, et al. Cyclosporine for SJS/TEN: a case series and review of the literature. Cutis 2011;87:24–9.

74. Schneck J, Fagot JP, Sekula P, et al. Effects of treatments on the mortality of Stevens-Johnson syndrome and toxic epidermal necrolysis: a retrospective study on patients included in the prospective EuroSCAR Study. J Am Acad Dermatol 2008;58(1):33–40. Available at: http://www.ncbi.nlm.nih.gov/pubmed/17919775. Accessed September 20, 2013.

75. Valeyrie-Allanore L, Wolkenstein P, Brochard L, et al. Open trial of cyclosporin treatment for Stevens-Johnson syndrome and toxic epidermal necrolysis. Br J Dermatol 2010;163(4):847–53. Available at: http://www.ncbi.nlm.nih.gov/pubmed/20500799. Accessed July 31, 2012.

Diagnosis and Management of Alopecia in Children

Leslie Castelo-Soccio, MD, PhD

KEYWORDS

- Alopecia areata • Telogen effluvium • Tinea capitis • Traction alopecia
- Trichotillomania/trichotillosis

KEY POINTS

- Alopecia in childhood is not uncommon.
- Tinea capitis is the most common cause of loss of hair in childhood and should be excluded in an evaluation.
- Clues to the type of hair loss include evidence of scale, hair breakage, and location of the hair loss.
- The age of the child and whether there are other comorbidities are additional clues to diagnosis.

INTRODUCTION
Overview

The ideal evaluation of a child with scalp hair loss should include a full history and physical examination with a detailed evaluation of the hair and scalp. In the pediatric office, it is usually possible to send dermatophyte screens or fungal cultures to rule out tinea as a source of alopecia, perform a hair pull test to see if hair is actively shedding, and assess overall pattern of hair loss and scalp health. A thorough history must include whether hair was never present/sparse after birth or whether hair was later lost in a localized manner or shed more diffusely. The history should also include diet and nutrition and underlying medical problems, with special attention to autoimmune disease. If medical providers suspect that alopecia is congenital, a detailed evaluation/history of teeth and tooth eruption, nails, skin, and the ability to sweat is needed. Congenital alopecia can be associated with general abnormalities of the ectoderm referred to as the broad category of diseases known as *ectodermal dysplasias*. Patients with ectodermal dysplasias will have long-term problems with dentition, hair, nails, sometimes heat regulation, and occasionally bones. In most cases, alopecia occurs after the development of full scalp hair and is related to infection, an autoimmune process, or trauma/traction.

Section of Dermatology, Department of Pediatrics, The Children's Hospital of Philadelphia, 3550 Market Street, 2nd Floor Dermatology, Philadelphia, PA 19104, USA
E-mail address: castelosocciol@email.chop.edu

Pediatr Clin N Am 61 (2014) 427–442
http://dx.doi.org/10.1016/j.pcl.2013.12.002
0031-3955/14/$ – see front matter © 2014 Elsevier Inc. All rights reserved.

Pathophysiology

All human hairs regularly cycle through anagen, the growth phase; telogen, the resting phase; and catagen, the transition phase.[1] The first anagen phase starts at about 18 to 20 weeks of gestation, with the first normal shedding period occurring sometime between 4 and 8 months of age. This period can occur as late as 1 year of age. This hair loss is the typical pattern hair loss seen in infants at their well visits. The occiput of the scalp differs in that it has expected telogen shedding that occurs earlier at about 2 to 3 months of age and accounts for the bald spot seen in the occiput of most infants around that time. Pressure and rubbing from sleeping on the back accentuate this hair loss. The number of hair follicles during the first 2 years does not change, but there is a transition from vellus hairs to terminal hairs.[2] Because terminal hairs are larger in caliber, the density of hair seems to increase. Hair darkens with age in most cases.

THE HISTORY AND PHYSICAL EXAMINATION

The most important question in the history is whether the hair loss is acute or gradual. Did the hair loss occur over months or within days? Alopecia areata (AA) will often occur with very rapid localized loss over days, whereas traction alopecia will occur slowly overtime with gradual thinning at the hairline or wherever there is tension on the hair. Telogen effluvium will start rapidly, but then the shedding stabilizes; there is increased but steady shedding over weeks to months. This type of shedding decreases with time until it shifts back to the patient's normal hair-shedding pattern.

Physical examination should evaluate all areas of the scalp in a systematic fashion. The scalp should be evaluated for localized or diffuse hair loss. The location of loss should be noted. Locations include periphery, occiput, vertex, temples, and parietal scalp. An evaluation should be performed for scale and redness of the scalp, which are signs of inflammation. In all cases, if redness or scale is present, tinea capitis should be ruled out. Scale can also be a sign of other inflammatory disorders like psoriasis, cutaneous lupus, eczema, or seborrheic dermatitis, which can lead to hair loss because of associated scale and inflammation. Clues to these other inflammatory disorders include cutaneous signs of inflammation in other parts of the body; previous atopic disease; or, in the case of cutaneous lupus, scarring on the scalp and a negative dermatophyte screen.

A hair pull test is a simple tool all pediatricians can use because it requires no special instruments. The hair pull test involves gently pulling 20 to 60 hairs between the thumb and forefinger in multiple locations of the scalp.[3] Anagen or growing hairs should remain rooted in place, whereas hairs in the telogen phase should come out easily. One can roughly estimate the number of hairs in telogen. If 2 hairs come out on a hair pull of approximately 20 hairs, telogen is about 10%. Normal telogen is between 10% and 20%. It is important to ask patients about when they last washed their hair. Ideally, it is the day before the examination. If it was the same day, you should expect fewer hairs to be shed. If it was 1 week before, you should expect more telogen hairs to be shed. Hairs from the pull test can be mounted and reviewed under microscope for hair shaft abnormalities as well as the phase of the cycle of the hair when practical. This practice is rare outside of specialist offices. A full skin examination including an evaluation of eyelashes, eyebrows, and nails should be completed. Evaluation of cervical chain lymphadenopathy should be performed and is often present in tinea capitis but can also be seen in other inflammatory disorders of the scalp, notably atopic dermatitis.

The history should include questions about general health; illness in the last 4 to 6 months, including illness with high fevers; and other stressors, including surgeries, new medications, and changes in school or home life. A good review of systems should be performed to look for concerns for hypothyroidism, anemia, diabetes, and other autoimmune disease. In children, this would include but is not limited to new constipation, fatigue, and increased nighttime urination. A family history of alopecia and autoimmune disease should also reviewed. Potential contacts at home or at school with alopecia should also be reviewed if there is concern for tinea capitis. Diet and nutrition should be reviewed, and risks for toxic exposures like lead should also be elicited.

REVIEW OF COMMON ALOPECIAS
Tinea Capitis

Overview
Tinea capitis is a dermatophyte infection that primarily affects children (**Fig. 1**, **Table 1**). Adult cases may be seen in the setting of immunosuppression.

Epidemiology
Children aged 3 to 7 years are the most commonly affected with slightly more cases in male patients. The epidemiology of tinea capitis varies within different geographic areas throughout the world. In inner-city schools in the United States, the prevalence of tinea capitis among African American children have been reported to be from 12% to as high as 30%, with higher numbers for younger grammar school children.[4] Infection rates for Hispanic and white children tend to be markedly lower, with an average prevalence of about 1% to 2%. Tinea may occur sporadically or epidemically and an increase in its incidence has been noted over the last few decades. Two species of dermatophyte are predominant in the United States. *Trichophyton tonsurans* is the most common cause of tinea capitis in children in the United States and is passed from human to human. *Microsporum canis* is the second most common and can be acquired from domestic pets. By some estimates, *Microsporum* accounts for less than 10% of all tinea capitis cases in the United States.[5]

Pathophysiology
Tinea capitis is caused by fungi of species of the genera *Trichophyton* and *Microsporum*. Through direct inoculation, the fungal hyphae grow centrifugally in the stratum corneum and into the hair follicle. The zone of involvement extends upward at the rate at which hair grows, and it is visible above the skin surface by days 12 to 14. Endothrix infections are characterized by arthroconidia (spores) within the hair shaft. The

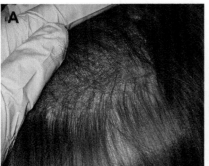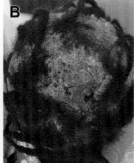

Fig. 1. (*A*) Scalp of child depicting scale and erythema representing tinea capitis. (*B*) Child with red and boggy scalp with thick, yellow scale characteristic of tinea capitis with a kerion.

Table 1
Summary of findings in common types of alopecia in children

Types of Alopecia	Definition	History	Physical Examination	Diagnosis	Treatment
Tinea capitis	Dermatophyte infection Can be scarring	Acute Can be recurrent Some chronic carriers	Scaly red alopecia patches Diffuse scale Broken hairs/black dots Cervical lymphadenopathy	Dermatophyte screen KOH microscopic examination	Oral antifungal medications Antifungal shampoos
AA	Autoimmune hair loss Nonscarring	Acute then chronic Episodes of activity and remission	Areata: round patches of smooth bald scalp Areata ophiasis: smooth hair loss on the periphery scalp Totalis: complete hair loss of scalp Universalis: complete hair loss on scalp, body Nail pitting, ridges Exclamation point hairs, lighter/thinner regrowing hairs	Smooth scalp Exclamation point hairs Fine regrowing hairs No lymphadenopathy No redness or scale	Topical/oral or intralesional corticosteroids Topical retinoids Contact irritants Systemic antiinflammatories Hair pieces/other cosmetic
Traction alopecia	Hair loss related to tension Can be scarring	Slow process, months to years	Decreased density of hair at areas of maximal tension Folliculitis (redness and pustules) around hair follicle White hair casts/pseudonits on hairs with increased tension	History of tension	Changing hair styles Decreasing friction
Telogen effluvium	Shedding of hair Nonscarring	Rapid shedding, weeks to months Occurs 3–4 mo after inciting event	Decreased density of hair throughout scalp Positive hair pull test	Positive hair pull test Shed hairs in telogen phase	Treat underlying cause Reassurance

cuticle is not destroyed. Ectothrix infections are characterized by hyphal fragments and arthroconidia outside the hair shaft, which lead to eventual cuticle destruction.

Clinical appearance
It invariably includes scale and some degree of redness and alopecia. It can be divided in diffuse scale, patch, black dot, diffuse pustular, and kerion varieties (see **Fig. 1**) Inflammation is more intense with zoophilic fungi. Kerions, which are swollen and sometimes purulent and boggy-appearing plaques, can occur with both zoophilic (fungi like *Microsporum* that prefer other animals to humans) and anthropophilic fungi (fungi like *Trichophyton* that prefer humans to other animals). Kerions are the body's unsuccessful attempt to clear tinea at the site of infection with increased inflammatory cells and soft tissue swelling. The actual kerion is often dermatophyte negative, but the increased inflammation can lead to scarring and alopecia.[6,7]

Differential diagnosis
Seborrheic and atopic dermatitis and psoriasis should be considered in the differential diagnosis of tinea capitis with diffuse scale and the patch variant. AA and trichotillo- mania are in the differential diagnosis of black dot tinea capitis. Bacterial folliculitis and dissecting folliculitis of the scalp should be considered in the differential diagnosis of diffuse pustular tinea capitis. Dissecting cellulitis is an inflammatory process considered part of the acne family whereby patients develop inflammatory papules and pustules in the scalp with accentuation in the occiput, which can lead to scarring. A cutaneous abscess and, less commonly, a neoplastic process like lymphoma are in the differential diagnosis for a kerion.

Prognosis
Most cases of tinea capitis can be successfully treated with the use of appropriate oral antifungal therapy and antifungal shampoos to prevent persistent shedding of spores. Extensive inflammation can lead to scarring, which leads to permanent localized alopecia. Recurrence can occur if hair grooming devices and other fomites are not cleaned properly.

Diagnostic studies
A dermatophyte culture will readily confirm the diagnosis of tinea capitis. Dermato- phyte cultures in contrast to fungal cultures are plated to look for specific causes of tinea and exclude other molds and yeasts that can be contaminants from the environ- ment. There will be a better yield and higher detection if a specific dermatophyte screen is performed. In order to properly obtain a specimen, an alcohol pad should be used to clean off any ointments or topical therapies previously applied to the scalp. A toothbrush or conventional bacterial swab can be used to plate material on Sabo- uraud agar containing antibiotics (penicillin/streptomycin or chloramphenicol) and cyclohexamide.[7,8] Many centers will send swabs or toothbrushes to the laboratories to be plated later.[9] Most dermatophytes can be identified within 2 weeks of plating. Standard potassium hydroxide (KOH) preparations for immediate microscope review can determine if tinea infection exists in many cases but are infrequently available in the pediatrician office. Conventional sampling of kerions often yield negative results because it mostly represents the inflammatory response to tinea; however, a moist- ened bacterial swab obtained from a pustular area and inoculated on a dermatophyte culture plate may yield a positive result, as may pressing the agar plate onto the kerion directly. Wood's lamp can be used to look for green fluorescence; however *Trichophy- ton* species, which are the most commonly isolated species in the United States, do not fluoresce. *Microsporum* species do fluoresce but are much less commonly seen.

Therapy

For infections involving *Trichophyton* species, terbinafine for 4 weeks and griseofulvin for 8 weeks show similar efficacy (**Table 2**). Itraconazole and fluconazole have also been used with high cure rates. Griseofulvin seems to be superior to terbinafine for cases caused by *Microsporum*. The addition of selenium sulfide or other antifungal shampoo used at minimum of 2 times a week for 4 weeks decreases the carriage of visible spores and is assumed to help prevent reinfection. Terbinafine is approved for tinea capitis infection in children older than 4 years. Griseofulvin is approved for the treatment of dermatophyte infections in children older than 2 years.[10–13] In children aged 1 month to less than 2 years, there is limited data for the use of griseofulvin; however, in practice, it is used frequently with few side effects and high efficacy. The most-cited data for this age group suggest that 10 mg/kg/d is safe and effective.[7] Many children under 1 year of age respond to topical therapy with azoles alone and do not need systemic medications. For the treatment of a kerion, the use of gentle soaks and/or keratolytic emollients can aid to remove crust. Some individuals advocate topical or oral steroids to decrease inflammation.

Other

Once treatment with appropriate systemic and adjuvant topical therapy has been commenced, the child can return to school. The definitive end point for adequate treatment is not the clinical response but the mycological cure. Repeat dermatophyte screening should be repeated at the end of therapy to confirm cure. Viable spores have been isolated from hairbrushes and combs. Cleansing these items with bleach or hot water (>100°C) can be used to destroy spores.[8]

Table 2
Systemic therapy for tinea capitis

Medication	Dosage		Duration (wk)
Griseofulvin			
Microsize[a]	20 mg/kg/d		6–8
Ultramicrosize	15–20 mg/kg/d (once a day or divided[b])		6–8
Terbinafine[c]	<20 kg	62.5 mg daily	4–6
	>20–<40 kg	125 mg daily	
	>40 kg	250 mg daily	
Itraconazole	5 mg/kg/d		2
Fluconazole	3–5 mg/kg/d		2–3

[a] Griseofulvin suspension 25 mg/mL is microsized. Tablets of 125 mg and 250 mg are usually ultra-microsized and can be crushed and put into soft foods.
[b] Griseofulvin in those less than 2 years of age consider 10 mg/kg/d.
[c] Terbinafine is approved by the Food and Drug Administration for tinea capitis in patients more than 4 years of age. Granules can be put into soft foods excluding acidic foods like applesauce.

AA

AA is a common type of nonscarring hair loss.

Epidemiology

There is a lifetime risk of about 1.5% to 1.7% in the general population. The lifetime risk increases to 6% in children of parents affected with alopecia areata. AA can affect any age; in 27% to 60% of patients, it has been shown to present before 20 years of age. One recent study showed the peak incidence for children aged between 1 and 5 years, though more studies show the peak incidence later in childhood.[14,15]

Pathophysiology

AA is considered an autoimmune disorder with a genetic basis and environmental triggers.[16] A genome-wide association study in a sample of 1054 patients with AA and 3278 controls showed associations with several genes that control the activation and proliferation of T cells, including interleukin-2 (IL-2) and its receptor, human leukocyte antigen, and the unique long 16 (UL16)- binding protein (ULBP) that encodes activating ligands of natural killer cells.[17] The association of AA with other autoimmune diseases, atopy, and the response to antiinflammatory therapies suggest the immune system has a key role in its pathogenesis.

Clinical appearance

AA manifests as a variety of clinical patterns.[14,18] The most common pattern is the sudden appearance of smooth, bald, round patches on the scalp that are asymptomatic and very occasionally mildly pruritic (**Fig. 2**A). Within the patches, exclamation point hairs can be seen by the naked eye or by dermoscopy (see **Fig. 2**B). These hairs are short hairs with dark, expanded tips that are markers of disease activity. Black dot hairs are hairs broken immediately at the surface of the scalp. The ophiasis pattern is a more extensive pattern of AA whereby hair is lost along the parietal scalp and the occiput (see **Fig. 2**C). This pattern has a less favorable prognosis. In rare cases, alopecia may be diffuse and look more like telogen effluvium. Some patients have total scalp hair loss (alopecia totalis), and some patients have total scalp and body hair loss (alopecia universalis) (see **Fig. 2**D). Only about 5% of patients who present with typical AA progress to alopecia totalis or universalis. As hairs grow, the hairs are often smaller in caliber and lighter in color. Hair color and diameter return with time. Nails may be involved, and many patients have pitting or vertical or longitudinal striations within the nails (**Fig. 5**).

Associations

AA can be associated with Hashimoto thyroiditis, diabetes mellitus, rheumatoid arthritis, pernicious anemia, lupus, celiac disease, and vitiligo. The prevalence of another autoimmune disease in patients with AA is 16%. Thyroid disease and vitiligo have the strongest relationship. A strong association of AA (10%) has been observed in patients with Down syndrome.[14,16]

Differential diagnosis

For localized AA, the main differential diagnoses are tinea capitis and trichotillomania. For diffuse AA, the main differential diagnoses are telogen effluvium and diffuse tinea capitis. For alopecia totalis and universalis, it is important to consider the possibility of ectodermal dysplasias, ichthyoses, or an underlying medical condition. In the setting of cutaneous features, such as diffuse scaling or xerosis or nail changes, a diagnosis of ectodermal dysplasias or ichthyoses should be considered. Although rare, in the setting of other autoimmune endocrinopathies, consider an autoimmune polyglandular syndrome (APS), such as APS type 1 (autoimmune polyendocrinopathy, candidiasis, ectodermal dystrophy). In the setting of a history of poor eating or failure to thrive, consider nutritional deficiencies, including zinc, iron, vitamin D, vitamin B, and protein deficiencies.

Prognosis

The course of AA is unpredictable. Hair loss and regrowth cycles can occur for years or for life. The prognosis is poorer if the age of onset is before puberty, there is

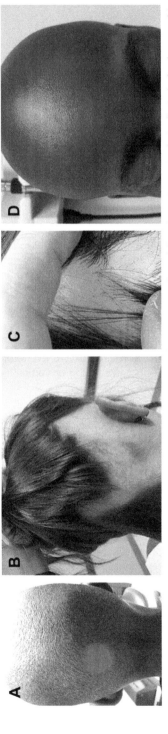

Fig. 2. (A) Child with single small, smooth, skin-colored, round, bald patch characteristic of AA. (B) Exclamation point hairs (hair shafts that are thinner closer to the scalp) that are characteristics of AA. (C) Smooth, bald patches extending from the parietal scalp to the occiput of the scalp and characteristic of the ophiasis pattern of AA. (D) Smooth, bald scalp of a child with complete scalp hair loss characteristic of alopecia totalis.

a positive family history, hair loss is extensive, there is history of atopic dermatitis, there is a history of long disease duration without regrowth, there are severe nail changes, and/or patients have Down syndrome.

Diagnostic studies

The diagnosis is usually a clinical one, though scalp biopsy will show an inflammatory lymphocytic infiltrate around the lower hair follicle. In most cases, biopsy is not necessary or recommended. Dermatophyte culture can rule out tinea capitis as a cause of the alopecia. Hair mounts can confirm normal hair shaft and normal proportion of anagen and telogen hairs when feasible. Dermoscopy (the evaluation of the skin with a dermatoscope) can also be useful. A dermatoscope is essentially a magnifier with a nonpolarized light source that can be placed on the skin to get a more detailed view. With dermoscopy of the scalp, one can identify characteristic exclamation point hairs as well as regrowing hairs. These hairs can be seen with good light without the aid of the dermatoscope. A good review of systems is essential. If there is concern for thyroid disease, anemia, or diabetes mellitus, screening thyroid stimulating hormone, free thyroxine, thyroid autoantibodies, fasting or random blood glucose, hemoglobin A1c, and complete blood count with differential and serum iron studies can be considered. Screening for thyroid dysfunction is not routine and should only be performed in the setting of signs and symptoms. In patients with significant disease, which includes alopecia totalis or universalis, and a strong autoimmune family history, some advocate obtaining thyroid autoantibodies to assess if screening needs to be performed more routinely for that individual patient. Routine testing of antinuclear antibody is not recommended.[14]

Therapies

Treatment of AA can be difficult. The most common treatment options for children less than 10 years of age include topical corticosteroids (class I–III) used alone or in combination with topical retinoids,[19–21] topical anthralin,[22,23] and rarely systemic steroids (pulse therapy).[24] Therapies are usually used for 6 to 8 weeks, with re-evaluation after that time period. Treatment in children more than 10 years of age includes those listed earlier but also includes topical sensitizers and intralesional corticosteroids. There are some children less than 10 years of age that tolerate intralesional steroid injection. There are limited data on the use of other systemic agents, including methotrexate,[25] hydroxychloroquine sulfate, and other immunomodulators. The use of ultraviolet B light phototherapy also has limited efficacy data. There has been no efficacy shown for the use of tacrolimus, tumor necrosis factor–alpha blockers,[26] topical latanoprost,[27] or 5-fluoruracil. The use of minoxidil is controversial. Several researchers describe positive effects on topical minoxidil in the treatment of AA. In placebo-controlled studies, the effect of minoxidil was not significant compared with placebo.[28] Therefore, minoxidil is not routinely recommended for children. Some children, in particular girls, wish to wear a hair piece; many children benefit from formal psychological support. Wigs for Kids and similar organizations can provide anatomically fitted hair prostheses at discounted rates based on financial need. The Child Alopecia Project also has support groups and can be helpful for children and parents adjusting to the diagnosis.

Traction Alopecia

Overview

Traction alopecia is a hair loss condition caused by damage to the hair follicle by constant pulling or tension over time. It often occurs in children and adults who wear tight braids, ponytails, or other tight hairstyles that lead to high tension, pulling, and breakage of hair. It can also occur in the setting of chemical processing of hair with dyes, other chemicals, or bleaches that damage the keratin of the hair and weaken the hair shaft, thus, further exacerbating traction- or tension-induced damage.[29,30]

Epidemiology
In the United States, traction alopecia is more common in children and teenagers in the African American population, likely because of hairstyling practices.

Pathophysiology
Constant pulling or tension on the hair follicle damages the dermal papilla, which is the source of new cells in the hair follicle to generate hair growth.

Clinical presentation
In traction alopecia, thinning of hair and alopecia are commonly located at the periphery of the scalp with accentuation of hair loss in the frontal and temporal regions. When hair is braided tightly in rows, hair loss occurs adjacent to the rows of braids. Often there will be a pustule around the hair follicle because tension can cause inflammation and a sterile folliculitis around pulled hairs (**Fig. 3**).

Differential diagnosis
Ophiasis pattern AA at early stages can mimic traction alopecia because, in this pattern, hair is lost at the periphery of the scalp. The ways to differentiate this from traction alopecia is that the history for autoimmune alopecia is generally an acute process. Trichotillomania can also mimic traction alopecia in the sense that patients may pull only at the periphery of the scalp; however, in trichotillomania, it is more common for hair to be lost on the top of the scalp, upper eyelashes, and eyebrows.

Diagnostic considerations
Perform a dermatophyte screen if any scale or redness and a bacterial swab for culture if there are any pustules.

Therapeutics
The key to treatment and reversal is identifying the problem early and not putting stress on the hair by keeping hairstyles loose and avoiding chemical treatment of the hair. In adulthood, some patients choose hair transplantation if hair loss is more permanent.[29,30]

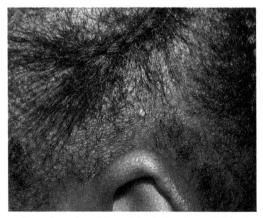

Fig. 3. Child with traction alopecia with a tight hairstyle and thinning of hair at tension sites. Depiction of pustule/folliculitis also observed in traction alopecia.

Prognosis

Prognosis is good if recognized early and hairstyling and treatment practices are changed. If scarring has occurred, there is no reversal of alopecia.

Telogen Effluvium

Overview

Telogen effluvium is a nonscarring alopecia that occurs when there is a shift of hair follicles from the anagen or growing phase abruptly to the telogen phase. These hairs are then synchronously shed after completion of telogen. Although typically only 10% to 15% of hairs are in telogen at one time, when this shift occurs, more than 20% to 50% of hairs on the scalp can be in telogen, resulting in a large degree of hair loss over a short amount of time.[31]

Epidemiology

This condition is quite common, but the exact prevalence is not known. Acute telogen effluvium can occur in either sex. Because hormonal changes in the postpartum period are a common cause of telogen effluvium, women may have a greater tendency to experience this condition. Children are as likely as adults to experience telogen effluvium.[32]

Pathophysiology

Stress occurs on the anagen hair follicle, which shifts it into the resting, or telogen, phase. Viruses, high fevers, other systemic illness, surgery, medications, nutritional deficiency (protein, iron, zinc, essential fatty acid), changes in thyroid function, and other traumatic events can all lead to the shift of a significant number of hair follicles to the telogen phase.

Clinical presentation

Patients experience a sudden increased shedding of hair diffusely over the scalp 3 to 4 months after the inciting event (**Fig. 4**). For some patients, the length of time that hair remains in telogen before shedding can be shorter or longer than 3 to 4 months. The telogen loss is followed by anagen regrowth over the next 6 to 12 months. If inciting events like hypothyroidism are not corrected, then, as new anagen hairs start to grow, they can be shifted back into telogen and shedding will continue.

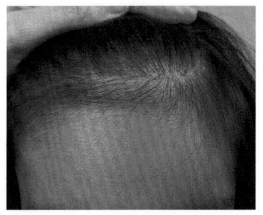

Fig. 4. Decreased density of hair and regrowing short, fine hairs at the frontal hairline in a child with telogen effluvium.

Differential diagnosis

The differential diagnosis for telogen effluvium includes diffuse AA, lead poisoning and nutritional deficiency. Nutritional deficiencies that lead to hair loss include zinc, iron, biotin, and protein deficiency. Testing lead levels, zinc levels, a complete blood count, ferritin, and complete metabolic panel are the first steps in evaluating these entities.[33]

Diagnostic considerations

The diagnosis can be made by finding a positive hair pull test where all examined hairs are in the telogen phase. Briefly, a hair pull test involves pulling 20 to 60 hairs and counting the number of hairs collected from the estimated total number of hairs pulled. This test gives you a rough telogen percentage. Normal telogen is between 10% and 20% of the hairs pulled. A history that elicits concern for protein malnutrition or other nutritional deficiency may trigger blood studies. Consider testing lead levels if suspicion is high. In cases when patients are on low-calorie diets or restricted diets because of a desire for weight loss/anorexia/bulimia or because of gastrointestinal disease or a food allergy, protein levels should be evaluated.[32]

Therapeutics

The treatment of any underlying disorders and correction of nutritional deficiencies are important. Otherwise, education about the condition and reassurance that hair regrowth will occur is all that is necessary. There are limited data on use of minoxidil in the treatment of telogen effluvium. Minoxidil is not recommended for use in children routinely.[34]

Prognosis

The prognosis is excellent because most patients regrow hair in 6 to 12 months.

Other

One clue to the diagnosis of telogen effluvium is that parents and patients often bring in large amounts of shed hair in a plastic bag, the *bag-of-hair sign*, to demonstrate the significant amount of hair that is being rapidly shed.

Trichotillomania/Trichotillosis

Overview

Trichotillomania is the compulsion to pull out one's hair. It is classified as an impulse control disorder. This type is a self-induced and recurrent type of hair loss. Many patients do not realize they are pulling their hair, and it is performed unconsciously while they are occupied with other activities like watching television and sometimes in their sleep. Some subdivide patients into *automatic* and *focused* hair pullers whereby those that are *automatic* perform the behavior in an *unconscious state*. Many children fall into this automatic hair pulling–behavior subgroup.[35,36]

Epidemiology

Although it can be seen in younger children, the behavior in children younger than 5 years is more similar to thumb-sucking behavior and usually resolves on its own. It is helpful to divide patients into 3 groups: preschool, preadolescent to young adult, and adults. These subgroups help inform the prognosis and treatment. Overall, the peak age in children is 9 to 13 years and may be triggered by depression, anxiety, or a significant life event. The lifetime prevalence is estimated to be between 0.6% and 4.0%.[36]

Pathophysiology
Trichotillomania falls under the obsessive-compulsive disorder spectrum. It is not clear what triggers the behavior. It is likely that multiple genes confer vulnerability to trichotillomania. One study identified mutations in the SLITRK1 (SLIT and NTRK [neutrophic tyrosinase kinase receptor, type1]) gene, and another study identified differences in the serotonin 2A receptor genes; mice with a mutation on the HOXB8 (homeobox-B8) gene showed abnormal behaviors, including hair pulling.[37] These data are preliminary but could indicate a genetic component in trichotillomania. Some of these genes have also been identified in other forms of obsessive-compulsive behavior.[38]

Clinical presentation
There is sudden onset of patchy hair loss with hairs of different lengths and often in geometric patterns. It can involve upper eyelashes, eyebrows, and pubic hair, in addition to scalp hair (see **Fig. 5**).

Differential diagnosis
AA and tinea capitis are the main diagnostic considerations. Usually with trichotillomania there are broken hairs of many lengths and regrowing hairs are coarse in contrast to AA whereby hairs are fine and light in color. In contrast to tinea capitis, there is little redness or scale with trichotillomania. Recurrent picking can lead to superficial bacterial infections, so this can complicate the picture.

Diagnostic considerations
The diagnosis can be difficult because many children are unaware or ashamed of the hair pulling behavior, and there are often problems with family denial or ignorance of

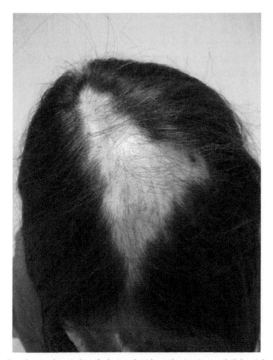

Fig. 5. Geometrically shaped patch of short, broken hairs in a child with trichotillomania.

the hair pulling. An accepting environment is critical to make the child and parent aware of the condition. In this condition, a hair pull test is negative. Dermoscopy can show broken hairs and flame hairs (hairs that show they have been stretched to point of breaking) and can be a tool to build the case for this diagnosis to the family.

Therapeutics

In preschool-aged children, management is conservative. Making the caregiver aware of the diagnosis and gently reminding children if the behavior is observed is usually sufficient. In most cases, it resolves within months. In preadolescents, teenagers, and adults, therapy usually involves behavioral therapy. Habit reversal training or acceptance and commitment training with the guidance of a psychologist/psychiatrist have been shown to be very effective but are intensive therapies.[39] Skilled therapists are sometime difficult to locate. In some studies, selective serotonin reuptake inhibitors and tricyclic antidepressants show improvement in symptoms, but overall the data for these agents in children are mixed. Anecdotal evidence and limited studies show N-acetylcysteine may be helpful in teenage and adult patients. One study in younger children did not show any benefit. From 600 mg to 1200 mg of N-acetylcysteine twice a day has been used. Support groups are often very helpful, especially for teenage patients.[40,41]

Prognosis

For preschool children, the hair pulling behavior usually resolves. In preadolescents, adolescents, and adults, it is often chronic and for some indicates a secondary underlying psychiatric disorder.

SUMMARY

Identifying and treating alopecia in children requires the astute clinician to differentiate between the common types of hair loss using a thorough history, review of systems, and systematic hair and scalp examination coupled with a comprehensive skin examination. Additionally, the ability to counsel patients and parents about the prognosis and treatment reduces anxiety.

REFERENCES

1. Paus R. Principles of hair cycle control. J Dermatol 1998;25(12):793–802.
2. Janniger CK, Bryngil JM. Hair in infancy and childhood. Cutis 1993;51(5):336–8.
3. Dhurat R, Saraogi P. Hair evaluation methods: merits and demerits. Int J Trichology 2009;1(2):108–19.
4. Mirmirani P, Tucker LY. Epidemiologic trends in pediatric tinea capitis: a population-based study from Kaiser Permanente Northern California. J Am Acad Dermatol 2013;69(6):916–21.
5. Higgins EM, Fuller LC, Smith CH. Guidelines for the management of tinea capitis. Br J Dermatol 2000;143:53–8.
6. Moriarty B, Hay R, Morris-Jones R. The diagnosis and management of tinea. BMJ 2012;345:e4380.
7. Trovato MJ, Schwartz RA, Janniger CK. Tinea capitis: current concepts in clinical practice. Cutis 2006;77(2):93–9.
8. Michaels BD, Del Rosso JQ. Tinea capitis in infants: recognition, evaluation and management suggestions. J Clin Aesthet Dermatol 2012;5(2):49–59.
9. Friedlander SF, Pickering B, Cunningham BB, et al. Use of the cotton swab method in diagnosing tinea capitis. Pediatrics 1999;104(2 Pt 1):276–9.

10. Friedlander SF, Aly R, Krafchik B, et al. Terbinafine in the treatment of Trichophyton tinea capitis: a randomized, double-blind, parallel-group, duration-finding study. Pediatrics 2002;109(4):602–7.
11. Gonzalez U, Seaton T, Bergus G, et al. Systemic antifungal therapy for tinea capitis in children. Cochrane Database Syst Rev 2009;17(4):CD004685.
12. Gupta AK, Cooper EA, Bowen JE. Meta-analysis: griseofulvin efficacy in the treatment of tinea capitis. J Drugs Dermatol 2008;7(4):369–72.
13. Fleece D, Gaughan JP, Aronoff SC. Griseofulvin versus terbinafine in the treatment of tinea capitis: a meta-analysis of randomized, clinical trials. Pediatrics 2004;114(5):1312–5.
14. Alkhalifah A, Alsantali A, Wang E, et al. Alopecia areata update: part II. Treatment. J Am Acad Dermatol 2010;62(2):191–202.
15. Mukherjee N, Burkhart CN, Morrell DS. Treatment of alopecia areata in children. Pediatr Ann 2009;38(7):388–95.
16. Petukhova L, Cabral RM, Mackay-Wiggin J, et al. The genetics of alopecia areata: what's new and how will it help our patients? Dermatol Ther 2011;24(3):326–36.
17. Petukhova L, Duvic M, Hordinsky M, et al. Genome-wide association study in alopecia areata implicates both innate and adaptive immunity. Nature 2010; 466(7302):113–7.
18. MacDonald Hull SP, Wood ML, Hutchinson PE, et al. Guidelines for the management of alopecia areata. Br J Dermatol 2003;149:692–9.
19. Das S, Ghorami RC, Chatterjee T, et al. Comparative assessment of topical steroids, topical tretinoin (0.05%) and dithranol paste in alopecia areata. Indian J Dermatol 2010;55:148–9.
20. Tosti A, Piraccini BM, Pazzaglia M, et al. Clobetasol propionate 0.05% under occlusion in the treatment of alopecia totalis/universalis. J Am Acad Dermatol 2003; 49:96–8.
21. Rigopoulos D, Gregoriou S, Korfitis C, et al. Lack of response of alopecia areata to pimecrolimus cream. Clin Exp Dermatol 2007;32:456–7.
22. Fiedler-Weiss VC, Buys CM. Evaluation of anthralin in the treatment of alopecia areata. Arch Dermatol 1987;123:1491–3.
23. Rokhsar CK, Shupack JL, Vafai JJ, et al. Efficacy of topical sensitizers in the treatment of alopecia areata. J Am Acad Dermatol 1998;39:751–61.
24. Sharma VK. Pulsed administration of corticosteroids in the treatment of alopecia areata. Int J Dermatol 1996;35:133–6.
25. Royer M, Bodemer C, Vabres P, et al. Efficacy and tolerability of methotrexate in severe childhood alopecia areata. Br J Dermatol 2011;165:407–10.
26. Strober BE, Siu K, Alexis AF, et al. Etanercept does not effectively treat moderate to severe alopecia areata: an open-label study. J Am Acad Dermatol 2005;52: 1082–4.
27. Roseborough I, Lee H, Chwalek J, et al. Lack of efficacy of topical latanoprost and bimatoprost ophthalmic solutions in promoting eyelash growth in patients with alopecia areata. J Am Acad Dermatol 2009;60:705–6.
28. Olsen EA, Carson SC, Turney EA. Systemic steroids with or without 2% topical minoxidil in the treatment of alopecia areata. Arch Dermatol 1992;128:1467–73.
29. Rodnet IJ, Onwudiwe OC, Callender VD, et al. Hair and scalp disorders in ethnic populations. J Drugs Dermatol 2013;12(4):420–7.
30. Samrao A, Price VH, Zedek D, et al. The "Fringe Sign"- a useful clinical finding in traction alopecia of the marginal hair line. Dermatol Online J 2011;17(11):1.
31. Headington JT. Telogen effluvium. New concepts and review. Arch Dermatol 1993;129(3):356–63.

32. Bedocs LA, Bruckner AL. Adolescent hair loss. Curr Opin Pediatr 2008;20(4): 431–5.
33. Trost LB, Bergfeld WF, Calogeras E. The diagnosis and treatment of iron deficiency and its potential relationship to hair loss. J Am Acad Dermatol 2006; 54(5):824–44.
34. Bardelli A, Rebora A. Telogen effluvium and minoxidil. J Am Acad Dermatol 1989; 21(3):572–3.
35. Huynh M, Gavino AC, Magid M. Trichotillomania. Semin Cutan Med Surg 2013; 32(2):88–94.
36. Panza KE, Pittenger C, Bloch MH. Age and gender correlates of pulling in pediatric trichotillomania. J Am Acad Child Adolesc Psychiatry 2013;52(3):241–9.
37. Chattopadhyay K. The genetic factors influencing the development of trichotillomania. J Genet 2012;91(2):259–62.
38. Gupta MA. Emotional regulation, dissociation, and the self-induced dermatoses: clinical features and implications for treatment with mood stabilizers. Clin Dermatol 2013;31(1):3–10.
39. Sarah HM, Hanam FZ, Hilary ED, et al. Habit reversal training in trichotillomania: guide for the clinician. Expert Rev Neurother 2013;13(9):1069–77.
40. Rodrigues-Barata AR, Tosti A, Rodriguez-Pichardo A, et al. N-Acetylcysteine in the treatment of trichotillomania. Int J Trichology 2012;4(3):176–8.
41. Bloch MH, Panza KE, Grant JE, et al. N-acetylcysteine in the treatment of pediatric trichotillomania: a randomized, double-blind, placebo-controlled add on trial. J Am Acad Child Adolesc Psychiatry 2013;52(3):231–40.

Superficial Fungal Infections in Children

Danielle M. Hawkins, MD*, Aimee C. Smidt, MD

KEYWORDS

• Tinea • Dermatophyte • Ringworm • Athlete's foot • Onychomycosis

KEY POINTS

- Dermatophyte infections are common in the pediatric population.
- Tinea infections are named by their anatomic location on the body.
- Dermatophyte infections are most often caused by *Trichophyton, Microsporum*, or *Epidermophyton* species.
- Most infections can be treated with topical therapy, with important exceptions being the face, scalp, and nails.

INTRODUCTION

Superficial fungal infections (mycoses) are caused by specific organisms with the ability to invade and proliferate in keratin-containing layers of the hair, skin, and nails. They are relatively common in the pediatric population. Some organisms induce little host response (such as *Malassezia*, the causative organism of tinea versicolor), whereas others (the dermatophytes) can lead to marked inflammation (tinea infections). Typical dermatophytes are members of 3 common genera: *Trichophyton, Microsporum*, and *Epidermophyton*.[1] The prevalence of certain dermatophytes can vary based on geographic location, whereas others exist worldwide. Infection can be acquired by contact with infected humans (anthrophilic), animals (zoophilic), or soil (geophilic).

Tinea infections are classified by their location on the body (**Table 1**). Dermatophytoses occur more commonly in children than adults, particularly tinea capitis. Although human immunodeficiency virus infection and immunosuppression can put patients at higher risk and can cause more severe infections, most affected children are healthy without underlying immunodeficiency. Superficial mycoses do not usually penetrate deeper than the superficial layers of skin, hair, and nails, but can lead to significant morbidity because of symptoms, concern for transmission, associated

Disclosures: None.
Department of Dermatology, University of New Mexico, 1021 Medical Arts Avenue Northeast, Albuquerque, NM 87131, USA
* Corresponding author.
E-mail address: dmhawkins@salud.unm.edu

Pediatr Clin N Am 61 (2014) 443–455
http://dx.doi.org/10.1016/j.pcl.2013.12.003   **pediatric.theclinics.com**
0031-3955/14/$ – see front matter © 2014 Elsevier Inc. All rights reserved.

Table 1
Classification of tinea infections based on anatomic location

Diagnosis	Location
Tinea corporis	Body
Tinea pedis	Foot
Tinea cruris	Groin
Tinea manuum	Hand
Tinea faciei	Face
Tinea capitis	Scalp
Tinea unguium (onychomycosis)	Nail

superinfections, and id reactions (discussed later). In this article, the most common manifestations of dermatophyte infections in children are first described, including diagnostic and treatment algorithms and associated phenomena. Clinical presentation and treatment options of superficial skin infections caused by noninflammatory fungal organisms, such as *Malassezia*, are also described.

INFECTION OF THE SKIN (TINEA)
Clinical Features

Tinea corporis
Tinea corporis refers to a dermatophyte infection of the skin on the trunk or extremities, with the exception of the palms or soles. It typically involves exposed areas, but can occur anywhere on the body. Worldwide, the most common causative agents are *Trichophyton rubrum* and *Trichophyton mentagrophytes.* Dermatophytes can be acquired from pets, or other animals, usually producing an inflammatory reaction. Close contact during sports, especially wrestling, can also spread organisms. Tinea corporis usually presents as an itchy, erythematous, classically annular plaque of varying size with active peripheral leading scale and central clearing (**Fig. 1**). Pustules may also be present. The amount of scale can be variable, especially if previously treated by topical corticosteroids, which suppress the host's local inflammatory response (so-called tinea incognito). Differential diagnosis includes nummular dermatitis and psoriasis, both of which are generally more diffusely distributed and are scaly

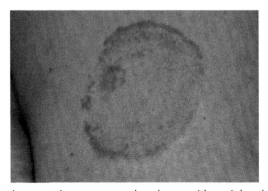

Fig. 1. Tinea corporis presenting as an annular plaque with peripheral leading scale and central clearing.

throughout the lesions. Granuloma annulare can mimic tinea corporis but is character-ized by an annular array of dermal, sometimes shiny papules without appreciable scale, often with a dusky or violaceous center, and is usually asymptomatic. A more complete differential diagnosis is presented in **Table 2**.

Clinical variants of tinea corporis: tinea profunda and Majocchi granuloma

Majocchi granuloma, typically caused by *Trichophyton rubrum*, is a dermatophyte infection involving the hair follicles on the body. An important clinical clue is the pres-ence of follicular-based pustules or granulomatous nodules (**Fig. 2**). It commonly occurs on the lower legs, especially in young women who shave, but can occur any-where that bears hair. It may also be propagated by the use of topical steroids. Tinea profunda is analogous to kerion of the scalp, with a robust inflammatory response to dermatophyte infection, leading to boggy, inflamed cutaneous plaques that can develop secondary abscesses.

Tinea pedis

Tinea pedis, or athlete's foot, commonly presents in adolescents but is rare in prepu-bertal children. Occlusive footwear (promoting a warm, moist environment) can pre-dispose patients to the development of fungal infection. Causative organisms also can be shed and transmitted on the floors of locker rooms, swimming pools, and households. There are 4 main clinical presentations: moccasin, interdigital, inflamma-tory, and ulcerative. The interdigital type is most common and consists of erythema, scaling, and maceration in the web spaces. The ulcerative subtype also has an inter-digital distribution, with more severe erosions and ulcers. Diffuse erythema and scaling of the plantar surfaces of the feet characterize the moccasin type (**Fig. 3**). In-flammatory tinea pedis (often acquired from animals) presents with vesicles, pustules, and blisters on the medial foot. All types can be pruritic, although subclinical disease is also possible. Tinea pedis can also be complicated by bacterial superinfection/impe-tiginization or cellulitis, and therefore treatment in the immunocompromised popula-tion is especially important.

Causative organisms include *Trichophyton rubrum*, *Trichophyton mentagrophytes*, and *Epidermophyton floccosum*. *Trichophyton tonsurans* is an especially common pathogen in children compared with adults.

Table 2
Differential diagnoses for tinea infections based on anatomic location

Tinea Corporis	Tinea Pedis	Tinea Cruris	Tinea Manuum	Tinea Faciei	Tinea Barbae
Granuloma annulare	Dyshidrotic eczema	Candidal intertrigo	Contact dermatitis	Granuloma annulare	Acne
Cutaneous lupus erythematosus	Contact dermatitis	Contact dermatitis	Dyshidrotic eczema	Cutaneous lupus erythematosus	Folliculitis
Atopic or nummular dermatitis	Bacterial or candidal infection	Psoriasis	Atopic dermatitis	Rosacea	Contact dermatitis
Pityriasis rosea	Psoriasis		Psoriasis	Sarcoidosis	Herpes zoster
Psoriasis	Pitted keratolysis			Seborrheic dermatitis	Herpes simplex
				Perioral dermatitis	Dental sinus tracts
				Atopic or nummular dermatitis	

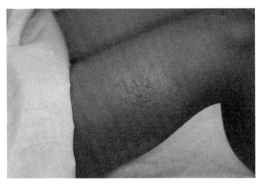

Fig. 2. Majocchi granuloma showing follicular-based pustules and granulomatous nodules.

Tinea cruris

Tinea cruris, also referred to as jock itch, is a superficial dermatophyte infection of the groin. It can occur in both sexes but is more frequent in males; in the pediatric population, it is most common in teenage boys. It often occurs in conjunction with tinea pedis, because the fungus is autologously spread upwards while putting on pants and undergarments. Other risk factors include both obesity and excessive sweating or participation in athletics, caused by the warm, moist environment this creates. Like tinea pedis, the most common causative organisms include *Trichophyton rubrum, Trichophyton mentagrophytes,* and *Epidermophyton floccosum.* Tinea cruris usually presents with erythematous to reddish-brown patches or thin plaques, with scaling and sharply demarcated borders. Pruritus is common. Unlike candidal intertrigo or psoriasis, tinea cruris generally spares the scrotum.

Tinea manuum

Tinea manuum is uncommon in childhood. It usually has a unilateral presentation and may occur in conjunction with tinea pedis in a 1 hand, 2 feet distribution. Onychomycosis/nail involvement of the affected hand may be a clue. It typically presents as mild erythema and diffuse scaling of the palmar surface of the hand, which may or may not be pruritic. Similar to tinea pedis, inflammatory dermatoses (such as dermatitis or psoriasis) may also be considered in the differential diagnosis (see **Table 2**).

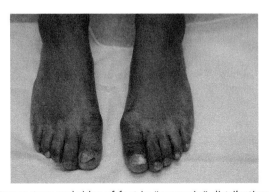

Fig. 3. Scaling between toes and sides of feet in "moccasin" distribution.

Tinea faciei

Tinea faciei is a dermatophyte infection of the face. Its presentation is similar to tinea corporis with erythematous annular plaques with scaly borders, but it can be masked by previous treatment with topical corticosteroids. It commonly begins with small scaly papules that may expand outwards in a ring, and subsequently develop hypopigmentation or hyperpigmentation in the center (**Fig. 4**). Pustules may also occur. The infrequent nature and variable appearance of tinea faciei make it frequently missed, with as many as 70% of patients being initially misdiagnosed with an inflammatory condition such as dermatitis.[2] Incomplete response or persistence/worsening after treatment with topical steroids should raise suspicion for dermatophyte infection.

Variants of tinea faciei

Tinea barbae is a dermatophyte infection of the beard or facial hair seen primarily in adolescent and adult males. Clinically, tinea barbae is characterized by folliculocentric papules, pustules, and possibly nodules. Causative agents typically involve zoophilic species, such as *Trichophyton mentagrophytes* and *Trichophyton verrucosum*.

Diagnostic Recommendations

In-office diagnosis can usually be established with potassium hydroxide (KOH) preparation of scrapings of affected skin; for best results, scraping of the active scale is important, and a glass slide may be used in place of a blade in children. It is helpful to inquire about history of previous treatments, because topical steroids may increase the number of organisms seen on KOH preparation, whereas recent use of topical antifungals may decrease organism load. Fungal cultures can be obtained safely in children by firm scraping of scale or hair with a disposable toothbrush, cytobrush, or sterile cotton swab, all of which should be premoistened with transport medium or tap water. Cultures may confirm the diagnosis but often take several weeks to grow and have a lower sensitivity than KOH preparation.[3] Sabouraud dextrose agar, Mycosel agar with chloramphenicol and cyclohexamide, and dermatophyte test medium are commonly used culture media; typical bacterial culture medium is not adequate. Infrequently, culture may return with a nondermatophyte mold, which usually represents contaminant (unless the patient is immunosuppressed). When a deeper infection (eg, tinea profunda, Majocchi granuloma) is in question, tissue biopsy for fungal culture may be necessary to aid in the definitive diagnosis.

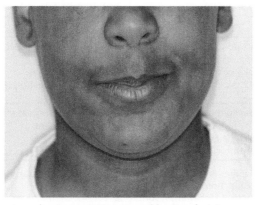

Fig. 4. Post-inflammatory dyspigmentation caused by tine faciei.

Therapeutic Recommendations

In most cases, topical antifungals are effective in treating tinea corporis and other superficial dermatophyte infections in non–hair-bearing areas. Prescription examples include ketoconazole, econazole, oxiconazole, sulconazole, clotrimazole, terbinafine, ciclopirox, and butenafine. Clotrimazole, terbinafine, miconazole, and tolnaftate are available over the counter. Nystatin is not effective for dermatophyte infections, and is primarily effective against *Candida* species. Topical medications are available in various vehicles, including creams, gels, sprays, and powders, and should be chosen based on ease of use for the anatomic location being treated. Medication should be applied to the affected area and 1 to 2 cm outward twice daily until resolved; some investigators advocate treating several days beyond clinical resolution. Because of their deeper/follicular involvement, tinea faciei, Majocchi granuloma, tinea barbae, and extensive or resistant infections generally require systemic therapy, such as oral terbinafine, fluconazole, or itraconazole (**Table 3** outlines recommended dosing regimens). Measures to prevent recurrence include concomitant treatment of any coexisting tinea pedis and proper foot hygiene.[4] Recommended hygiene practices include keeping feet clean and dry, wearing breathable cotton socks, avoiding tight-fitting footwear, keeping toenails short, and using separate nail clippers for infected and healthy toenails.

INFECTION OF THE SCALP/HAIR (TINEA CAPITIS)
Introduction

Tinea capitis (ringworm of the scalp) occurs commonly in children and rarely in adults. The estimated prevalence in inner-city school-age children is 3% to 8%.[5] Risk factors

Table 3
Recommended dosing regimens for pediatric tinea capitis

Drug	Recommended Dosing	Monitoring	Available Formulations
Griseofulvin	20–25 mg/kg/d (microsize suspension) x 6–8 wk 10–15 mg/kg/d (ultramicrosize suspension) for 6–8 wk	No monitoring generally necessary	Tablets Liquid
Terbinafine	125 mg (<25 kg) 187.5 mg (25–35 kg) 250 mg (>35 kg) every day × 3–4 wk	Discuss risk-benefit profile with individual patient/family, advise as to signs/symptoms of hepatotoxicity Baseline LFTs and repeat after 1 mo of treatment	Tablets Granules
Fluconazole	6 mg/kg/d for 3–6 wk or 6 mg/kg once weekly for 8–12 wk	Periodic liver function tests (AST/ALT, alkaline phosphatase), renal function tests, electrolytes, CBC, platelets	Tablets Liquid
Itraconazole	3–5 mg/kg/d for 4–6 wk or 5 mg/kg daily for 1 wk each month for 2–3 mo	Baseline LFTs and repeat after 1 mo of treatment	Tablets Liquid

Abbreviations: ALT, alanine aminotransferase; AST, aspartate aminotransferase; CBC, complete blood count; LFTs, liver function tests.

Adapted from Bolognia JL, Schaffer JV, Jorizzo JL, editors. Dermatology. 3rd edition. London: Mosby; 2012.

include crowded living quarters and low socioeconomic status.[6] Transmission can occur by indirect contact with hairs, brushes/combs, headwear, and epithelial cells of an infected person, although transmission from animals is also possible. Adults may be asymptomatic but contagious carriers or may have evidence of tinea infections of the skin instead of hair. *Trichophyton* and *Microsporum* species are the causative organisms. *Trichophyton tonsurans* is the most common cause of tinea capitis in the United States.[7] *Microsporum canis,* the second most common pathogenic organism in the United States, can be transmitted by dogs, cats, and rodents.

Clinical Features

Clinical presentation varies based on the causative organism and on the host immune response. The most common presentation of tinea capitis is a scaly, circumscribed plaque of alopecia with broken hairs resembling black dots (**Fig. 5**). Other presentations can include widespread scaling of the scalp, patchy alopecia, or diffuse pustules (**Table 4**). Wood lamp examination can help identify *Microsporum* species, which emit a bright green fluorescence in a completely dark room. Posterior cervical or occipital lymphadenopathy can be an important clue. When the infection is more advanced or accompanied by a robust immune reaction, a markedly inflamed, boggy plaque with pustules, tenderness and lymphadenopathy can develop (kerion formation).

Differential Diagnosis

Differential diagnosis of tinea capitis can be broad and includes alopecia areata, traction alopecia, trichotillomania, syphilis, Langerhans cell histiocytosis, and inflammatory alopecias such as lichen planopilaris or dissecting folliculitis (rare in children). Seborrheic dermatitis (cradle cap) can produce scaling, erythema, and pruritus of the scalp but is more diffuse compared with the usually focal nature of tinea capitis and it does not generally lead to hair loss. Other inflammatory conditions such as psoriasis, bacterial folliculitis, and impetigo can mimic the kerion presentation. A careful history focused on previous medical conditions, external trauma/manipulation of the scalp, and the presence/absence of affected contacts can help to differentiate these conditions. A detailed skin examination should also be performed to look for manifestations of the other possible conditions (eg, nail pitting in alopecia areata, greasy scale in the ears or body folds for psoriasis and seborrheic dermatitis). Again, posterior cervical, occipital, or postauricular lymphadenopathy is suggestive, although not pathognomonic.[8]

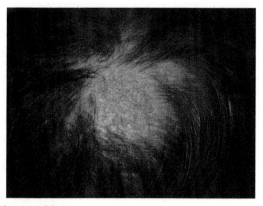

Fig. 5. 'Black dot' tinea capitis.

Table 4
Clinical presentations of dermatophyte infections of the scalp

Presentation	Description
Black dot	Caused by endothrix infection (*Trichophyton tonsurans* most common)
Kerion	Boggy, tender, inflamed hairless plaque Advanced disease with robust host response
Gray patch	More subtle presentation Patchy alopecia with scale ± erythema
Diffuse scale	Widespread scaling of the scalp
Diffuse pustular	Scattered pustules with scale, alopecia, often lymphadenopathy
Favus	Most severe Usually caused by *Trichophyton schoenleinii* Thick yellow crusts (scutula) around hairs

Adapted from Higgins EM, Fuller LC, Smith CH. British Association of Dermatologists. Guidelines for the management of tinea capitis. Br J Dermatol 2000;143(1):53–8; with permission.

Diagnostic Recommendations

As discussed earlier, Wood lamp examination can be helpful to evaluate for *Microsporum* species. Clinical suspicion of tinea capitis should be confirmed by KOH preparation or fungal culture. Scale from the affected area of the scalp should be scraped with a sterile number 15 surgical blade or glass slide for KOH preparation. As discussed earlier, scalp brushings and hairs collected with a dampened swab, cytobrush, or disposable toothbrush can be sent for fungal culture. The presence or absence of fungi can usually be confirmed within a few days, but organism identification by fungal culture may take several weeks. Treatment of clinically obvious cases should not wait for fungal culture confirmation, but therapy may need to be modified to target a specific organism once it is identified.

Therapeutic Recommendations

Systemic antifungals are the mainstay of treatment of all types of tinea capitis, because topical medications alone do not penetrate effectively into the hair follicles. Patients should be reevaluated every 6 weeks to determine need for continued treatment and should show consistent improvement in alopecia, scale, erythema, and inflammation. Therapy should be continued until all signs of inflammation and active hair loss have subsided. In cases of kerion formation, scarring alopecia may be a permanent complication.[9] Oral griseofulvin for a minimum of 6 to 8 weeks remains the treatment of choice for tinea capitis caused by *Microsporum* species in children. The duration of treatment may need to be extended to 3 months or more for more recalcitrant cases. Griseofulvin is generally well tolerated, with rare side effects including headache, abdominal pain, photosensitivity, and cutaneous drug eruptions. Contraindications include porphyrias, pregnancy, and hepatic failure.[10] Terbinafine produces superior cure rates for *Trichophyton* species and may be more effective than griseofulvin in a shorter period.[11] Because *Trichophyton* is a more common pathogen in the United States, many investigators recommend this as first-line therapy for children with tinea capitis. Side effects of terbinafine include headache, and gastrointestinal symptoms; hepatotoxicity is a rare but potentially serious complication. Recommended treatment regimens and laboratory monitoring guidelines are outlined in **Table 3**.

Adjunctive treatment with antifungal shampoos such as ketoconazole 2% or selenium sulfide shampoo is sometimes recommended. Physically cutting the affected hair is not necessary. Any combs/brushes, hats, and headwear should be washed or discarded and sharing of such items among family members discouraged until the infection is fully resolved. Affected siblings or other family members should be treated as well to prevent reinfection.[1]

INFECTION OF THE FINGERNAILS OR TOENAILS (TINEA UNGUIUM OR ONYCHOMYCOSIS)
Introduction

Onychomycosis is the broad category of infections of the nail unit caused by yeasts and molds. Tinea unguium refers to dermatophyte infections of the nail unit. Although the infection is more common in adults, the number of cases in children is increasing.[12] Many affected children have first-degree relatives with onychomycosis or tinea pedis. The most common causative dermatophytes are *Trichophyton rubrum, Trichophyton mentagrophytes,* and *E floccosum.*[10]

Clinical Features

Onychomycosis is generally asymptomatic, but patients may complain of pain or itching of the affected nails or surrounding skin. It most commonly affects the toenails and less so the fingernails. It is rarely symmetric; involvement of all nails points to alternative diagnoses such as nail psoriasis, lichen planus, or trachyonychia, as seen with alopecia areata.[10] Clinically, onychomycosis can be divided into 3 types: distal lateral subungual onychomycosis, proximal subungual onychomycosis, and superficial white onychomycosis.[13] Distal lateral subungual onychomycosis is the most common type seen in children.[14]

Distal lateral subungual mycosis begins with yellow to white discoloration on a corner of the affected nail, which spreads proximally toward the proximal nail fold. Subungual debris causes significant thickening of the nail, which may break off and expose the nail bed. Proximal subungual onychomycosis begins with proximal discoloration, which then spreads distally. Superficial white onychomycosis begins with white, soft areas on the nail plate, which can spread to involve the entire nail.

Differential Diagnosis

Conditions that mimic onychomycosis are listed in **Box 1**. Careful history and skin examination for signs of other conditions (eg, typical psoriatic plaques on elbows and knees or patchy smooth alopecia suggestive of alopecia areata) can assist practitioners in establishing the cause of onychodystrophy. Suspected cases should have laboratory confirmation before initiating treatment (see later discussion).

Box 1
Differential diagnosis for suspected onychomycosis

Psoriasis

Traumatic, medication-induced, or postinfectious onycholysis

Subungual verrucae (warts)

Pachyonychia congenita

Trachyonychia

Chronic paronychia

Graft-versus-host disease

Diagnostic Recommendations

Suspected cases should be confirmed by histopathologic examination or fungal culture to avoid unnecessary exposure to systemic antifungals and their potential side effects. Clippings or curettage of the affected nail(s) for periodic acid-Schiff staining can establish a diagnosis. Fungal culture can identify the causative agent and assist in selecting the appropriate treatment. Samples should be taken from subungual debris, the underside of the nail plate, or clippings of the affected free edge of the nail.

Therapeutic Recommendations

Systemic antifungal therapy is the most effective treatment of onychomycosis as topical medications usually do not adequately penetrate through the nail. The exception is in cases involving a solitary nail not involving the nail matrix (clinically, the lunula, the white half-moon at the cuticle), in which topical ciclopirox can be considered.[4] Ciclopirox solution is painted on the entire affected nail nightly. Patients should be instructed to file the affected nail and remove the medication with nail polish remover once a week until resolved.

Historically, griseofulvin has been the standard recommended treatment in children with onychomycosis; however, it is associated with lower cure rates when used for nail disease compared with other medications. Therefore, current guidelines typically suggest oral terbinafine as first line for this indication.[15] Recommended treatment duration is 6 weeks for fingernails and 3 months for toenails. Recurrence rates are high, and complete cure rates for systemic antifungals are estimated to be 70%.[16] Patients should be educated specifically on recommended foot hygiene practices, as detailed earlier. **Table 5** outlines suggested treatment regimens. Monitoring guidelines are the same for this indication as for tinea capitis, as discussed earlier.

ID REACTIONS

The dermatophytid or id reaction is a diffuse hypersensitivity response to a primary dermatosis elsewhere on the body. This reaction can frequently occur in the setting of a dermatophytosis but may also occur with concomitant allergic contact dermatitis or superficial bacterial infection. The hallmark features of an id reaction include the generalized, symmetric distribution of monomorphic juicy papules (and even, sometimes, vesicles), which can last several weeks or longer. Itching may be severe, but the child is clinically otherwise well.

Table 5
Treatment recommendations for onychomycosis

Medication	Dosing	Duration
Terbinafine	<20 kg: 62.5 mg/d 20–40 kg: 125 mg/d >40 kg: 250 mg/d	6 wk of continuous treatment of fingernails 12 wk of continuous treatment of toenails
Itraconazole	<20 kg: 5 mg/kg/d 20–40 kg: 100 mg/d 40–50 kg: 200 mg/d >50 kg: 200 mg twice a day	Daily for 1 wk per month × 2 mo for fingernails, 3 mo for toenails
Fluconazole	3–6 mg/kg once weekly	12–16 wk for fingernails 18–26 wk for toenails

An id reaction can also occur after initiating systemic antifungal treatment (typically, griseofulvin) and is often misdiagnosed as a drug reaction in this context. In this setting, the antifungal treatment should be continued and the id reaction treated with topical corticosteroids and oral antihistamines for symptomatic relief. Eradication of the fungal infection as the triggering process remains the mainstay of treatment.

PITYRIASIS (TINEA) VERSICOLOR
Introduction

Pityriasis versicolor (also known as tinea versicolor) is a superficial mycosis caused by organisms in the *Malassezia* genus, most commonly *Malassezia globosa, Malassezia sympodialis,* and *Malassezia furfur.*[17] These organisms are naturally found on human skin but cause clinical manifestations when the yeast form transforms to the mycelial form.[1] Risk factors include warm temperatures, high humidity, immunosuppression, malnutrition, oily skin, excessive sweating, and corticosteroid use. It is most common in tropical climates and primarily affects adolescents and young adults. It has been reported in prepubertal children, although in these cases, the possibility of precocious puberty should be explored.[18]

Clinical Features

The most common sites of involvement are the upper trunk and shoulders. Patients have multiple monomorphic, round to oval, sharply demarcated macules, papules, patches, or plaques, with mild scaling and hypopigmentation or hyperpigmentation, hence the name versicolor (**Fig. 6**). A pink to red undertone can occur with heat and exercise, and is more prominent in white skin. Sun exposure and darker skin types can predispose to more pronounced dyspigmentation.

Differential Diagnosis

Please refer to **Box 2** for differential diagnosis.

Diagnostic Recommendations

KOH preparation of scrapings of affected skin shows short fungal hyphae and spores in clusters resembling spaghetti and meatballs. Fungal culture usually is not helpful because *Malassezia furfur* is a component of normal skin flora; therefore, diagnosis

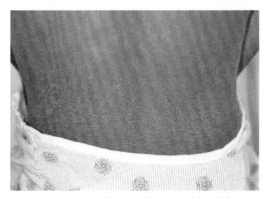

Fig. 6. Pityriasis versicolor showing patches or plaques with mild scaling.

> **Box 2**
> **Differential diagnosis of tinea versicolor**
>
> Vitiligo
>
> Pityriasis alba
>
> Postinflammatory dyspigmentation
>
> Pityriasis rosea
>
> Confluent and reticulated papillomatosis
>
> Atopic or nummular dermatitis
>
> Cutaneous T-cell lymphoma (mycosis fungoides)

is usually made on clinical grounds. Biopsy is usually not necessary, unless the eruption is not responding to typical treatment.[10]

Therapeutic Recommendations

Tinea versicolor can be treated with topical selenium sulfide or ketoconazole as a shampoo or a cream preparation. The shampoo should be left on the affected areas for 10 to 15 minutes before rinsing to obtain maximal benefit. Systemic therapy may be indicated for widespread or recalcitrant disease. Fluconazole or itraconazole administered as a single dose is effective (**Box 3**). Oral ketoconazole, previously a treatment of choice for tinea versicolor, is no longer recommended as first line for dermatophyte or candidal infections because of its potential to cause life-threatening hepatotoxicity (http://www.fda.gov/Drugs/DrugSafety/ucm362415.htm). If prescribed for short-term use (which may limit risk overall), the dose should be taken followed by exertional physical activity leading to sweating, which causes secretion of the drug into the sweat glands. Sweat should be allowed to evaporate and showering delayed for at least several hours to keep the medication on the skin. The dose can be repeated after 7 days. Topical medications can be used for adjunctive/preventative purposes, because recurrence is common.

> **Box 3**
> **Treatment of tinea versicolor**
>
> *Suggested treatment regimens for tinea versicolor*
>
> Topical
>
>   Ketoconazole 2% shampoo: daily application for 3 days; can use 2 to 3 times/wk for maintenance/prevention
>
>   Selenium sulfide 2.5% shampoo: daily application while bathing for 1 to 2 weeks, can use 2 to 3 times/wk for maintenance/prevention
>
> Systemic
>
>   Fluconazole: 300 mg single dose; repeat 14 days after initial dose
>
>   Itraconazole: 400 mg single dose or 200 mg daily for 7 days
>
> *Data from* Paller AS, Mancini AJ. Hurwitz's pediatric dermatology. 4th edition. London: Elsevier; 2011.

SUMMARY

Superficial fungal infections are common in children and adolescents in the United States and worldwide and are usually caused by dermatophyte species, which lead to a host inflammatory response. Tinea infections are classified by anatomic location on the body and can often be treated with topical agents (with some important exceptions). Infection of the face, scalp, and nails usually warrants systemic therapy. Awareness of risk factors for infection, causative organisms, and clinical presentations is paramount to recognizing superficial fungal infections. Appropriate timely diagnosis and effective treatment practices can decrease morbidity, prevent further transmission, and positively affect patients' quality of life.

REFERENCES

1. Elewski BE, Hughey LC, Sobera JO, et al. Fungal diseases. In: Bolognia JL, Jorizzo JL, Schaffer JV, editors. Dermatology. 3rd edition. London: Mosby; 2012.
2. Shapiro L, Cohen HJ. Tinea faciei simulating other dermatoses. J Am Med Assoc 1971;217:828.
3. Karimzadegan-Nia M, Mir-Amin-Mohammadi A, Bouzari N, et al. Comparison of direct smear, culture and histology for the diagnosis of onychomycosis. Australas J Dermatol 2007;48(1):18–21.
4. Friedlander SF, Chan YC, Chan YH, et al. Onychomycosis does not always require systemic treatment for cure: a trial using topical therapy. Pediatr Dermatol 2013;30:316–22. http://dx.doi.org/10.1111/pde.12064.
5. Lorch Dauk KC, Comrov E, Blumer JL, et al. Tinea capitis: predictive value of symptoms and time to cure with griseofulvin treatment. Clin Pediatr (Phila) 2010;49(3):280–6.
6. Elewski BE. Tinea capitis: a current perspective. J Am Acad Dermatol 2000;42:1–20.
7. Seebacher C, Bouchara JP, Mignon B. Updates on the epidemiology of dermatophyte infections. Mycopathologia 2008;166(5–6):335–52.
8. Hubbard TW. The predictive value of symptoms in diagnosing childhood tinea capitis. Arch Pediatr Adolesc Med 1999;153(11):1152.
9. Pride HB, Tollefson M, Silverman R. What's new in pediatric dermatology? part II. Treatment. J Am Acad Dermatol 2013;68(6):899.e1–11.
10. Paller AS, Mancini AJ. Hurwitz's pediatric dermatology. 4th edition. London: Elsevier; 2011.
11. Gupta AK, Drummond-Main C. Meta-analysis of randomized, controlled trials comparing particular doses of griseofulvin and terbinafine for the treatment of tinea capitis. Pediatr Dermatol 2013;30:1–6.
12. Gupta AK, Skinner AR. Onychomycosis in children: a brief overview with treatment strategies. Pediatr Dermatol 2004;21:74–9.
13. Zaias N. Onychomycosis. Arch Dermatol 1972;105:263–74.
14. Gupta AK, Sibbald G, Lynde CW, et al. Onychomycosis in children: prevalence and treatment strategies. J Am Acad Dermatol 1997;36:395–402.
15. Baran R, Hay RJ, Garduno JI. Review of antifungal therapy, part II: treatment rationale, including specific patient populations. J Dermatolog Treat 2008;19(3):168–75.
16. Gupta AK, Paquet M. Systemic antifungals to treat onychomycosis in children: a systematic review. Pediatr Dermatol 2013;30:294–302. http://dx.doi.org/10.1111/pde.12048.
17. Prohic A, Ozegovic L. Malassezia species isolated from lesional and non-lesional skin in patients with pityriasis versicolor. Mycoses 2007;50:58–63.
18. Jena DK, Sengupta S, Dwari BC, et al. Pityriasis versicolor in the pediatric age group. Indian J Dermatol Venereol Leprol 2005;71:259–61.

Cutaneous Bacterial Infections Caused by *Staphylococcus aureus* and *Streptococcus pyogenes* in Infants and Children

Beatriz Larru, MD, PhD, Jeffrey S. Gerber, MD, PhD*

KEYWORDS

- Skin and soft tissue infection • *Staphylococcus aureus* • *Streptococcus pyogenes*
- MRSA • Cellulitis • Abscess

KEY POINTS

- Purulent lesions (eg, abscesses) are generally caused by *Staphylococcus aureus*; nonpurulent infections (eg, cellulitis, erysipelas) are usually caused by *Streptococcus pyogenes*.
- The increase in skin and skin structure infection (SSSI) rates is largely attributed to the emergence of methicillin-resistant *S aureus*.
- Careful history and examination and close clinical monitoring are needed to identify severe infections or uncommon causes.
- Antibiotics are often unnecessary for management of uncomplicated skin abscesses if incision and drainage are performed.
- Blood cultures are rarely helpful for uncomplicated infections. Their yield is higher in severe disease and can help with antibiotic selection.
- Management of SSSI should target the most likely organism(s) and minimize both the spectrum and duration of antibiotic therapy.

INTRODUCTION

Acute skin and skin structure infections (SSSIs) are among the most common bacterial infections in children. SSSIs account for nearly 25% of pediatric clinical encounters, most occurring in the outpatient office or emergency department (ED).[1–4]

SSSIs represent a wide spectrum of disease severity, from impetigo to necrotizing fasciitis. Prompt recognition coupled with timely and judicious antimicrobial use

Disclosure of Funding: None.
Division of Infectious Diseases, The Children's Hospital of Philadelphia, Perelman School of Medicine, University of Pennsylvania, 3615 Civic Center Boulevard, Philadelphia, PA 19104-4318, USA
* Corresponding author. Center for Pediatric Clinical Effectiveness, The Children's Hospital of Philadelphia, 3535 Market Street, Philadelphia, PA 19104.
E-mail address: gerberj@email.chop.edu

Pediatr Clin N Am 61 (2014) 457–478
http://dx.doi.org/10.1016/j.pcl.2013.12.004   pediatric.theclinics.com
0031-3955/14/$ – see front matter © 2014 Elsevier Inc. All rights reserved.

optimizes patient outcomes and minimizes the occurrence of adverse drug effects and the emergence of antimicrobial resistance.[5,6]

Because specimens for culture are not obtained for many SSSIs, treatment is often empiric and chosen based on the clinical presentation (eg, erysipelas vs abscess) and local microbial epidemiology.[7-10] *Staphylococcus aureus* and *Streptococcus pyogenes* are the most common causes of community-onset SSSI.[11-16]

This article describes the epidemiology, clinical presentation, and management of common cutaneous bacterial infections most often caused by *S aureus* and *S pyogenes* in children.

CURRENT EPIDEMIOLOGY OF *S AUREUS* AND *S PYOGENES*
S aureus

S aureus is the most common culture-confirmed pathogen from SSSIs in the United States.[17-20] *S aureus* has a propensity to cause abscesses in any tissue/organ, most commonly the skin. Approximately 25% to 40% of the US children and adults are permanently colonized or are transient carriers of *S aureus*. Children presenting with purulent SSSIs have a high rate of *S aureus* nasal colonization.[21-24] The medical burden of SSSIs, particularly abscesses, has increased nationwide since the emergence of community-acquired (CA) methicillin-resistant *S aureus* (MRSA).[25-30] This seems to be driven by additional MRSA cases as opposed to replacement of methicillin-sensitive *S aureus* (MSSA) with MRSA.[31,32] In the United States, the predominant clone is USA300, which has now spread from the community into hospitals.[33,34] US pediatric hospital admissions for SSSIs doubled (0.46% vs 1.01%) from 1997 to 2009, elevating SSSIs from the 21st most common pediatric discharge in 1997 to ninth most common in 2009.[35,36] ED visits for SSSIs have also increased, from 1.2 million visits in 1993 to 3.4 million in 2005.[4,37,38]

S pyogenes

Just as *S aureus* represents the dominant cause of cutaneous abscesses, *S pyogenes* causes most nonpurulent SSSIs, such as cellulitis or erysipelas. Infections with *S pyogenes* are frequent in daily practice but often underrepresented in epidemiologic studies because mild or superficial streptococcal cellulitis is often managed in the outpatient setting without culture confirmation.[37,39] According to the SENTRY antimicrobial surveillance program (covering both the United States and Canada), beta-hemolytic *Streptococcus* represents the seventh most common cause (4.1% of isolates) of SSSI in the United States (*S aureus* accounted for 44.6% of isolates, 35.9% of which were MRSA).[1,26] However, since the 1980s, severe *S pyogenes* necrotizing fasciitis has been increasingly reported in the United States and worldwide.[5,27]

PATHOGENESIS OF SSSI

The main determinant of cutaneous infection is the balance between the virulence of the organism and the host defense. For example, compromised cutaneous barrier function, such as in patients with chronic dermatitis or in premature infants, or immune compromising states, such as children undergoing cancer chemotherapy, can heighten the risk and severity of SSSI.[7,9,40]

S aureus

CA-MRSA is not a single microbiological entity but the term for a collection of *S aureus* clones containing the mobile genetic element, staphylococcal chromosome cassette (SSC) carrying the gene (*mecA*) encoding an altered penicillin binding protein conferring resistance to methicillin and antistaphylococcal β-lactams.[11,41] CA-MRSA also commonly contains the *lukS-PV* and *lukF-PV* genes encoding the Panton-Valentine leukocidin (PVL), a pore-forming toxin associated with deep-seated tissue infection and necrotizing pneumonia. PVL is found less commonly among HA-MRSA or MSSA strains, and might contribute to disease pathogenesis.[21,23,24,42]

S pyogenes

S pyogenes (group A *Streptococcus*) is distinguished from other beta-hemolytic streptococci by its carbohydrate cell wall antigens. Subtypes of *S pyogenes* can be distinguished by the M protein antigens (encoded by the *emm* gene) in its cell wall, which serve as virulence factors. Most cases of *S pyogenes* SSSI are caused by strains producing at least one streptococcal pyrogenic exotoxin (A, B, or C).[25,42,43] Despite these known virulence factors, the wide spectrum of disease severity associated with *S pyogenes* suggests that differences in host defense mechanisms likely play a major role in the development of invasive disease.[5,25,41]

CLINICAL AND DIAGNOSTIC APPROACH

Infections of the skin and soft tissues can be broadly classified based on the extent of tissue involvement and the specific anatomic site of infection. Superficial infections involve the epidermis, the dermis, or both. Deep infections involve the hypodermis, fascia, and muscle. Superficial infections usually evolve from local spread of organisms, typically without systemic symptoms; less commonly, small, superficial infections can elicit a robust systemic response caused by elaboration of toxins. Deeper infections tend to arise by the hematogenous spread of organisms from a distant site.[6,35,44] SSSIs can also be classified as uncomplicated or complicated, based on the severity of illness and the vulnerability of the host. However, this division is artificial and subjective because of the spectrum of SSSI presentations and patient comorbidities.[37,38,43]

Although the cause of SSSI is often elusive, this article focuses on SSSIs typically caused by *S aureus* or *S pyogenes* (**Table 1**). Obtaining a detailed history, including the epidemiologic setting and immune status of the child, is key to refining the differential diagnosis and appropriate index of suspicion for specific causal agents (**Fig. 1**).[25,37,45]

Cutaneous Abscess

Cutaneous abscesses are localized collections of pus in cavities formed by necrosis or disintegration of tissue within the dermis and subcutaneous fat. They are painful, tender nodules progressing to fluctuant protruding pustules, often surrounded by a rim of erythematous swelling. Buttock abscesses are most frequently encountered in preschool children, whereas extremity abscesses are most frequently found in older children.[26,44,46] *S aureus*, especially CA-MRSA, is now the most common cause of cutaneous abscesses in the United States.[27,47]

Folliculitis, Furuncles, and Carbuncles

Folliculitis results from inflammation of hair follicles, manifesting as clusters of small erythematous papules or pustules.[39,40,48] Inflammation is superficial and pus is only present in the epidermis. The sites most commonly affected include the scalp, extremities, and perioral and paranasal regions, as well as areas of the skin that are occluded or prone to moisture and friction, such as the axillae or medial thighs.[41,49] Sycosis barbae is a severe, painful, deep, recurrent form of facial folliculitis caused by *S aureus*

Table 1
Causes of SSSI

Disease	Key Features	Most Common Causes	Less Common Causes[a]/Other Considerations
Abscess	Discrete collection of pus surrounded by a fibrinoid wall within the dermis and subcutaneous tissues	MRSA, MSSA, *S pyogenes* less common	Enterobacteriaceae, anaerobes, *Pseudomonas* spp, *Mycobacterium* spp
Folliculitis	Papular/pustular inflammation of the hair follicle within the epidermis	MRSA, MSSA	*Pseudomonas* spp (hot-tub folliculitis), *Malassezia* spp, *Klebsiella* spp, *Enterobacter* spp, *Escherichia coli*, *Proteus* spp
Furuncle	Painful, firm/fluctuant lesion originating from a hair follicle extending through the dermis	MRSA, MSSA	Consider underlying immunodeficiency (eg, chronic granulomatous diseases, hyper-IgE syndrome) if poorly responsive to appropriate therapy or persistent recurrence
Carbuncle	Organized collection of adjacent furuncles connected by sinus tract with multiple drainage points	MRSA, MSSA	
Impetigo	Large vesicles and/or honey-crusted lesions	Nonbullous: MRSA, MSSA, *S pyogenes* Bullous: MRSA, MSSA	Clinical appearance overlaps with Herpes simplex virus, Varicella-Zoster virus reactivation
Ecthyma	Crusted ulcer penetrating into the dermis with black eschar and elevated margins	MRSA, MSSA, *S pyogenes*	Ecthyma gangrenosum associated with *Pseudomonas aeruginosa* bacteremia
Staphylococcal scalded skin syndrome	Local or generalized skin blistering and exfoliation	MSSA, MRSA	Important to differentiate from Stevens-Johnson syndrome and toxic epidermal necrolysis (more serious conditions involving mucous membranes)
Cellulitis	Painful, erythematous infection of deep skin with poorly demarcated borders	*S pyogenes*, MRSA, MSSA	*Pasteurella* spp, *Capnocytophaga canimorsus* (animal bites), *Aeromonas hydrophila* (freshwater immersion), *Erysipelothrix rhusiopathiae* (fisherman), *Haemophilus influenzae*, *Streptococcus pneumoniae* (periorbital, facial), *Pseudomonas aeruginosa*, *Cryptococcus neoformans* (immunosuppression)

(continued on next page)

Table 1
(continued)

Disease	Key Features	Most Common Causes	Less Common Causes[a]/ Other Considerations
Erysipelas	Superficial inflammation of the dermis with sharply demarcated borders and lymphatic involvement	*S pyogenes*	Group B, C, and G *Streptococcus*
Intertrigo	Erosion of skin in deep skin folds	*S pyogenes*	*Candida albicans*
Paronychia	Inflammation of the soft tissue surrounding the nail bed	MRSA, MSSA, *S pyogenes*	Mixed aerobic and anaerobic flora (*Eikenella corrodens, Bacteroides* spp, *Fusobacterium* spp)
Dactylitis	Inflammation of the distal volar pad of the phalanges	MRSA, MSSA, *S pyogenes*	Group B *Streptococcus* (rarely)
Necrotizing fasciitis	Infection of the deeper layer of the superficial fascia with major destruction of tissue	Type II necrotizing fasciitis: *S pyogenes* MRSA, MSSA	Type I necrotizing fasciitis: mixed flora (anaerobes, GNB, *Enterococcus* spp) Gas gangrene: *Clostridium* spp Anaerobic cellulitis: *Clostridium* spp Meleney synergistic gangrene: MRSA, MSSA, microaerophilic streptococci
Pyomyositis	Acute infection of muscle with abscess formation	MRSA, MSSA	*S pyogenes* (necrotizing myositis), *Clostridium* spp (clostridial myonecrosis)

Abbreviations: GNB, gram-negative bacilli; IgE, immunoglobulin E.

[a] Children and adolescents with immunodeficiency are at higher risk for uncommon causes of SSSI that can have a fulminant course.

Data from Shah S. Pediatric practice infectious diseases. New York: McGraw Hill Professional; 2009.

that occurs mainly in young African American men. Inflammation involves the entire depth of the hair follicle. Painful papules and pustules can coalesce into plaques that recur after healing with scarring.[35,43,50,51]

Furuncles (or boils) result from folliculitis that extends through the dermis into the subcutaneous tissue. Furunculosis is uncommon in early childhood but the incidence increases in adolescents, particularly those living in crowed conditions with poor hygiene. These painful abscesses can occur anywhere on hairy skin, and are most often located on the scalp, buttocks, or extremities. Severe lesions may heal with scarring (**Fig. 2**A).[25,33,43]

Carbuncles consist of groups of furuncles characterized by multiple drainage points and inflammatory changes in the surrounding connective tissue. Carbuncles are commonly found on areas of thickening skin such as the nape of the neck, the back, or the thighs. Fever and systemic symptoms are often present and lesions usually heal with scarring.[42–44]

History: specific exposures, skin trauma, healthcare contact, presence of comorbidities (including immune status)

Physical examination
- Extent and location of erythema, edema, warmth or tenderness
- Presence of fluctuance, purpura, bullae, crepitus, necrosis, systemic signs, lymphangitic spread and depth of infection

Surgical consultation if severe and deep tissue infection is suspected

Laboratory studies
- Uncomplicated, purulent SSSI/abscesses
    - culture pus if available and if etiology/resistance pattern uncertain
- Complicated SSSI, consider:
    - complete blood count with differential
    - basic metabolic panel
    - C-reactive protein
    - creatine phosphokinase
    - blood culture: yield 12.5% in complicated STTI (<1% in uncomplicated STTI)
    - Gram stain and culture of needle aspiration or punch biopsy specimens*
        - punch biopsy higher yield (20% to 30%) than swab/aspiration of non-purulent cellulitis (<10%)
    (*Obtain cultures from skin under a crust or eschar or from an eroded area or vesicle/bullae and not only from pus)

Imaging studies
- Can be helpful to determine the depth of the infection for severe/complicated disease
- Image should never delay surgical evaluation and debridement in critical illness
    - plain radiographs: gas or periosteal elevation/pus
    - ultrasound: abscess
    - CT or MRI to delineate fascial planes for potentially deeper infection

Fig. 1. Approach to the diagnosis of SSSI. (*Adapted from* Rajan S. Skin and soft-tissue infections: classifying and treating a spectrum. Cleve Clin J Med 2012;79(1):57–66.)

Impetigo

Impetigo is a common and highly contagious bacterial infection of the superficial layers of the epidermis. Peak incidence is in children aged 2 to 5 years, although older children may also be affected. It occurs most frequently among economically disadvantaged children in hot and humid regions but is also prevalent in northern climates,

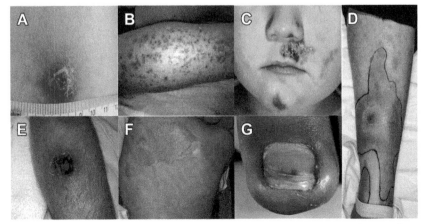

Fig. 2. Common SSSI. (*A*) Furuncle, (*B*) Non-bullous impetigo, (*C*) Impetiginized herpetic lesions, (*D*) Cellulitis, (*E*) Ecthyma, (*F*) Staphylococcal Scalded Skin Syndrome, (*G*) Acute paronychia.

particularly in the summer and late fall. Colonization of skin (S pyogenes) or nares (S aureus) typically precedes the development of impetigo. It usually occurs on exposed areas of the body, such as the face and extremities. Although regional lymphadenitis might occur, systemic symptoms are usually absent.[42,43] Impetigo is most often caused by S aureus and S pyogenes; there are no discerning features distinguishing these organisms. Diagnosis can be confirmed by culture of the base of the lesion after removal of the crust or from the intact bullae (see **Fig. 2**B, C).[25,41,52]

Suppurative complications of streptococcal impetigo are uncommon (2%–5% of cases). Cutaneous infections with nephritogenic strains of S pyogenes are the major antecedent of poststreptococcal glomerulonephritis; however, there are no conclusive data that treatment of streptococcal pyoderma prevents nephritis.[6,44,53] Acute rheumatic fever is not a sequela of impetigo.

Nonbullous impetigo accounts for almost 70% of cases, most commonly on the face and limbs. The predominant overall cause is S aureus, and S pyogenes is particularly unusual in children younger than 2 years of age.[10,43] Lesions begin as papules that rapidly evolve into vesicles surrounded by an area of erythema progressing to the characteristic honey-crusted exudate. Lesions are usually painless and gradually enlarge and break down over a period of 4 to 6 days to form thick crusts. If left untreated the lesions heal slowly, resolving in approximately 2 weeks without scaring.[25,45,54]

Bullous impetigo can appear as clusters of bullae or as a solitary, exudative lesion. Bullous impetigo is caused by toxin-producing strains of S aureus, usually from a strain producing exfoliative exotoxin A and B, which can be isolated from bullous lesions. At first, superficial vesicles rapidly enlarge to form flaccid bullae filled with clear yellow fluid, which can darken to become turbid and sometimes purulent. Lesions often coalesce to form large, reddish plaques, particularly around the oronasal orifices. Bullae may rupture, often leaving a thin brown crust resembling lacquer. Constitutional symptoms are more likely to occur than with nonbullous impetigo.[44,46,49,55]

Cellulitis

Cellulitis is an acute infection involving primarily the dermis and subcutaneous tissues. S pyogenes was classically reported as the main cause but over the past decade numerous reports have noted the increasing prevalence of MRSA, particularly when associated with furuncles, carbuncles, or abscess (ie, purulent cellulitis).[43,47] Streptococci cause diffusely spreading infections, whereas S aureus cellulitis tends to be more localized, often surrounding a purulent lesion (see **Fig. 2**D).[39,41,48]

Lesions are characterized by edema, pain, tenderness, warmth, erythema, and spreading with irregular margins. Cellulitis may be accompanied by lymphangitis and lymphadenopathy.[49,56] Most commonly, cellulitis occurs in the lower extremities preceded by clinically unapparent local skin trauma. In children, approximately 25% of cellulitis cases are associated with abscess and roughly 1% with osteomyelitis. Vesicles, bullae, and cutaneous hemorrhagic manifestations such as petechiae or ecchymoses may develop on the inflamed skin. If widespread and associated with systemic toxicity, a deeper infection such as necrotizing fasciitis should be considered (**Box 1**).[35,42,50,51]

Although cellulitis can occur at virtually any cutaneous surface, there are specific anatomic locations that result in characteristic infections with shared epidemiology, pathophysiology, and clinical presentation:

- Perianal cellulitis is associated with rectal pain, pruritus, and sharply circumscribed perianal erythema. It is most often caused by S pyogenes and has a

> **Box 1**
> **Clinical features suggesting deep necrotizing infection**
>
> - Severe, excruciating pain
> - Wooden-hard feel of lesion
> - Systemic toxicity: fever, leukocytosis, thrombocytopenia, hypotension/shock, altered mental status, renal failure
> - Presence of bullae (related to occlusion of deep blood vessels)
> - Ecchymosis preceding skin necrosis
> - Presence of gas in soft tissues detected by palpation (crepitus) or imaging
> - Edema extending beyond the margin of erythema
> - Cutaneous anesthesia
> - Rapid spread despite initiation of appropriate antibiotic therapy
>
> *Data from* Stevens DL, Bisno AL, Chambers HF, et al. Practice guidelines for the diagnosis and management of skin and soft-tissue infections. Clin Infect Dis 2005;41(10):1373–40.

peak incidence between the ages of 3 and 5 years.[25,43] Perianal cellulitis can be complicated by abscess formation and development of anal fissures. Perianal streptococcal dermatitis has been reported to be an infectious trigger for guttate psoriasis; patients presenting with guttate psoriasis should be examined for asymptomatic *S pyogenes* infection.[6,43,44]

- Periorbital (preseptal) cellulitis is an infection of tissues anterior to the orbital septum characterized by periorbital edema, erythema, warmth, and tenderness. Periorbital cellulitis is typically caused by *S pyogenes* or *S aureus*. This condition is to be differentiated from orbital cellulitis, which is an extension of bacterial sinusitis involving postseptal tissues, typically caused in vaccinated children by *Streptococcus pneumoniae*, *Haemophilus influenzae*, *Moraxella catarrhalis*, or anaerobic cocci, and characterized by chemosis, painful limited extraocular movements, proptosis, and reduced visual acuity.[43] Complications of orbital cellulitis include loss of vision, retrobulbar abscess, subperiosteal abscess, osteomyelitis, meningitis, and cavernous sinus thrombosis.[25,40,52,57]

Cellulitis remains a clinical diagnosis and its pathophysiology is still largely unknown.[35,53] Microbiological diagnosis of cellulitis is elusive. If blood culture is considered the gold standard for microbiological diagnosis, *S pyogenes* accounts for most cases. However, blood cultures are reported positive in less than 1% of uncomplicated SSSI and in only 12.5% of complicated SSSI, which might bias these distinctions.[10,58] However, if lesions are subjected to needle aspiration or punch biopsy, then *S aureus* is recovered most frequently (although at most one-third of such samples recover any pathogen).[43,54] Given these data coupled with clinical response to various antimicrobial treatment regimens (discussed later), beta-hemolytic streptococci remain the most likely pathogen for nonpurulent cellulitis.[35,49,55]

Erysipelas

Erysipelas is a painful, well-demarcated, superficial infection of the dermis that involves the cutaneous lymphatics. Erysipelas occurs most often in young children and older adults. In neonates, erysipelas can originate from the umbilical stump and spread into the abdominal wall.[40,43] Although mainly caused by *S pyogenes*, similar lesions can be caused by group C or G streptococci, *Streptococcus agalactiae*, or *S aureus*.[41,43] Erysipelas manifests as an abrupt, intensely erythematous lesion raised above the level of the surrounding skin with characteristic sharply demarcated borders. It most commonly involves the legs or face. Patients are typically febrile; adenopathy and lymphangitis may also be present. Severe pain and/or systemic symptoms may suggest deeper infection or toxic shock syndrome (TSS).[38,56]

Ecthyma

Ecthyma is a deep, ulcerative infection of the skin. Ecthyma can initially resemble impetigo but progresses to deeper penetration into the dermis, evolving into a crusted ulcer up to 4 cm in diameter with a black eschar and elevated margins.[5,42,59] Lesions are usually located in the legs in association with minor trauma or pruritic conditions such as insect bites or scabies. Lymphangitis, cellulitis, and poststreptococcal glomerulonephritis are potential complications of ecthyma.[6,43] In contrast with the isolated, outside-to-inside progression of typical ecthyma, ecthyma gangrenosum refers to the systemic spread of bacteria with multiple similar-appearing lesions resulting from necrotizing bacterial vasculitis. This condition is often associated with *Pseudomonas aeruginosa* bacteremia, especially in immunocompromised patients, but can also involve other pathogens, including *S aureus* (see **Fig. 2E**).[6,38]

Staphylococcal Scalded Skin Syndrome

Staphylococcal scalded skin syndrome (SSSS) is a toxin-mediated epidermolytic disease resulting in severe skin blistering and exfoliation caused by circulation of staphylococcal exfoliative toxins A and B.[43,60] This condition predominantly occurs in children less than 6 years of age, most commonly in young infants (who have decreased renal excretion of toxin because of immature renal function).

The inciting infection usually occurs in the eye or nasopharynx. SSSS can be limited to a few localized blisters that burst and leave a tender erythematous base (manifesting as localized bullous impetigo in older children), but exfoliation may involve the entire body surface (Ritter disease in neonates).

The hallmark of SSSS is the presence of midepidermal separation at the zona granulosa (Nikolsky sign); with friction, the epidermis peels off easily, often in large sheets. Healing typically occurs without scarring (see **Fig. 2F**).[25,40,43,57]

Intertrigo

Intertrigo is created by friction of opposing skin surfaces exacerbated by moisture trapped in deep skin folds. Young infants are especially susceptible because of their abundant deep skin folds. Secondary infections with *S pyogenes*, *S aureus*, *Candida* spp, or other pathogens can occur and can be difficult to differentiate.[5,25,35] Intertrigo manifests as intensely erythematous, well-demarcated patches. Associated foul smell; presence of thick, red, macerated, or scaly plaque-type lesions; or presence of low-grade fever or fussiness are typical of *S pyogenes* intertrigo, whereas satellite lesions favor *Candida* spp. Recurrence requiring retreatment is common.[6,43,58] If the eruption persists, more invasive diagnostic procedures such as skin biopsy should be considered to rule out less common causes, including atopic or seborrheic dermatitis, scabies, erythrasma, contact dermatitis, inverse psoriasis, Langerhans cell histiocytosis, or acrodermatitis enteropathica.[35,43]

Acute Paronychia

Acute paronychia is an infection of the soft tissue fold surrounding a fingernail or toenail resulting from minor trauma facilitating bacterial entry into the cuticle or nail fold. Acute paronychia is most often caused by *S aureus*, whereas chronic paronychia is most often caused by *Candida* spp.[35] Risk factors for paronychia include dermatitis, nail biting, and chronic thumb or finger sucking. Paronychia presents with erythema, edema, and tenderness of the proximal and lateral nail fold or may extend beneath the nail and suppurate (see **Fig. 2**G).[40,43]

Blistering Distal Dactylitis

Blistering distal dactylitis is typically seen in children aged 2 to 16 years and is most often caused by *S pyogenes* (less commonly by *S aureus*). It manifests as a tense, nontender bulla with an erythematous base involving the distal volar fat pad of the phalanges. One or more digits can be affected (particularly in *S aureus* infections) and systemic symptoms are generally absent.[43]

Necrotizing Fasciitis

Necrotizing fasciitis is an uncommon, severe SSSI characterized by rapidly evolving soft tissue necrosis and pain out of proportion to the physical findings involving the deeper layer of the superficial fascia but largely sparing the adjacent skin, deep fascia, and muscle.[38] *S pyogenes* is often implicated, although *S aureus*, including CA-MRSA, is increasingly recognized as a cause of necrotizing fasciitis in the United States. Between roughly 30% and 55% of necrotizing fasciitis cases are polymicrobial.[5,59] Necrotizing fasciitis may follow minor trauma or surgery, but in approximately half of cases no visible skin lesion is present. Early in the infection, distinguishing between simple cellulitis and necrotizing fasciitis can be difficult (see **Box 1**).[6] Thus, a high clinical suspicion is paramount; most patients with necrotizing fasciitis are not diagnosed at hospital admission.[38] Necrotizing fasciitis is a medical emergency requiring prompt surgical debridement; if necrotizing fasciitis is suspected on clinical grounds, surgical intervention should not be delayed while awaiting confirmation by laboratory testing or imaging studies.[60]

TSS

TSS is a severe, life-threatening, systemic infection resulting from toxin elaboration by *S aureus* or *S pyogenes*, often associated with minor or occult cutaneous infection.[43] Staphylococcal TSS is caused by a staphylococcal superantigen (usually TSS-1) that stimulates overproduction of inflammatory mediators leading to capillary leak, hypotension, and multiorgan failure. CA-MRSA rarely produce TSS toxin. Streptococcal TSS is caused by toxin-producing *S pyogenes* strains with multisystem clinical manifestations that are similar to those of staphylococcal TSS. The initial clinical presentation of streptococcal TSS is often localized to the primary infection site; however, *S pyogenes* TSS can occur without an identifiable focus of infection.[5,25] Diagnosis of TSS is mainly clinical (**Fig. 3**); blood cultures are positive in less than 5% of cases.

Pyomyositis

Pyomyositis refers to abscess development within skeletal muscle. It can occur secondary to trauma (minor or major), varicella infection, or vigorous exercise. A male predominance (2:1) as well as a seasonal variability (warmer months) has been described. *S aureus*, including CA-MRSA, is typically implicated, but *S pyogenes* is an increasingly important cause of pyomyositis.[6,43] Large muscle groups of the thighs and buttocks, followed by the spine or shoulder muscle groups, are most commonly affected. Untreated infection evolves from nonspecific muscle cramping with low-grade fever to more localized muscle pain with pronounced systemic symptoms. The overlying skin

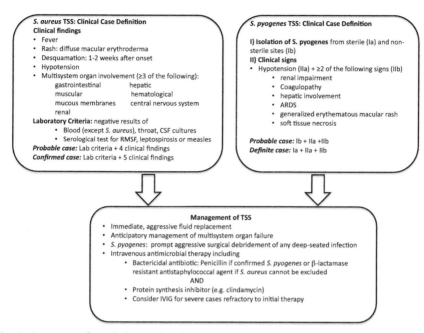

Fig. 3. Summary of staphylococcal and streptococcal TSS. ARDS, acute respiratory distress syndrome; CSF, cerebrospinal fluid; IVIG, intravenous immunoglobulin; RMSF, rocky mountain spotted fever. (*Adapted from* Pickering LK, Baker CJ, Kimberlin DW, et al, editors. Red Book: 2009 Report of the Committee on Infectious Diseases. 28th edition. Elk Grove Village (IL): American Academy of Pediatrics; 2009.)

varies from mild warmth to erythema with exquisite tenderness. Children with pyomyositis can have concomitant osteomyelitis (41%) or septic arthritis (7%).[35]

THERAPY

Management of SSSI depends on the specific disease process and severity of illness. Therapy consists of nonantimicrobial measures as well as topical and systemic antimicrobial regimens. For abscesses, incision and drainage are paramount. For an isolated abscess, incision (with disruption of septations in loculated collections) and complete drainage are often sufficient (**Table 2**); for purulent SSSIs with a combination of cellulitis, myositis, or fasciitis, incision and drainage of large or loculated collections are often required as an adjunct to systemic antimicrobial therapy for timely and complete resolution of infection. For early, superficial SSSIs with localized induration but minimal fluctuance, warm compresses can help mature the abscess before incision and drainage.[2–4,34,61]

As with any bacterial infection, empiric antimicrobial therapy should consider the most likely causative pathogens and, if available, culture results should direct definitive therapy with the ultimate goal of targeting the organism while limiting exposure to unnecessary broad-spectrum agents (**Tables 3** and **4**).[6,53,62–66]

In general, empiric antimicrobial therapy should target *S pyogenes* for nonpurulent SSSIs such as uncomplicated cellulitis, and *S aureus* for purulent SSSIs such as abscesses.[8,10,67–69] In the past, empiric antibiotic prescribing for these sometimes-overlapping conditions was simple: choosing a narrow-spectrum antistaphylococcal agent (eg, first-generation cephalosporin or a β-lactam/β-lactamase combination)

Table 2
Summary of studies evaluating the need for antimicrobials in uncomplicated SSSI in children

Study	Year	N	Type	Comparison	Outcome
Dallas (US)[81]	2004	69	Prospective observational	None ID in 96%	No significant differences between children who received effective antibiotics and those who did not Lesion >5 cm was significant predictor of hospitalization
Saint Louis (US)[82]	2009	161	Randomized double blind	Placebo or TMP-SMX after ID	Antibiotic Tx decreased new lesion development at 10 d No significant difference between 2 groups in new lesion development at 3-mo follow-up
Philadelphia (US)[84]	2009	2096	Retrospective nested case control	β-Lactam vs clindamycin vs TMP-SMX	Compared with β-lactams, clindamycin conferred no benefit for nondrained, noncultured SSSI treated as an outpatient TMP-SMX associated with increased risk of Tx failure
Taiwan[76]	2009	197	Retrospective cohort	None 80.4% ID	91% of children who did not receive appropriate antibiotic achieved clinical cure
Maryland (US)[78]	2010	200	Randomized control trial	Cephalexin vs clindamycin	No difference between cephalexin and clindamycin for uncomplicated SSSI Close follow-up and fastidious wound care of appropriately drained lesions likely more important than initial antibiotic choice
Philadelphia (US)[83]	2011	148	Retrospective cohort	None	Rate of ED treatment failure was low (7.6%) and was irrespective of methicillin resistance or appropriate antibiotic therapy
Tennessee (US)[80]	2011	47,501	Retrospective cohort	β-Lactam vs clindamycin vs TMP-SMX	Compared with clindamycin, TMP-SMX or β-lactam use associated with increased risk of treatment failure and recurrence Effect most significant among children who underwent ID
Boston (US)[77]	2013	153	Randomized multicenter double blind	Cephalexin + TMP-SMX vs cephalexin + placebo	Among patients diagnosed with uncomplicated cellulitis without abscess, the addition of TMP-SMX to cephalexin did not improve outcomes

Abbreviations: ED, emergency department; ID, incision and drainage; SMX, trimethoprim-sulfamethoxazole; TMP, trimethoprim; Tx, treatment.

Table 3
Commonly used antimicrobials for *S aureus* and *S pyogenes* SSSI

Antimicrobial	Spectrum			Pediatric Dose
	GAS	MSSA	MRSA	
Amoxicillin	++	−	−	40–90 mg/kg/d q8–q12h PO
Amoxicillin/ clavulanate	++	++	−	25 mg/kg/d of amoxicillin component q12h PO
Ampicillin/ sulbactam	++	++	−	100–400 mg/kg/d of ampicillin component q6h IV (max 8 g ampicillin component/d)
Cefazolin	++	++	−	50–100 mg/kg/d q8h IV (max 6 g/d)
Cephalexin	++	++	−	50–100 mg/kg/d q6h PO (max 4 g/d)
Clindamycin[a]	+	+	+[b]	15–30 mg/kg/d q8h PO (max 1.8 g/d) or 25–30 mg/kg/ d q8h IV (max 2.7 g/d)
Dicloxacillin	++	++	−	25–50 mg/kg/d q6h PO
Doxycycline	+/−	+	+	Not recommended <8 y ≤45 kg: 4.4 mg/kg in 2 divided doses on day 1, then 2.2 mg/kg q24 divided in 1 or 2 doses, PO or IV >45 kg: 100 mg q12h on day 1 followed by 100 mg q24h, PO or IV
Linezolid	++	++	++	10 mg/kg/dose q12 (preterm neonates and children) or q8h (term neonates), PO or IV
Nafcillin	++	++	−	100–200 mg/kg/d q4–q6h IV (max 12 g/d)
Oxacillin	++	++	−	150–200 mg/kg/d q4–q6 IV (max 2 g every 4–6 h)
Penicillin G aqueous	++	−	−	100–400 KU/kg/d divided q4–q6h IV (max 20 KU/d)
Penicillin V potassium	++	−	−	15–50 mg/kg/d divided q6–q8h PO (max 3 g/d)
TMP-SMX	+/−	++	++	6–12 mg/kg/d (based on TMP component) q12, PO
Vancomycin	++	++	++	10–15 mg/kg/d q6h, IV
Newer Antimicrobials				
Daptomycin[c]	++	++	++	Adult: 4–6 mg/kg/dose q24h, IV Neonates (GA ≥32 wk): 6 mg/kg/dose q12h, IV (limited data available) Children 2–6 y: 8–10 mg/kg/dose q24h, IV (limited data available) Children ≥6 y to <12 y: 7 mg/kg/dose q24h, IV (limited data available) Children >12 y: 4–6 mg/kg/dose q24h, IV
Ceftaroline[c]	++	++	++	Adult: 600 mg q12 h, IV Safety and efficacy not established for children <18 y
Telavancin[c]	++	++	++	Adult: 10 mg/kg q24h, IV Safety and efficacy not established for children <18 y
Tigecyline[c]	++	++	++	Adult: 100 mg initial followed by 50 mg q12h, IV Children ≥12 y: 1.5 mg/kg initial as a single dose followed by 1 mg/kg/dose q12h (limited experience)
Quinupristin/ dalfopristin[c]	++	++	++	Adult: 7.5 mg/kg q12h, IV Safety and efficacy not established for children <18 y

++, >95% susceptible; +, usually susceptible; +/−, variably susceptible/resistant; −, usually resistant.

Abbreviations: GAS, group A *Streptococcus* (*S pyogenes*); IV, intravenous route; PO, oral route; q6h, every 6 hours; q8h, every 8 hours.

[a] D-test should be performed to exclude inducible clindamycin resistance for *S aureus*.
[b] Varies significantly by region.
[c] Not US Food and Drug Administration approved for children less than 18 years old.

Table 4 Considerations for the treatment of SSSI	
Impetigo	Removal of crust and application of topical antibiotics (bacitracin, neomycin, polymyxin B, mupirocin[a], retapamulin) may eradicate localized nonbullous diseases Systemic antimicrobial therapy targeting both S aureus and S pyogenes should be used for: 1. Multiple or widespread lesions 2. Face, eyelid, or perioral lesions 3. Nonbullous impetigo in multiple family members or sport team players
Folliculitis	Recurrent/uncomplicated superficial folliculitis: antibacterial soaps and good hygiene; consider topical antibiotics Refractory or deeper infections: systemic antibiotics
Intertrigo	Simple intertrigo typically responds to measures that minimize moisture and reduce friction Consider topical antibiotics
SSSS	Dehydration and superinfection can occur with extensive exfoliation IV antistaphylococcal therapy +/− protein synthesis inhibitor (topical antibiotics are not useful)
Ecthyma	Mild cases are often treatable with topical antibiotics More severe cases require systemic antibiotics targeting both S pyogenes and S aureus
Erysipelas	PO or IV penicillin depending on clinical severity Antistaphylococcal therapy should be considered in patients who fail to improve with penicillin or have features suggestive of S aureus such as bullous erysipelas
Acute paronychia	Warm compress often curative for superficial lesions If oral flora suspected (nail biting, finger sucking), consider antibiotic with anaerobic activity
Dactylitis	ID +/− antimicrobial therapy
Necrotizing fasciitis	Serial surgical debridement often required; amputation may be necessary for severe cases Areas where debridement is more challenging (neck, abdomen, head, thorax) are associated with higher mortality IV broad-spectrum antibiotics until microbiology data available Clindamycin, a protein synthesis inhibitor, used for its bacteriostatic effects (not cell wall dependent, like β-lactam agents) to combat organisms in stationary phase of growth (Eagle effect) as well as the theoretic advantage of interrupting toxin production; linezolid might share this beneficial effect but there are few data to support this Supportive care is crucial; patients usually require early care in intensive care unit Despite treatment, high mortality (up to 45%), especially with delayed surgical treatment
Pyomyositis	Drainage of purulent collections coupled with systemic antimicrobial therapy

[a] Inappropriate long or intermittent use of mupirocin has been associated with mupirocin-resistant staphylococci, particularly in patients with severe skin and soft tissue infection.

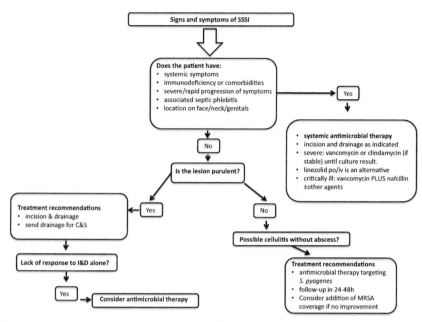

Fig. 4. Outpatient approach to management of SSSI. C&S, culture and sensitivities; I&D, incision and drainage. (*Adapted from* NeVille-Swensen M, Clayton M. Outpatient management of community-associated methicillin-resistant Staphylococcus aureus skin and soft tissue infection. J Pediatr Health Care 2011;25(5):308–15.)

provided adequate coverage for both S pyogenes and S aureus. The emergence of MRSA complicates this approach.[12,13,70–74] For example, clindamycin usually covers S pyogenes, but activity against MRSA varies by geographic region and is declining. Although trimethoprim (TMP)-sulfamethoxazole (SMX) has excellent MRSA activity, its S pyogenes coverage is less reliable. Recent data support the concept that is probably not necessary to cover MRSA in otherwise healthy outpatients with uncomplicated, nonpurulent cellulitis.[15,75–84]

However, predicting MRSA infections is difficult. MRSA colonization of skin or nares does not always correlate with the presence of MRSA in wound isolates.[12,15,18,20,85–88] Moreover, a recent study shows that it is common for patients with MRSA SSSIs to have subsequent MSSA SSSIs.[22,89]

Duration of antibiotic treatment generally depends on the extent of infection, adequate drainage (for abscesses), host immune status, and initial clinical response. For uncomplicated SSSI requiring antibiotic treatment, short courses (5–7 days) are generally sufficient. Progression despite receiving antibiotics could be caused by infection with resistant microbes or by a deeper, more serious infection. Patients with progressing or severe infection despite antimicrobial therapy should be hospitalized and treated more aggressively.[26–30,90]

If S aureus is suspected or confirmed, an agent effective against MRSA should be used in regions where the incidence of MRSA is high (**Fig. 4**).[3,13,31,32,91] Vancomycin or linezolid should be considered for severe infections before identification and susceptibly.[36,92] Treatment with other agents such as TMP-SMX, clindamycin, or tetracycline (for children ≥8 years) is reasonable for empiric treatment of less severe infections and for step-down therapy based on results from susceptibility testing.[4,93–96] Since the emergence of CA-MRSA, clindamycin is the most commonly prescribed antibiotic for *S aureus* SSSI in hospitalized children.[39,97]

SUMMARY

Acute SSSIs are common bacterial infections of children and include generally benign conditions such as impetigo and uncomplicated cellulitis as well as severe, life-threatening infections such TSS. Diagnosis is largely based on clinical grounds and antimicrobial therapy is often empiric. *S pyogenes* typically causes nonpurulent SSSIs (cellulitis) and *S aureus* accounts for most purulent SSSIs. The emergence CA-MRSA has increased the prevalence of, and complicated antibiotic choice for, skin and soft tissue infections. For abscesses, incision and drainage are critical and might obviate antimicrobial therapy.

REFERENCES

1. Moet GJ, Jones RN, Biedenbach DJ, et al. Contemporary causes of skin and soft tissue infections in North America, Latin America, and Europe: report from the SENTRY Antimicrobial Surveillance Program (1998-2004). Diagn Microbiol Infect Dis 2007;57(1):7–13. http://dx.doi.org/10.1016/j.diagmicrobio.2006.05.009.
2. Hersh AL, Chambers HF, Maselli JH, et al. National trends in ambulatory visits and antibiotic prescribing for skin and soft-tissue infections. Arch Intern Med 2008;168(14):1585–91. http://dx.doi.org/10.1001/archinte.168.14.1585.
3. Qualls ML, Mooney MM, Camargo CA, et al. Emergency department visit rates for abscess versus other skin infections during the emergence of community-associated methicillin-resistant *Staphylococcus aureus*, 1997-2007. Clin Infect Dis 2012;55(1):103–5. http://dx.doi.org/10.1093/cid/cis342.
4. Pallin DJ, Egan DJ, Pelletier AJ, et al. Increased US emergency department visits for skin and soft tissue infections, and changes in antibiotic choices, during the emergence of community-associated methicillin-resistant *Staphylococcus aureus*. Ann Emerg Med 2008;51(3):291–8. http://dx.doi.org/10.1016/j.annemergmed.2007.12.004.
5. Wong CJ, Stevens DL. Serious group A streptococcal infections. Med Clin North Am 2013;97(4):721–36. http://dx.doi.org/10.1016/j.mcna.2013.03.003.
6. Stevens DL, Bisno AL, Chambers HF, et al. Practice guidelines for the diagnosis and management of skin and soft-tissue infections. Clin Infect Dis 2005;41(10):1373–406. http://dx.doi.org/10.1086/497143.
7. Larson AA, Dinulos JG. Cutaneous bacterial infections in the newborn. Curr Opin Pediatr 2005;17(4):481–5.
8. Sadow KB, Chamberlain JM. Blood cultures in the evaluation of children with cellulitis. Pediatrics 1998;101(3):E4.
9. Miller LS, Cho JS. Immunity against *Staphylococcus aureus* cutaneous infections. Nat Rev Immunol 2011;11(8):505–18. http://dx.doi.org/10.1038/nri3010.
10. Malone JR, Durica SR, Thompson DM, et al. Blood cultures in the evaluation of uncomplicated skin and soft tissue infections. Pediatrics 2013;132(3):454–9. http://dx.doi.org/10.1542/peds.2013-1384.
11. Britton PN, Andresen DN. Paediatric community-associated *Staphylococcus aureus*: a retrospective cohort study. J Paediatr Child Health 2013;49(9):754–9. http://dx.doi.org/10.1111/jpc.12255.

12. Ray GT, Suaya JA, Baxter R. Diagnostic microbiology and infectious disease. Diagn Microbiol Infect Dis 2013;76(1):24–30. http://dx.doi.org/10.1016/j.diagmicrobio.2013.02.020.

13. Ray GT, Suaya JA, Baxter R. Incidence, microbiology, and patient characteristics of skin and soft-tissue infections in a U.S. population: a retrospective population-based study. BMC Infect Dis 2013;13(1):252. http://dx.doi.org/10.1186/1471-2334-13-252.

14. Tattevin P, Schwartz BS, Graber CJ, et al. Concurrent epidemics of skin and soft tissue infection and bloodstream infection due to community-associated methicillin-resistant *Staphylococcus aureus*. Clin Infect Dis 2012;55(6):781–8. http://dx.doi.org/10.1093/cid/cis527.

15. Pallin DJ, Espinola JA, Leung DY, et al. Epidemiology of dermatitis and skin infections in United States Physicians' Offices, 1993–2005. Clin Infect Dis 2009; 49(6):901–7. http://dx.doi.org/10.1086/605434.

16. Faden H, Rose R, Lesse A, et al. Clinical and molecular characteristics of staphylococcal skin abscesses in children. J Pediatr 2007;151(6):700–3. http://dx.doi.org/10.1016/j.jpeds.2007.07.040.

17. Paintsil E. Pediatric community-acquired methicillin-resistant *Staphylococcus aureus* infection and colonization: trends and management. Curr Opin Pediatr 2007;19(1):75–82. http://dx.doi.org/10.1097/MOP.0b013e32801261c9.

18. Moran GJ, Abrahamian FM, Lovecchio F, et al. Acute bacterial skin infections: developments since the 2005 Infectious Diseases Society of America (IDSA) guidelines. J Emerg Med 2013;44(6):e397–412. http://dx.doi.org/10.1016/j.jemermed.2012.11.050.

19. Taylor AR. Methicillin-resistant *Staphylococcus aureus* infections. Prim Care 2013;40(3):637–54. http://dx.doi.org/10.1016/j.pop.2013.06.002.

20. Mistry RD. Skin and soft tissue infections. Pediatr Clin North Am 2013;60(5): 1063–82. http://dx.doi.org/10.1016/j.pcl.2013.06.011.

21. Shallcross LJ, Fragaszy E, Johnson AM, et al. The role of the Panton-Valentine leucocidin toxin in staphylococcal disease: a systematic review and meta-analysis. Lancet Infect Dis 2012;13(1):43–54. http://dx.doi.org/10.1016/S1473-3099(12)70238-4.

22. Kaplan SL. Implications of methicillin-resistant *Staphylococcus aureus* as a community-acquired pathogen in pediatric patients. Infect Dis Clin North Am 2005;19(3):747–57. http://dx.doi.org/10.1016/j.idc.2005.05.011.

23. Diep BA, Gillet Y, Etienne J, et al. Panton-Valentine leucocidin and pneumonia. Lancet Infect Dis 2013;13(7):566. http://dx.doi.org/10.1016/S1473-3099(13)70102-6.

24. Ladhani S, Garbash M. Staphylococcal skin infections in children: rational drug therapy recommendations. Paediatr Drugs 2005;7(2):77–102.

25. Baker CJ, Kimberlin DW. Red book. American Academy of Pediatrics; 2009.

26. Karamatsu ML, Thorp AW, Brown L. Changes in community-associated methicillin-resistant *Staphylococcus aureus* skin and soft tissue infections presenting to the pediatric emergency department: comparing 2003 to 2008. Pediatr Emerg Care 2012;28(2):131–5. http://dx.doi.org/10.1097/PEC.0b013e318243fa36.

27. Holsenback H, Smith L, Stevenson MD. Cutaneous abscesses in children: epidemiology in the era of methicillin-resistant *Staphylococcus aureus* in a pediatric emergency department. Pediatr Emerg Care 2012;28(7):684–6. http://dx.doi.org/10.1097/PEC.0b013e31825d20e1.

28. Edelsberg J, Taneja C, Zervos M, et al. Trends in US hospital admissions for skin and soft tissue infections. Emerg Infect Dis 2009;15(9):1516–8. http://dx.doi.org/10.3201/eid1509.081228.

29. Cohen PR. Community-acquired methicillin-resistant *Staphylococcus aureus* skin infections: implications for patients and practitioners. Am J Clin Dermatol 2007;8(5):259–70.
30. Gosbell IB. Methicillin-resistant *Staphylococcus aureus*: impact on dermatology practice. Am J Clin Dermatol 2004;5(4):239–59.
31. Dukic VM, Lauderdale DS, Wilder J, et al. Epidemics of community-associated methicillin-resistant *Staphylococcus aureus* in the United States: a meta-analysis. Otto M. PLoS One 2013;8(1):e52722. http://dx.doi.org/10.1371/journal.pone.0052722.t001.
32. Iwamoto M, Mu Y, Lynfield R, et al. Trends in invasive methicillin-resistant *Staphylococcus aureus* Infections. Pediatrics 2013;132(4):e817–24. http://dx.doi.org/10.1542/peds.2013-1112.
33. Demos M, McLeod MP, Nouri K. Recurrent furunculosis: a review of the literature. Br J Dermatol 2012;167(4):725–32. http://dx.doi.org/10.1111/j.1365-2133.2012.11151.x.
34. Pottinger PS. Methicillin-resistant *Staphylococcus aureus* infections. Med Clin North Am 2013;97(4):601–19. http://dx.doi.org/10.1016/j.mcna.2013.02.005.
35. Shah S. Pediatric practice infectious diseases. McGraw Hill Professional; 2009.
36. Lopez MA, Cruz AT, Kowalkowski MA, et al. Trends in resource utilization for hospitalized children with skin and soft tissue infections. Pediatrics 2013;131(3):e718–25. http://dx.doi.org/10.1542/peds.2012-0746.
37. Rajan S. Skin and soft-tissue infections: classifying and treating a spectrum. Cleve Clin J Med 2012;79(1):57–66. http://dx.doi.org/10.3949/ccjm.79a.11044.
38. Napolitano LM. Severe soft tissue infections. Infect Dis Clin North Am 2009;23(3):571–91. http://dx.doi.org/10.1016/j.idc.2009.04.006.
39. Jeng A, Beheshti M, Li J, et al. The role of β-hemolytic streptococci in causing diffuse, nonculturable cellulitis. Medicine 2010;89(4):217–26. http://dx.doi.org/10.1097/MD.0b013e3181e8d635.
40. Hedrick J. Acute bacterial skin infections in pediatric medicine: current issues in presentation and treatment. Paediatr Drugs 2003;5(Suppl 1):35–46.
41. Esposito S, Bassetti M, Borre S, et al. Diagnosis and management of skin and soft-tissue infections (SSTI): a literature review and consensus statement on behalf of the Italian Society of Infectious Diseases and International Society of Chemotherapy. J Chemother 2011;23(5):251–62.
42. Torok ME, Conlon CP. Skin and soft tissue infections. Medicine 2009;37(11):603–9. http://dx.doi.org/10.1016/j.mpmed.2009.08.007.
43. Long SS, Pickering LK, Prober CG. Principles and practice of pediatric infectious disease. Revised Reprint. Saunders; 2008.
44. Vayalumkal JV, Jadavji T. Children hospitalized with skin and soft tissue infections: a guide to antibacterial selection and treatment. Paediatr Drugs 2006;8(2):99–111.
45. Sladden MJ, Johnston GA. Current options for the treatment of impetigo in children. Expert Opin Pharmacother 2005;6(13):2245–56. http://dx.doi.org/10.1517/14656566.6.13.2245.
46. Bernard P. Management of common bacterial infections of the skin. Curr Opin Infect Dis 2008;21(2):122–8. http://dx.doi.org/10.1097/QCO.0b013e3282f44c63.
47. Chira S, Miller LG. *Staphylococcus aureus* is the most common identified cause of cellulitis: a systematic review. Epidemiol Infect 2009;138(03):313. http://dx.doi.org/10.1017/S0950268809990483.
48. Phoenix G, Das S, Joshi M. Diagnosis and management of cellulitis. BMJ 2012;345:e4955. http://dx.doi.org/10.1136/bmj.e4955.

49. Gunderson CG. Cellulitis: definition, etiology, and clinical features. Am J Med 2011;124(12):1113–22. http://dx.doi.org/10.1016/j.amjmed.2011.06.028.
50. N SM. Cellulitis-2004. N Engl J Med 2004;350:904–12.
51. Dawson AL, Dellavalle RP, Elston DM. Infectious skin diseases: a review and needs assessment. Dermatol Clin 2012;30(1):141–51. http://dx.doi.org/10.1016/j.det.2011.08.003.
52. Seltz LB, Smith J, Durairaj VD, et al. Microbiology and antibiotic management of orbital cellulitis. Pediatrics 2011;127(3):e566–72. http://dx.doi.org/10.1542/peds.2010-2117.
53. Chambers HF. Editorial commentary: cellulitis, by any other name. Clin Infect Dis 2013;56(12):1763–4. http://dx.doi.org/10.1093/cid/cit126.
54. Patel Wylie F, Kaplan SL, Mason EO, et al. Needle aspiration for the etiologic diagnosis of children with cellulitis in the era of community-acquired methicillin-resistant Staphylococcus aureus. Clin Pediatr 2011;50(6):503–7. http://dx.doi.org/10.1177/0009922810394652.
55. Gunderson CG, Martinello RA. A systematic review of bacteremias in cellulitis and erysipelas. J Infect 2012;64(2):148–55. http://dx.doi.org/10.1016/j.jinf.2011.11.004.
56. Bonnetblanc JM, Bédane C. Erysipelas: recognition and management. Am J Clin Dermatol 2003;4(3):157–63.
57. Kress DW. Pediatric dermatology emergencies. Curr Opin Pediatr 2011;23(4):403–6. http://dx.doi.org/10.1097/MOP.0b013e3283483efd.
58. Honig PJ, Frieden IJ, Kim HJ, et al. Streptococcal intertrigo: an underrecognized condition in children. Pediatrics 2003;112(6 Pt 1):1427–9.
59. Fung HB, Chang JY, Kuczynski S. A practical guide to the treatment of complicated skin and soft tissue infections. Drugs 2003;63(14):1459–80.
60. Dryden MS. Complicated skin and soft tissue infection. J Antimicrob Chemother 2010;65(Suppl 3):iii35–44. http://dx.doi.org/10.1093/jac/dkq302.
61. Liu C, Bayer A, Cosgrove SE, et al. Clinical practice guidelines by the Infectious Diseases Society of America for the treatment of methicillin-resistant Staphylococcus aureus infections in adults and children. Clin Infect Dis 2011;52(3):e18–55. http://dx.doi.org/10.1093/cid/ciq146.
62. Ruhe JJ, Smith N, Bradsher RW, et al. Community-onset methicillin-resistant Staphylococcus aureus skin and soft-tissue infections: impact of antimicrobial therapy on outcome. Clin Infect Dis 2007;44(6):777–84. http://dx.doi.org/10.1086/511872.
63. Hsiao CB, Dryja D, Abbatessa L, et al. Staphylococcus aureus antimicrobial susceptibility of abscess samples from adults and children from the Kaleida Health System in western New York State, 2003 to 2006. J Clin Microbiol 2010;48(5):1753–7. http://dx.doi.org/10.1128/JCM.01065-08.
64. Jones H. Systemic antibiotic treatment of skin, skin structure, and soft tissue infections in the outpatient setting. Adv Skin Wound Care 2012;25(3):132–40. http://dx.doi.org/10.1097/01.ASW.0000412918.04324.77 [quiz: 141–2].
65. Jenkins TC, Sabel AL, Sarcone EE, et al. Skin and soft-tissue infections requiring hospitalization at an academic medical center: opportunities for antimicrobial stewardship. Clin Infect Dis 2010;51(8):895–903. http://dx.doi.org/10.1086/656431.
66. Guay DR. Treatment of bacterial skin and skin structure infections. Expert Opin Pharmacother 2003;4(8):1259–75. http://dx.doi.org/10.1517/14656566.4.8.1259.
67. Eells SJ, Chira S, David CG, et al. Non-suppurative cellulitis: risk factors and its association with Staphylococcus aureus colonization in an area of endemic community-associated methicillin-resistant S. aureus infections. Epidemiol Infect 2010;139(04):606–12. http://dx.doi.org/10.1017/S0950268810001408.

68. Schmitz GR. Best clinical practices. J Emerg Med 2011;41(3):276–81. http://dx.doi.org/10.1016/j.jemermed.2011.01.027.

69. Wells RD, Mason P, Roarty J, et al. Comparison of initial antibiotic choice and treatment of cellulitis in the pre- and post-community-acquired methicillin-resistant *Staphylococcus aureus* eras. Am J Emerg Med 2009;27(4):436–9. http://dx.doi.org/10.1016/j.ajem.2008.03.026.

70. Meddles-Torres C, Hu S, Jurgens C. Changes in prescriptive practices in skin and soft tissue infections associated with the increased occurrence of community acquired methicillin resistant *Staphylococcus aureus*. J Infect Public Health 2013;6(6):423–30. http://dx.doi.org/10.1016/j.jiph.2013.04.010.

71. Mistry RD, Weisz K, Scott HF, et al. Emergency management of pediatric skin and soft tissue infections in the community-associated methicillin-resistant *Staphylococcus aureus* era. Acad Emerg Med 2010;17(2):187–93. http://dx.doi.org/10.1111/j.1553-2712.2009.00652.x.

72. Eady EA, Cove JH. Staphylococcal resistance revisited: community-acquired methicillin resistant *Staphylococcus aureus*–an emerging problem for the management of skin and soft tissue infections. Curr Opin Infect Dis 2003;16(2):103–24. http://dx.doi.org/10.1097/01.aco.0000065071.06965.ca.

73. Walraven CJ, Lingenfelter E, Rollo J, et al. Diagnostic and therapeutic evaluation of community-acquired methicillin-resistant *Staphylococcus aureus* (MRSA) skin and soft tissue infections in the emergency department. J Emerg Med 2012;42(4):392–9. http://dx.doi.org/10.1016/j.jemermed.2011.03.009.

74. Bocchini CE, Mason EO, Hulten KG, et al. Recurrent community-associated *Staphylococcus aureus* infections in children presenting to Texas Children's Hospital in Houston, Texas. Pediatr Infect Dis J 2013;32(11):1189–93. http://dx.doi.org/10.1097/INF.0b013e3182a5c30d.

75. Phillips S, MacDougall C, Holdford DA. Analysis of empiric antimicrobial strategies for cellulitis in the era of methicillin-resistant *Staphylococcus aureus*. Ann Pharmacother 2006;41(1):13–20. http://dx.doi.org/10.1345/aph.1H452.

76. Teng CS, Lo WT, Wang SR, et al. The role of antimicrobial therapy for treatment of uncomplicated skin and soft tissue infections from community-acquired methicillin-resistant *Staphylococcus aureus* in children. J Microbiol Immunol Infect 2009;42(4):324–8.

77. Pallin DJ, Binder WD, Allen MB, et al. Clinical trial: comparative effectiveness of cephalexin plus trimethoprim-sulfamethoxazole versus cephalexin alone for treatment of uncomplicated cellulitis: a randomized controlled trial. Clin Infect Dis 2013;56(12):1754–62. http://dx.doi.org/10.1093/cid/cit122.

78. Chen AE, Carroll KC, Diener-West M, et al. Randomized controlled trial of cephalexin versus clindamycin for uncomplicated pediatric skin infections. Pediatrics 2011;127(3):e573–80. http://dx.doi.org/10.1542/peds.2010-2053.

79. Cadena J, Sreeramoju P, Nair S, et al. Diagnostic microbiology and infectious disease. Diagn Microbiol Infect Dis 2012;74(1):16–21. http://dx.doi.org/10.1016/j.diagmicrobio.2012.05.010.

80. Williams DJ, Cooper WO, Kaltenbach LA, et al. Comparative effectiveness of antibiotic treatment strategies for pediatric skin and soft-tissue infections. Pediatrics 2011;128(3):e479–87. http://dx.doi.org/10.1542/peds.2010-3681.

81. Lee MC, Ríos AM, Aten MF, et al. Management and outcome of children with skin and soft tissue abscesses caused by community-acquired methicillin-resistant *Staphylococcus aureus*. Pediatr Infect Dis J 2004;23(2):123–7. http://dx.doi.org/10.1097/01.inf.0000109288.06912.21.

82. Duong M, Markwell S, Peter J, et al. Randomized, controlled trial of antibiotics in the management of community-acquired skin abscesses in the pediatric patient. Ann Emerg Med 2010;55(5):401–7. http://dx.doi.org/10.1016/j. annemergmed.2009.03.014.

83. Mistry RD, Scott HF, Zaoutis TE, et al. Emergency department treatment failures for skin infections in the era of community-acquired methicillin-resistant *Staphylococcus aureus*. Pediatr Emerg Care 2011;27(1):21–6. http://dx.doi.org/10. 1097/PEC.0b013e318203ca1c.

84. Elliott DJ, Zaoutis TE, Troxel AB, et al. Empiric antimicrobial therapy for pediatric skin and soft-tissue infections in the era of methicillin-resistant *Staphylococcus aureus*. Pediatrics 2009;123(6):e959–66. http://dx.doi.org/10.1542/peds.2008-2428.

85. Chen AE, Cantey JB, Carroll KC, et al. Discordance between *Staphylococcus aureus* nasal colonization and skin infections in children. Pediatr Infect Dis J 2009;28(3):244–6. http://dx.doi.org/10.1097/INF.0b013e31818cb0c4.

86. Skov R, Christiansen K, Dancer SJ, et al. Update on the prevention and control of community-acquired methicillin-resistant *Staphylococcus aureus* (CA-MRSA). Int J Antimicrob Agents 2012;39(3):193–200. http://dx.doi.org/10.1016/j. ijantimicag.2011.09.029.

87. Bar-Meir M, Tan TQ. *Staphylococcus aureus* skin and soft tissue infections: can we anticipate the culture result? Clin Pediatr 2010;49(5):432–8. http://dx.doi.org/ 10.1177/0009922809350496.

88. Reber A, Moldovan A, Dunkel N, et al. Should the methicillin-resistant *Staphylococcus aureus* carriage status be used as a guide to treatment for skin and soft tissue infections? J Infect 2012;64(5):513–9. http://dx.doi.org/10.1016/j.jinf. 2011.12.023.

89. Patel AB. Reversion of methicillin-resistant *Staphylococcus aureus* skin infections to methicillin-susceptible isolates. JAMA Dermatol 2013;149(10):1167. http://dx.doi.org/10.1001/jamadermatol.2013.4909.

90. NeVille-Swensen M, Clayton M. Outpatient management of community-associated methicillin-resistant *Staphylococcus aureus* skin and soft tissue infection. J Pediatr Health Care 2011;25(5):308–15. http://dx.doi.org/10.1016/j. pedhc.2010.05.005.

91. Awad SS, Elhabash SI, Lee L, et al. Increasing incidence of methicillin-resistant *Staphylococcus aureus* skin and soft-tissue infections: reconsideration of empiric antimicrobial therapy. Am J Surg 2007;194(5):606–10. http://dx.doi. org/10.1016/j.amjsurg.2007.07.016.

92. Itani KM, Biswas P, Reisman A, et al. Clinical efficacy of oral linezolid compared with intravenous vancomycin for the treatment of methicillin-resistant *Staphylococcus aureus*–complicated skin and soft tissue infections: a retrospective, propensity score-matched, case-control analysis. Clin Ther 2012;34(8):1667–73.e1. http://dx.doi.org/10.1016/j.clinthera.2012.06.018.

93. Morgan M. Treatment of MRSA soft tissue infections: an overview. Injury 2011; 42(S5):S11–7. http://dx.doi.org/10.1016/S0020-1383(11)70127-9.

94. Lawrence KR, Golik MV, Davidson L. The role of primary care prescribers in the diagnosis and management of community-associated methicillin-resistant *Staphylococcus aureus* skin and soft tissue infections. Am J Ther 2009;16(4): 333–8. http://dx.doi.org/10.1097/MJT.0b013e31817fdea8.

95. Wood JB, Smith DB, Baker EH, et al. Has the emergence of community-associated methicillin-resistant *Staphylococcus aureus* increased trimethoprim-sulfamethoxazole use and resistance?: a 10-year time series analysis. Antimicrobial Agents Chemother 2012;56(11):5655–60. http://dx.doi.org/10.1128/AAC.01011-12.

96. Schmitz GR, Bruner D, Pitotti R, et al. Randomized controlled trial of trimethoprim-sulfamethoxazole for uncomplicated skin abscesses in patients at risk for community-associated methicillin-resistant *Staphylococcus aureus* infection. Ann Emerg Med 2010;56(3):283–7. http://dx.doi.org/10.1016/j.annemergmed.2010.03.002.

97. Herigon JC, Hersh AL, Gerber JS, et al. Antibiotic management of *Staphylococcus aureus* infections in US Children's Hospitals, 1999-2008. Pediatrics 2010;125(6):e1294–300. http://dx.doi.org/10.1542/peds.2009-2867.

Index

Note: Page numbers of article titles are in **boldface** type.

Moving?

Make sure your subscription moves with you!

To notify us of your new address, find your **Clinics Account Number** (located on your mailing label above your name), and contact customer service at:

Email: journalscustomerservice-usa@elsevier.com

800-654-2452 (subscribers in the U.S. & Canada)
314-447-8871 (subscribers outside of the U.S. & Canada)

Fax number: 314-447-8029

Elsevier Health Sciences Division
Subscription Customer Service
3251 Riverport Lane
Maryland Heights, MO 63043

*To ensure uninterrupted delivery of your subscription, please notify us at least 4 weeks in advance of move.

Printed and bound by CPI Group (UK) Ltd, Croydon, CR0 4YY

03/10/2024

01040494-0009